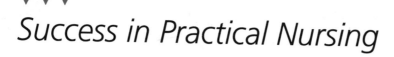

Success in Practical Nursing

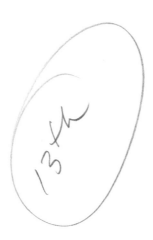

13th

Signe S. Hill, BSN, MA, RN

Formerly, Instructor, Practical Nurse Program
Northeast Wisconsin Technical College
Green Bay, Wisconsin

Helen A. Howlett, BSN, MS, RN

Instructor, Practical Nurse Program
Northeast Wisconsin Technical College
Green Bay, Wisconsin

Success in
Practical Nursing

▼▼▼

Personal and Vocational Issues *Third Edition*

W.B. Saunders Company
A Division of Harcourt Brace & Company
Philadelphia London Toronto Montreal Sydney Tokyo

W.B. SAUNDERS COMPANY
A Division of Harcourt Brace & Company

The Curtis Center
Independence Square West
Philadelphia, Pennsylvania 19106

Library of Congress Cataloging-in-Publication Data

Hill, Signe S.
    Success in practical nursing: personal and vocational issues   /
Signe S. Hill, Helen A. Howlett. — 3rd ed.

        p.   cm.

    ISBN 0–7216–6877–1

    1. Practical Nursing—Vocational guidance.   I. Howlett, Helen A.
II. Title.

RT62.H45   1997

610.73'06'93—dc20

DNLM/DLC   96–35766

SUCCESS IN PRACTICAL NURSING   ISBN 0–7216–6877–1
Personal and Vocational Issues
Third Edition

Printed in the United States of America.

Last digit is the print number: 9   8   7   6   5   4   3   2   1

▼▼▼

*To my children Michael, Keith, Valerie and Marla,
who have provided my greatest lessons in life.*
—Signe S. Hill

*To my son Matthew Stephen Christian Howlett, the
spice of my life, and Holly Collar, a supportive friend.*
—Helen A. Howlett

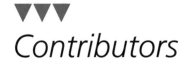

Contributors

Judith A. Mix, *MSN, EdD*

Associate Dean Health Occupations,
Northeast Wisconsin Technical College,
Green Bay, Wisconsin

Michael S. Hill, *MS, CRC, CCM, QRC*

Vocational Consultant
Employee Development Corporation
New Brighton, Minnesota

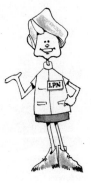

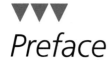

Preface

Dear Student Practical Nurse and Instructor,

The feeling of kinship and partnership with you continues. Many of you took the time to respond to our request for feedback. It is this feedback plus recent legal changes/clarifications for the practical nurse that became the basis for the third edition.

The third edition is designed to assist students to get through a challenging year of study. Critical thinking is encouraged as well as active participation in problem solving in personal and academic life. Excellent resources for the postgraduate student, especially in leadership and management areas, are included.

Both Judith Mix and Michael Hill responded to our request to update the chapters they wrote for the second edition. Dr. Mix expanded on the basics of communication needed to be successful in your chosen vocation. Mr. Hill reached into predictions for the year 2005 to assist you in finding the job you wish to have.

Most of all we continue to be partners with you in both learning and facilitating the learning process. Send your comments to us in care of the Nursing Books Division, W.B. Saunders Company. We look forward to hearing from you.

Signe S. Hill
Helen A. Howlett

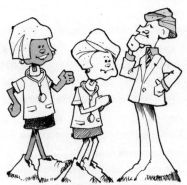

*Illustrations by
Robert Yancey,
Luxemburg, Wisconsin.*

▼▼▼
Acknowledgments

Making additions and revisions for the third edition was influenced directly and indirectly by numerous persons and we want to acknowledge the following: Ilze Rader, our editor at W.B. Saunders Company; Marie Thomas, editorial assistant, for responding to our numerous requests and making them seem rational; former and present students of practical nursing, the instructors who challenge their students to think critically; Mona Kempfert, a special friend for her computer skill; Mary Parrott, manager of the Learning Resource Center at the Northeast Wisconsin Technical College, and her staff, who keep us up to date on journals and periodicals; and the following instructors who reviewed this revision: Barbara Biles, BSN, RN, Southern Westchester BOCCES, School of Practical Nursing, Valhalla, New York; Monica G. DeCarlo, MSN, RN, C, Indiana County Area Vocational-Technical School, School of Practical Nursing, Indiana, Pennsylvania; Laurelle S. Fuselier, RN, ADRN, Louisiana Technical College, Acadian Campus, School of Practical Nursing, Crowley, Louisiana; Julie Blaine Guppy, BSN, RN, Joplin R-VIII School of Practical Nursing, Franklin Technical School at MSCC, Joplin, Missouri; Genevieve Lucenti, RN, BS, CIV, Southern Westchester BOCCES, School of Practical Nursing, Valhalla, New York; Marlene I. Martenson, BSN, RN, South Central Area Practical Nursing School, West Plains, Missouri; and Joyce A. Wilson, RN, BA, South Plains College, School of Vocational Nursing, Levelland, Texas. Finally, we acknowledge each other, colleagues and still friends. Mutual respect, honest feedback, unwavering support, and sharing of current materials provide the tether.

▼▼▼
Contents

Who You Are

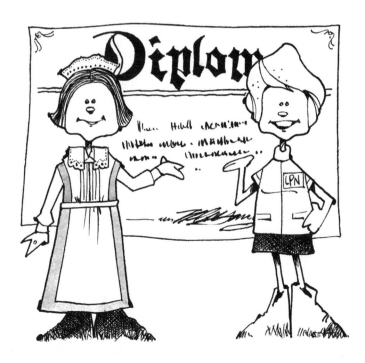

How Practical Nursing Evolved

▼▼▼ O U T L I N E

Early Western Cultures
Age of Christianity
The Renaissance
Age of Industrialization
Seventeenth and Eighteenth Centuries

Nineteenth Century
First School of Nursing
Florence Nightingale
Civil War

Formal Training: Practical Nursing
Twentieth Century: Organization/ Law/Licensing
You Have Come a Long Way

▼▼▼ K E Y   T E R M S

self proclaimed nurse
Phoebe
Sisters of Charity
Semmelweis
almshouses

Sairey Gamp
Betsy Prig
Florence Nightingale
Dorothea Lynnde Dix
Clara Barton

Lillian Wald
Mississippi, 1914
NAPNES
NFLPN

▼▼▼ O B J E C T I V E S

Upon completing this chapter you will be able to:

1. Describe the role of self-defined practical nurses throughout history.

2. Discuss four major events that influenced changes in practical nursing.

3. Identify the year in which the first school of practical nursing was founded.

4. Name the year in which licensing for practical nursing first began.

5. Present the rationale for your personal stand on entry into nursing practice.

The length of the course for the modern trained practical (or vocational) nurse* is approximately one year in most states, with some variation in the actual number of weeks. Historically speaking, nurses had less educational preparation for their work than do current trained practical nurses.

In reviewing the varied and colorful evolution of this vocation, practical nurses are referred to in a broad sense as those who from the beginning of time chose to or were appointed to care for individuals who were ill, injured, dying, or having babies. Names used to designate this person have included attendant, wet nurse, self-proclaimed nurse, midwife, trained nurse, and practical nurse. Most often, the individual doing this work was someone who seemed to have a "gift" or "touch" for helping others during a medical crisis. Some "nurses" learned from others in an apprenticeship setting, and others extended their "mothering" skills to the care of the sick. The practical nurse was the original home health nurse and visiting nurse. Much of the care was offered in the home. They were on call for the needy. It is worth noting that as early practical nurse training programs became available, they carefully limited their teaching to what would be known by a good homemaker or a competent maid. Training included information that would in no way compete with that of the physicians of the time, who themselves had limited knowledge and training. It is also interesting to realize that nursing history does not parallel medical history. When medicine advanced, nursing did not. When medical advances slowed down, nursing progressed.

Nursing has experienced many changes throughout its history, and the changes are not yet over. A major change that has occurred in practical nursing is a gradual increase in the required formal knowledge base and a requirement for licensing to practice practical nursing. Unlike the historically untrained or poorly trained practical nurse, who had unlimited and unsupervised freedom to practice, the present practical nurse is now often a hybrid who is being taught basic skills during the educational program. After graduation, the licensed practical/vocational nurse (LP/VN) is permitted to perform complex nursing skills as delegated by the registered nurse (RN) and allowed by the nurse practice act. Delegation is allowed as long as the RN is willing to teach the skill, observe the return demonstration, and document the teaching or learning process for the LP/VN's file in the place of employment. In addition, most nurse practice acts call for *direct* supervision by RNs for all complex nursing tasks delegated by them. See Chapter 19 for information on delegation.

Reading about nursing history can be enjoyable and can help you see your place among the many centuries of women and men who have given care, relief, and support to the sick. In this chapter we provide a broad overview of the role of nursing during different periods of history. *By knowing about the changes that occurred in nursing in the past, you will be ready to better understand and adapt to possible changes in the future.*

▼▼▼
Early Western Cultures

Recorded nursing history is about one and a half centuries old, but it is interesting to speculate about what might have occurred before that time. It is known that primitive cultures looked on illness as a direct reflection of a personal relationship with the gods. Ill fortune, as it applied to health, was regarded as a sign of disfavor because of behavior that was not pleasing to the gods. Among these cultures there was generally a wise person (medicine man) who possessed magical powers that allowed him to get in touch with and deal with the angered gods. For example, some pagan cultures had a shaman (holy man) who would go into a trance. While in the trance he would "slip into a crack in the earth" to travel down the river to the "valley of the dead." There he would bargain with the gods to find out what was needed from the one who was ill or if indeed the ill person would die. Stories of these customs were passed on through song.

---

* The term licensed vocational nurse is the legally recognized term in California and Texas; all other states in the United States use the term licensed practical nurse.

▽▽▽
Ancient Egypt

Although no direct evidence exists of nursing in Egypt, written records of procedures used in ancient Egypt were probably those of the attendants (nurses) who assisted the priests in caring for the ill. Temples erected to honor the god Apollo, worshipped as the god of medicine, became sanitariums where diseased people were treated. It is thought that Egyptian physicians and attendants 4000 years ago had an extensive list of treatments for specific illnesses. They differed rather remarkably from medicines used today. Interesting evidence was found in the tomb of an eleventh-dynasty queen, whose tomb included a medicine chest complete with vases, spoons, medicines, and herbs. "Lizard's blood, swine's ears and teeth, putrid meat and fat, tortoise brains, old books boiled in oil, milk of a lying-in woman, water of a chaste woman, lice and excreta of men, donkeys, dogs, lions and cats are examples of some of the ingredients that were used" (Kalish and Kalish, 1978, p. 3). Egyptian physicians were considered skillful at treating fractures. There is evidence of detailed instructions for daily nursing care, which included recording the pulse, using splints and bandages, and using hollow reeds for urinary catheters.

▽▽▽
Ancient Hebrews

The ancient Hebrews had houses for the sick and homes for the aged and began many practices of personal hygiene and public sanitation. Once again, the close association between religion and medicine was seen, as priests functioned in the role of major health officer.

The Old Testament often refers to nursing functions: "Many passages refer to wet nurses, and those who nursed the sick or acted as companions. Numbers 11:12, Exodus 2:7, 2:9, II Kings 4:4, Genesis 24:59, 35:8" (Becker and Fendler, 1990, p. 28).

▽▽▽
Ancient Greece

In the fifth century BC, the greatest civilization of all, the Greeks, gave the world *Hippocrates, Socrates, Plato,* and *Aristotle* and a system of logical thought that paved the way for rational treatment of illness, rather than seeing illness as god-inflicted. Hippocrates, the "father of modern medicine," translated teachings, once the secrets of priests, into a textbook of medicine and introduced a system of observing symptoms and applying carefully reasoned principles to care. These observations replaced the superstitions and illogical concepts of primitive medicine. However, many of Hippocrates' teachings were discarded because of the previously established beliefs. The Hippocratic oath is the ethical code of modern medical practice. Aristotle provided additional knowledge about the heart and blood vessels, but because it was forbidden to touch the dead, his knowledge was not widely used.

Women did not become trained nurses in Greece because they occupied a low position in society. They were not considered worthy to be trained in medicine or nursing. Household nursing and child care was done by domestics or servants. The Hippocratic nursing procedures for the sick were carried out by the physician or the physician's students.

▼▼▼
Age of Christianity

Greece's power and prestige declined. The Roman empire was the dominant power at the time of Christ's birth. Rome established military hospitals, and much of the practical nursing of the day was done by relatives and friends. Much of the knowledge medicine and nursing gained in the Greek era of power was lost. Few could read and understand the works of Hippocrates and other great thinkers of his time.

As Christianity grew through the centuries, nursing developed as a form of Christian charity. Christian nurses included both men and women, each caring for members of their own sex. St. Paul, of Biblical fame, introduced a woman named Phoebe, an ordained deaconess, to Rome about 30 years after the Crucifixion. *Phoebe,* a practical nurse, is known as the *first visiting nurse.* In addition to the order founded by the deaconess, other orders were founded that ministered to the sick and the poor.

▽▽▽
Dark Ages and Middle Ages

When the power of the Roman empire declined, invading tribes brought violence and chaos to Europe. The period from 400 to 1000 A.D. has been called the Dark Ages to reflect the loss of widespread education and learning in Europe. The Christian church retreated behind the walls of convents and monasteries. It was within these walls that learning was kept alive. In the Middle Ages (1000–1450) both men and women were involved in nursing because monks and nuns continued to do the practical necessary nursing of that time. One of the more interesting groups of monks was the *Knights Hospitalers,* who were a military order trained to fight as well as to tend the sick and wounded.

One of the nursing brotherhoods founded during this time was the *Alexian Brothers,* which continues to exist in a dual religious and nursing role. The history of nursing during this period includes stories of highborn women who renounced their heritage to care for the sick. Someone needed to do the nursing because the Middle Ages was a time of horrible epidemics. Among the epidemics was the infamous bubonic plague that killed millions of people. At the end of the Middle Ages, Europe seemed to be old and worn out. Religious fervor was replaced by cynicism and despair. Religious orders no longer assumed as much responsibility for care of the sick.

▼▼▼
The Renaissance

The Renaissance (1450–1650) was a time of rebirth of learning. The information of the ancient Greeks and Romans was sought and put to use.

The scientific method of the Greeks was employed again. The disciplines of anatomy, physiology, and scientific healing were developed. Nursing declined and was all but forgotten until the nineteenth century. It is thought that the religious reformation, in which the church split into Catholic and Protestant factions, contributed to the decline in organized nursing. In Protestant countries, such as England and Germany, monasticism nearly ended, and with it, nursing. Greater

personal freedom may have been achieved during the Renaissance, but with it the tradition of unselfish service to humanity almost disappeared. It was a cruel age, marked by neglect of the poor, homeless, and ill. It is worth noting that one man, *St. Vincent de Paul,* almost single-handedly organized the *Sisters of Charity* in France to care for the poor and nurse the sick.

▼▼▼
Age of Industrialization

As industrialization became more widespread in the eighteenth century, so did problems with disease. The movement of people to cities, the unhealthy working conditions, child labor, and overcrowding all had an impact on health care during the Industrial Revolution. Hospitals did not meet the needs of patients, but they grew in number, as did their mortality rates. Many patients shared the same bed and unsanitary conditions. Medical and nursing knowledge did not include the practice of asepsis. Once inside the hospital, patients frequently contracted more diseases than those they had when they came to the hospital. Home care continued without benefit of training, although the chances for survival were probably better in the home than in the hospital. In Vienna during this time, women in labor begged to be allowed to deliver in the street rather than in the hospital. To be admitted meant sure death because the mortality rate at times was 100%. It was not until 1847 that *antiseptic methods* were first developed and used. **Ignaz Philipp Semmelweis,** a Hungarian obstetrician, began to study what was called *childbed fever.* When a physician friend died following a cut on the finger during an autopsy, Semmelweis recognized that his friend had died from essentially the same disease that killed women who had babies. He identified the cause of the childbed (puerperal) fevers as septic materials carried to the mothers on the hands of medical students directly from the autopsy room. As a result, he insisted that medical students and physicians wash their hands in a solution of *chloride of lime* before entering the obstetrics ward. Antisepsis soon included the instruments and utensils used in the ward. As a result, the rate of death from childbed fever dropped dramatically in that ward.

▼▼▼
Seventeenth and Eighteenth Centuries

Meanwhile, back in the North American colonies, during the seventeenth and early eighteenth centuries, hospital care did not exist for those without families to care for them. (Illustrations in this chapter depict historical nursing settings.) What did exist were alms-houses for the poor and pesthouses for those with contagious diseases. The motivation for building the pesthouses was to protect the public, not to treat the sick. Medicine in America was less developed than that in Europe. Colonial physicians were poorly trained except for the few who obtained their education in England. Nursing continued to be done by untrained persons as well as those in a few religious orders whose mission was to care for the sick. The *first real hospital in America* was built in Philadelphia in the mid-1700s at the urging of *Benjamin Franklin*. All of the early American hospitals emulated French and English hospitals and made hospitalization available to the poor for a small fee. Hospitals obtained medical services by permitting teaching on the wards. Medical advances were slow. The treatment of choice for many diseases was brandy, whiskey, emetics, purgatives, and bleeding.

▼▼▼
Nineteenth Century

Early nineteenth-century American hospitals were places of confinement where one picked up additional diseases. The hospital wards were dirty, unventilated, and filled with patients with discharging wounds. Perfume was used to cover up offensive odors. Nurses of that time used snuff as a way of trying to make their work conditions bearable. Pain, hemorrhage, infections, and gangrene were the order of the day. Nursing was considered an inferior, undesirable occupation. Religious attendants (nurses) were replaced by lay people often drawn from the criminal population. They exploited and abused patients. Supervision was nonexistent, and there was little or no nursing service at night, unless a delivery or a death was expected. For that, a "watcher" was hired.

Nurses were often widows with large families. Drinking on duty and accepting bribes from patients and families were commonplace. "Vice was rampant among these women, who sometimes aided the dying by removing pillows and bed clothes and by performing other morbid activities to hasten the end" (Kalish and Kalish, 1978).

In Europe, nursing in secular institutions had

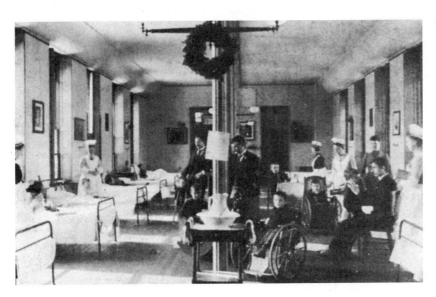

Figure 1–1
A pediatric unit under the aegis of the Connecticut Training School (ca. 1878). Note that there are two faculty members supervising three students. (Courtesy of Yale Medical Library.) (From Dolan JA, Fitzpatrick ML, Herrmann EK. *Nursing in Society: A Historical Perspective.* 15th ed. Philadelphia: W.B. Saunders, 1983.)

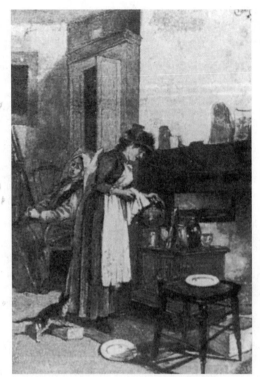

Figure 1–2

Caring for a sick person in a tenement house. (From Dolan JA, Fitzpatrick ML, Herrmann EK. *Nursing in Society: A Historical Perspective.* 15th ed. Philadelphia: W.B. Saunders, 1983.)

become nonexistent, especially in Protestant countries, where the services of the Sisters of Charity were not available. Typical of the hospital nurse at the time were the ignorant, gin-soaked nurse midwives such as Sairey Gamp and Betsy Prig in Charles Dickens' 1849 novel, *Martin Chuzzlewit.*

Nursing care in America was every bit as bad. An excerpt describing the cholera epidemic in the Philadelphia General Hospital in 1833 painted a picture of overcrowding and demands for increased wages. Nurses drank the stimulants intended for the sick and were seen drunk and fighting over the dead. Finally, an appeal was made to the Bishop for the services of the Sisters of Charity. They came, restored order, and nursed the sick.

▼▼▼
First School of Nursing

It was not until 1836 that the *first real school of nursing* was founded. In that year a German pastor established a hospital in his parish in *Kaiserswerth, Germany*. The purpose of the program was to teach the Lutheran Order of Deaconesses principles of nursing care. Many of the graduates of the Kaiserswerth Deaconess Institute settled in other parts of the world and established similar programs. The most famous pupil was Florence Nightingale, founder of modern nursing, who attended the school for three months.

▼▼▼
Florence Nightingale

Shortly after the start of the 1853 *Crimean War* (in which Britain, France, and Turkey fought against Russia for control of access to the Mediterranean from the Black Sea), information about the neglect and poor care of casualties began to reach England. A correspondent for the London *Times* wrote vivid accounts of the deplorable conditions and lack of medical and nursing care for the British troops. He noted that Russian troops were tended by the Sisters of Mercy, the French were tended by the Sisters of Charity, and the wounded of England were almost completely neglected. So persistent were his charges that a commission was sent to investigate. As a result, the Secretary of War decided that England, too, should have a group of women nurses to tend the war casualties. He contacted Florence Nightingale, explaining the situation to her. Because she had both nursing and administrative experience, the Secretary of War perceived her as the one nurse in England capable of organizing and supervising care. Florence Nightingale had an unusual background for a nurse of that period. She had wealthy, influential parents, was well educated before pursuing nursing, and had been presented at court, indicating her social standing. She had to beg her parents to be permitted to take nurses' training because nursing was seen as a profession suitable only for the Sairey Gamp type of woman.

Being appointed to the task of organization and

supervision of nurses during the Crimean War gave Miss Nightingale an unexpected opportunity for achievement. She left England for Crimea with 38 self-proclaimed nurses of limited experience, of which 24 were nuns.

Florence Nightingale and her nurses arrived to find overcrowded, filthy hospitals with no beds, no furniture, no eating utensils, no medical supplies, no blankets, no soap, no linens, and no lamps. The barracks

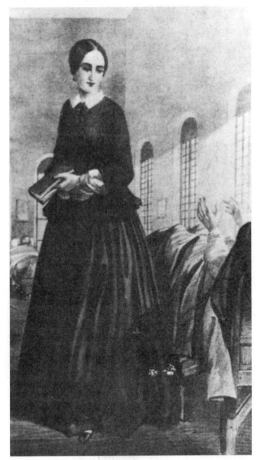

Figure 1–3
Florence Nightingale carrying out the "nursing process." (Nursing Mirror photograph.) (From Dolan JA, Fitzpatrick ML, Herrmann EK. *Nursing in Society: A Historical Perspective.* 15th ed. Philadelphia: W.B. Saunders, 1983.)

hospital, meant for 1700 patients, packed in 3000 to 4000 patients.

The wounded lay on the floor in their battle uniforms, in filth. Florence Nightingale took charge, using the supplies she had, and personally raised funds to purchase supplies that the doctors could not obtain for the army. She hired people to clean up the "hospitals" and established laundries to wash linens and uniforms. She expected a great deal of herself and those who worked with her. It was not an easy task, and a major prejudice that had to be overcome was that of the medical officers, who considered the nurses intruders. The hours were long and difficult for Miss Nightingale and her nurses. She was concerned too that sometimes the nurses became more involved in converting patients to their particular faith than in giving general care. She believed that the best nurses were those who were of good character, experienced a sense of calling, and were well trained to meet the physical needs of patients. Often after hours, it is said that Miss Nightingale could be seen making additional rounds with her lamp to check on the patients, earning her the title "the lady with the lamp."

By the end of six months, it was obvious that the efforts of Miss Nightingale and her nurses were paying off. The death rate among the wounded dropped from 420 per 1000 to 22 deaths per 1000 casualties. She stayed through the war and was the last to leave. Many of her nurses had become ill during the war and were sent home to recover. Miss Nightingale herself became ill with Crimean fever, probably typhus, and almost died. When she returned home she was decorated by Queen Victoria.

*Santa Filomena**
Whene'er a noble deed is wrought,
Whene'er is spoken a noble thought,
    Our hearts, in glad surprise,
    To higher levels rise.
The tidal wave of deeper souls
Into our inmost being rolls,
    And lifts us unawares

---

* Henry Wadsworth Longfellow (His tribute to Florence Nightingale, "Saint of the Crimea." Published in the first number of the *Atlantic Monthly,* November, 1857.)

Out of all meaner cares.
Honour to those whose words or deeds
Thus help us in our daily needs,
    And by their overflow
    Raise us from what is low!
Thus thought I, as by night I read
Of the great army of the dead,
    The trenches cold and damp,
    The starved and frozen camp—
The wounded from the battle plain,
In dreary hospitals of pain—
    The cheerless corridors,
    The cold and stony floors.
Lo! in that house of misery,
A lady with a lamp I see
    Pass through the glimmering gloom,
    And flit from room to room.
And slow, as in a dream of bliss,
The speechless sufferer turns to kiss
    Her shadow, as it falls
    Upon the darkening walls.
As if a door in heaven should be,
Opened, and then closed suddenly,
    The vision came and went—
    The light shone and was spent.
On England's annals, through the long
Hereafter of her speech and song,
    That light its rays shall cast
    From portals of the past.
A lady with a lamp shall stand
In the great history of the land,
    A noble type of good,
    Heroic womanhood.
Nor even shall be wanting here
The palm, the lily, and the spear,
    The symbols that of yore
    Saint Filomena bore.

One of Florence Nightingale's major goals was to establish a school of nursing in England. An overwhelming number of physicians opposed such a school on the basis that "because nurses occupied much the same positions as housemaids, they needed little instruction beyond poultice making, the enforcement of cleanliness and attention to their patients' personal needs" (Kalish and Kalish, 1978, p. 43). Miss Nightingale believed nurses should work only in hospitals, not on private duty. She did establish a school of nursing in 1860 in England and wrote several books on nursing. Her most famous book was *Notes on Nursing.* She emphasized high moral character in addition to technical skills. The core of her spirituality was a belief in perfection. To her, nursing was a sacred calling, a commitment to work for mankind, not a business. Other Victorian women like her shared the sense of the sacredness of time and the belief that wasting it was a sin. Nursing became a way for Florence Nightingale to work toward the perfection of mankind and her personal salvation. She was against licensure because she thought it was too much like a union. Her major contributions were the elimination of prejudice against a better class of women entering nursing and the generation of a push toward development of nursing as a respectable vocation. She was intelligent, well educated, and skeptical. This combination made her the foremost critical thinker in nursing, of its meaning and its role.

In the spring of 1989, the Florence Nightingale Museum opened in London, England on the grounds of St. Thomas Hospital, the site of the Nightingale School of Nursing. The Museum is a tribute to this nursing leader despite the fact that she wrote before her death: "I do not wish to be remembered when I am gone" (quote from Miss Nightingale's personal journal as found in the museum). In spite of her great and courageous contributions to nursing, Florence Nightingale saw only her own faults and her failures.

> *What would Florence Nightingale say to nursing applicants today who say they are entering nursing to "help" people, to get a job, or to make money? Have we matured as a vocation or as a profession? What do you think?*

▼▼▼
Civil War

During the same time period in America, when the country began the Civil War in 1861, there was no such thing as a trained nurse. In the South, especially, there was a great deal of prejudice toward women working in hospitals. There was general male opposition, but especially opposition from the medical profession. As a southern woman put it, "It seems strange that what the aristocratic women of Great Britain have done with honor is a disgrace for their sisters on this side of the Atlantic to do" (Kalish and Kalish, 1978).

Casualties were high on both sides.[12] Many died right on the field. Others died because of a poorly trained medical corps. Southern women offered their services as volunteers, but most of the nursing was done by infantrymen assigned to do a task they did not want to do. It was well into the war before southern women were recognized by the Confederate government for their contribution.

In the North, women offered their services as nurses to the government. One hundred women were selected to take a short training course from doctors in New York City. **Dorothea Lynnde Dix,** a teacher by profession and a long-time advocate for better conditions for mental patients, was appointed Superintendent of Nurses. Her task was to organize a corps of female nurses. She requested women under 30, plain-looking, wearing simple brown or black dresses and no bows, curls, jewelry, or hoop skirts. Women who did not meet the criteria nursed anyway but without official recognition or pay from the government. Eventually, through Miss Dix's efforts, the first hospitals for the mentally ill were also established.

In evaluating the nursing of the Civil War, doctors decided that the nursing system was defective. They did not approve of the women. However, it was a success in the eyes of the wounded soldiers.

Clara Barton, a teacher by profession, was one of the first civilians in the Civil War to round up army supplies. She rented a warehouse, filled market baskets, and encouraged friends to send comforts for the soldiers. Her efforts resulted in her being appointed Superintendent of the Department of Nurses for the Army in 1864. Clara Barton's efforts frequently found her on the front lines, and she nearly lost her life on two occasions. After the war, President Johnson commissioned her to do what she wanted to do—find missing prisoners of war. Later, while visiting in Europe for health reasons, she met *J. Henri Dunant,* founder of the *International Red Cross.* He asked her help in introducing the Red Cross to America. Finally in 1881, through Clara Barton's efforts, the first chapter of the *American Red Cross* was established in Danville, New York.

As often happens, something good emerges out of something not so good. Many of Florence Nightingale's books and ideas had made their way to America but had been ignored. The Civil War experience was the force needed to develop nurse training schools. The first training schools were separate from hospitals, the intent being to educate nurses. Soon, hospital-based schools of nursing sprang up. In many hospitals, schools became a cost-effective way of providing a nursing labor force, that is, free. After graduation, nurses generally worked in patients' homes.

Being a student nurse in the 1870s was a difficult experience. Living conditions, working hours, and responsibilities required a great deal of physical and emotional endurance. Not only did these students work long hours, they were also required to sign contracts in return for a course of lectures, on-the-job training, and minimal allowances.

▼▼▼
Formal Training: Practical Nursing

The *first* class for formal training of practical nurses was offered in 1892 *at the YWCA* in Brooklyn, New York. The focus was on training nurses to offer home health care for patients with chronic illness, the aged, and children. The course was three months in length. It was considered successful, and because of this, other similar programs were developed. Identified programs included an 1892 course in Boston, offered by the Massachusetts Emergency and Hygiene Association, the *Ballard School in New York in 1897,* and the *Brattleboro School in Vermont in 1907.* The course of study included cooking, care of the house, dietetics, simple science, and simple nursing procedures.

Until World War I most nursing done by practical nurses was home nursing, primarily because most people were cared for in the home. Even surgery was performed in the home. There is some truth in the way old Western movies portrayed surgery being done on the kitchen table. The nurse's 24-hour schedule included such procedures as cupping and applying *leeches,* preparing *stupes* for relief of abdominal distention, *mustard plasters* for relief of congestion, and

Table 1–1
Practical Nursing Milestones

Period in History	Event
Ancient Egypt	Untrained attendants assisted priests in caring for the ill
Ancient Hebrew	Wet nurses and attendants nursed the sick and acted as companions
Ancient Greece (fifth century BC)	Household nursing and child care was done by domestics and servants
Age of Christianity	Both men and women were nurses; each cared for members of own sex. *Phoebe*—The first visiting nurse
Dark Ages (400–1000)	Monks and nuns continued to do practical nursing
	Knights Hospitalers—A military order trained to fight as well as to tend the sick and wounded
Middle Ages	Time of epidemics. Highborn women renounced their heritage to care for the sick
	Alexian Brothers founded—A nursing brotherhood that still exists in a dual religious and nursing role
	At the end of the Middle Ages religious orders no longer assumed as much responsibility for care of the sick
Renaissance (1450–1650)	Scientific methods of Greeks were employed again, but nursing declined until the 19th century
Age of Industrialization (18th century)	Deplorable, unsanitary conditions
	Untrained care givers
	Semmelweiss—Developed antiseptic methods (1847)
17th- and 18th-century colonies	Almshouses and pesthouses. Nursing done by untrained persons
19th-century America	Nursing considered an inferior, undesirable occupation. Care given by untrained lay people often drawn from the criminal population
	Charles Dickens' novel *Martin Chuzzlewit* (1849) introduced Sairey Gamp and Betsy Prig as the nurse prototype of that period
1836	First real school of nursing, in Kaiserwerth, Germany. *Florence Nightingale* attended for three months
	Eighteen years later, after start of Crimean War, she nursed wounded with 38 self-identified (untrained) nurses
1860	*Florence Nightingale* established a school of nursing in England. She wrote several books. The most famous was *Notes on Nursing*
Civil War (1861)	In the South: Most nursing done by infantrymen assigned to task. Southern women volunteered services.
	In the North: *Dorothea Lynde Dix,* a teacher, was appointed Superintendent of Nurses and organized a corps of female nurses (untrained)
1864	*Clara Barton,* a teacher, collected supplies for soldiers. Led to her appointment as Superintendent of the Department of Nurses for the Army.
1881	*Clara Barton* established the first chapter of the *American Red Cross* in Danville, New York
1892	First class for formal training of practical nursing: YWCA, Brooklyn, New York

Table 1–1
Practical Nursing Milestones (Continued)

Period in History	Event
1893	*Henry Street Settlement* founded by *Lillian Wald,* a social worker, who graduated from a nursing program.
	Practical nurses pioneered in this new public health movement. They went into homes and taught to families in New York slums the basics of cleanliness and control of communicable diseases
1914	*Mississippi* is the first state to pass a law to *license practical nurses*
1917	*Standardization* of nursing requirements for practical nursing by *National League of Nursing Education*
World War I	Shortage of practical nurses. Army School of Nursing established. *Smith Hughes Act* of 1917 provided money for developing additional schools of practical nursing
1920s	Acute shortage of practical nurses. Many did not return to nursing after the war
1920–1940	Most practical nursing limited to Public Health Agencies and Visiting Nurse Associations
World War II	At home, practical nurses worked in clinics, health departments, industries, hospitals. In the war, ventured into hardship tours in Europe, North Africa, and the Pacific. Number of practical nurses peaked in 1940 at 159,009
1941	*NAPNES* (National Association of Practical Nurse Education and Service), the nation's professional organization dedicated exclusively to practical nursing, was founded
End of World War II	Nursing shortage saw movement of practical nurses into hospitals and gradually increasing responsibilities
1944	Comprehensive study of practical nursing by U.S. Department of Vocational Education. This was the first time that tasks of practical nursing were agreed upon
1949	Joint Committee on Practical Nurses and Auxiliary Workers in Nursing Services recommended use of title licensed practical nurse and differentiated between tasks of registered nurses and licensed practical nurses
1952	Approximately 60% of the nurse work force was made up of practical nurses
1960s	ANA (American Nurses Association) first moves toward two distinct levels in nursing—professional and technical
1980s	Resurgence of ANA's move toward two distinct levels of nursing. This resulted in some states adopting two levels of nursing and then rescinding their decision because of the nursing shortage
	The American Medical Association (AMA) initiated and subsequently dropped the Registered Care Technician (RCT) proposal.
1990s	No acute shortage exists at this time. Unlicensed personnel are used for patient care. The number of hospital jobs have decreased. The primary employment site has moved into the community

poultices for drawing out pus from infections, and administering *enemas*. These were often nutritive enemas containing eggnog with brandy or chicken broth. Remember, there were no intravenous solutions then. Some practical nurses also assumed the then-accepted role of midwife and taught new mothers the basics of cleanliness, diet, and care of the child. In New York City in 1919 approximately 1700 midwives attended 30% of all births in the city.

By the end of the nineteenth century there was a renewed interest in charitable work and concern for the sick. Practical nursing began to expand from home nursing to public health nursing, care of patients in the slums, school nursing, industrial nursing, and well-baby care. Once again, practical nurses pioneered in this new public health movement. One of the best-known centers in 1893 was the Henry Street Settlement in New York. It was founded by Lillian Wald, a social worker who graduated from nursing and intended to become a doctor. She taught home nursing to immigrants and was so impressed by their need for medical care that she left medical school to begin a nursing service, The Henry Street Settlement. Practical nurses who were members of the Henry Street Settlement taught families in New York slums the basics of cleanliness and control of communicable diseases. There was a decrease in school absenteeism because the spread of childhood illness was reduced. School nurses visited schools and new mothers and their babies. They taught mothers the basics of preventing the summertime killer of infants—cholera infantum. It was estimated that their efforts resulted in survival of 1200 more babies than usual during the summer heat wave. Another original contribution of the nurses was the development of "Little Mother Leagues" in the slums, in which all girls over eight years old were taught to take care of their younger siblings, including the infants.

▼▼▼
Twentieth Century: Organization/Law/Licensing

By 1903, states began to take steps that ultimately led to monitoring of practical nursing. It was during this period that nursing organizations were developed. Certainly the most influential step was taken by the *National League of Nursing Education* (now the National League for Nursing, or NLN), which in 1917 developed a nationwide system of standardization of nursing requirements for practical nursing.

In 1914, *Mississippi* was the first state to pass a law licensing practical nurses. This was an important event because the public had no way of knowing who was giving them nursing care. Remember that for centuries self-proclaimed nurses were responsible for the majority of the nursing that was done. Licensing, however, was not mandatory, and by 1938 New York was the *only state to have mandatory licensure.*

> **Does your state have mandatory licensure? What year did it begin?**

At the onset of World War I, there were few practical nurses and few schools of practical nursing. Hurriedly "trained" nurses were rushed to the battle-front. An army school of nursing was established to combat the severe nursing shortage and to improve the overall quality of care. Many nurses looking for glamour and excitement found superhuman demands made of them during the war.

The home front was facing a battle of its own in 1917–1918, with a major epidemic of pneumonia in 1917 and a worldwide epidemic of Spanish influenza in 1918. The mortality rate was high, especially in 1918. The *Smith Hughes Act of 1917* did provide money for developing additional schools of practical nursing. However, the new schools could not supply enough nurses quickly enough to meet the severe shortage in the United States.

After the war, many nurses did not continue nursing. There was an acute shortage of nurses in the 1920s. Many more hospitals opened schools of nursing, but their real purpose was to provide staffing. Hospitals without schools were staffed heavily with untrained help.

In the period between the two World Wars, 1920–1940, six states had laws licensing practical nurses, but there were few practical nursing schools throughout the country. Much of their work continued to be done in public health agencies and in visiting nurse associations.

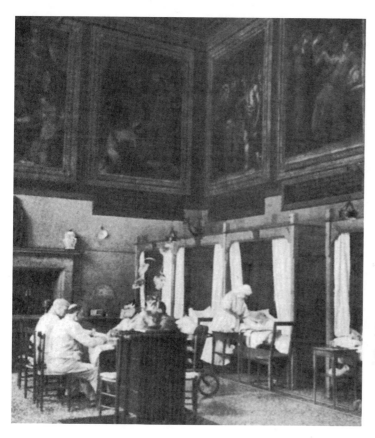

Figure 1–4

A Sister at the Hotel Dieu in Beaune giving care to a patient in a room compartment. Ambulatory patients enjoy meals at the table in the center. Note the works of art. (From Dolan JA, Fitzpatrick ML, Herrmann EK. *Nursing in Society: A Historical Perspective.* 15th ed. Philadelphia: W.B. Saunders, 1983.)

During the depression of the 1930s, many nurses lost their jobs or worked in hospitals for room and board rather than a salary. When it became fairly obvious that America was becoming involved in World War II, nursing leaders began to prepare for the need for all kinds of nurses. They did not want to face the nursing shortage experienced during World War I. This was a monumental task because nursing had decreased in popularity as a vocation. Much of the dialogue heard then sounded a great deal like that of the mid-1980s. For example, a hospital executive was quoted as saying, "Nurses should either get off their high horses and do the physical work they started out to do or move over and let others do it. There is too much talk about 'high professional standards' and not enough about taking care of the sick" (Kalish and Kalish, 1978). In the 1990s, nursing continues to search for its role both as a vocation and as a profession.

Practical nurses played a significant role both at home and in the war. At home, practical nurses worked in clinics, in health departments, in industry, and in hospitals. In the war, nurses could be found in Europe, North Africa, and the Pacific. One of the most widespread diseases they battled was malaria in the East Indies, the Philippines, and the southern Asiatic countries. The number of practical nurses in America peaked in 1940 at 159,009 and by 1944 was already experiencing a decline.

The National Association for Practical Nurse Education and Service, Inc. (NAPNES) was founded in 1941. The multidisciplinary composition of its membership includes licensed practical nurses, registered nurses, physicians, hospital and nursing-home administrators, students, and public members.

This association was the first to be recognized by the U.S. Department of Education as an official accrediting agency for schools of practical nursing. For the past several years, NAPNES has no longer accredited practical nursing programs.

The end of World War II saw a continuing shortage of nurses. It was this shortage that helped practical nurses play an important part in hospital nursing. Most hospitals gradually increased the responsibilities designated for the practical nurse.

In 1944, the U.S. Department of Vocational Education made a comprehensive study of practical nursing. This was the first time that the tasks of practical nursing were agreed upon. Extensive specific duties were outlined with an emphasis on maintaining aseptic technique. The terms "to judge," "to appraise," "to recognize," and "to determine" were often used to describe the scope of the practical nurse's job.

Other important changes followed. In 1949, the Joint Committee on Practical Nurses and Auxiliary Workers in Nursing Services recommended use of the title licensed practical nurse. Furthermore, the Committee differentiated between the tasks of the RN and the LPN and saw the LPN as being under the supervision of the RN. The Committee also suggested that practical nurses organize to make decisions on their salary, working conditions, and employment standards.

Because of the work of the Joint Committee, many practical nursing programs were strengthened with regard to content and focused for the first time on the preparation of practical nursing instructors. Up to this point, any graduate nurse was eligible to teach practical nursing.

By 1952, almost 60% of the nursing work force was made up of practical nurses. In many instances, RNs expressed bitterness because hospitals, clinics, and other agencies were hiring practical nurses for less money and assigning tasks to them beyond their educational level. They also expressed concern that the public was unable to differentiate between the levels of nurses because both wore the same type of white uniforms, caps, and pins. Many practical nurses quickly stopped wearing the practical nursing insignia, which was meant to identify the practical nurse. In many agencies, pay continued to be poor, and practical nurses

alternately performed tasks belonging to the RN one day and those belonging to nursing aides, for lesser compensation, on other days. Many practical nurses felt trapped in such situations because of their need for employment.

In 1961, the *National League for Nursing (NLN)* established a separate department of practical nursing programs. A major breakthrough was the development of a system for *accrediting schools* of practical nursing. This was supported by the *American Nurses Association (ANA)* and the *National Federation of Licensed Practical Nurses (NFLPN)*. To be accredited by the NLN, a school had to meet standards set by the NLN. With the exception of programs receiving federal funds, it was not, nor is it now, mandatory for schools to be accredited by the NLN because the major responsibility for approval of nursing programs rests with each state board of nursing. The NLN continues to accredit nursing programs while it challenges the U.S. Department of Education's recommendation to withdraw the NLN's recognition as an accrediting agency. The 1960s brought a move by the ANA to streamline nursing into two distinct levels: the two-year technical and the four-year professional nurse.

In 1975 there were 1337 practical nursing programs, graduating a total of 46,080 practical nurses. Approximately two-thirds of the practical nurses were employed in hospitals, 17.3% in nursing homes, 7.5% in private duty, and 6.5% in doctors' offices, clinics, and dental offices. Admission standards in most schools increased, as did the difficulty of the curriculum.

In the 1980s a resurgence of the ANA movement toward establishing two levels of nursing temporarily gained momentum. Some states worked toward adoption of the ANA recommendation. Because a serious nursing shortage developed in the late 1980s, the ANA movement stalled.

With the goal of easing the nursing shortage, the American Medical Association in the summer of 1989 proposed a new health care worker, the Registered Care Technologist (RCT). The RCT would be trained in one- and two-year programs. Because this new level of health care worker correlated with existing personnel, the practical nurse and the associate-degree nurse, the RCT proposal was not successful. This event is a gentle reminder for practical nurses to be strong, organized, and vigilant as a group. As we approach the twenty-first century, no acute nursing shortage exists, and some researchers predict surpluses. Unlicensed personnel and "crosstrained" allied health workers are being used for patient care in creative ways. Changes in the health care system are occurring daily, as are changes in opportunities for LPNs.

In 1993 there were 1098 practical nursing programs (Nursing Data Source, 1994). A survey of 1993 LP/VNs showed that 38.7% worked in hospitals, 48.6% worked in long-term care facilities, and 12.7% were employed in community or home care settings (Nursing Data Source, 1994). Home health care is once again becoming important because of shortened hospital stays.

Practical nurses are also finding employment in insurance companies that handle medical claims, in wellness and diet centers, in veterinarian's offices, as industrial nurses, as private nurses for physicians, and in the armed forces. It is clear that the practical nurse continues to be needed to provide skilled, technical care to patients in many areas.

▽▽▽
Important Influences in Nursing History

Many RNs influenced the course of nursing and practical nursing history. Table 1-2 identifies some of those registered nurses.

▼▼▼
You Have Come a Long Way

As a final note, it may be interesting to compare present practical nursing tasks with those that you would have been expected to perform in 1887. Practical nursing has indeed come a long way.

The following job description was given to floor nurses by a hospital in 1887 (author unknown):

In addition to caring for your 50 patients, each nurse will follow these regulations:

1. Daily sweep and mop the floors of your ward, dust the patient's furniture, and window sills. Maintain an even temperature in your ward by bringing in a scuttle of coal for the day's business.
2. Light is important to observe the patient's condition. Therefore, each day fill kerosene lamps, clean chimneys, and trim wicks. Wash the windows once a week.
3. The nurse's notes are important in aiding the physician's work. Make your pens carefully; you may whittle nibs to your individual taste.
4. Each nurse on day duty will report every day at 7 A.M. and leave at 8 P.M., except on the Sabbath, on which day you will be off from 12 noon to 2 P.M.
5. Graduate nurses in good standing with the director of nurses will be given an evening off each week for courting purposes or two evenings a week if you go regularly to church.
6. Each nurse should lay aside from each pay day a goodly sum of her earnings for her benefits during her declining years so that she will not become a burden. For example, if you earn $30 a month you should set aside $15.
7. Any nurse who smokes, uses liquor in any form, gets her hair done at a beauty shop, or frequents dance halls will give the director of nurses good reason to suspect her worth, intentions, and integrity.
8. The nurse who performs her labors and serves her patients and doctors without fault for five years will be given an increase of five cents a day, providing there are no hospital debts outstanding.

Table 1–2
Some Persons/Events in Nursing History

Mary Robinson	1859	First visiting nurse
Linda Richards	1873	America's first professionally trained nurse; organized other training schools
Euphemia Van Rensselaer	1876	Introduced first uniform—apron and cap (Bellevue Training School for Nurses)
Mary E.P. Mahoney	1879	First black graduate nurse
Elizabeth Weston	1888	First Native American nurse. Graduate of Training School of the University of Pennsylvania. Came from Lincoln School for Indian girls in Philadelphia. After graduation returned to care for her people on a Sioux reservation in North Dakota
Emily L. Loveridge	1890	Graduate of Bellevue Training School for Nurses. Went west to establish first school of nursing in northwest at Good Samaritan Hospital, Portland, Oregon
Isabel Hampton Robb	1893	Wrote first substantial nursing text: *Nursing: Its Principles and Practice for Hospital and Private Use*
Lillian Wald, Mary Brewster	1893	First visiting nurse service for the poor: Nurses Settlement House in slum section, lower east side, New York City. Later moved to Henry Street and name changed to Henry Street Settlement House
Lavinia L. Dock	1896	First president of forerunner of ANA (Nurses Associated Alumnae of the United States and Canada). Outlined principles on which ANA was founded
Dita H. Kinney	1901	First nurse Superintendent of Nurses of Army Nurse Corps
Mrs. Bedford Fenwick (Great Britain)	1901	First president of International Council of Nurses. Proposed state registration of nurses
Adelaide Nutting	1907	First graduate of Johns Hopkins Training School for Nurses. First nurse in the world to hold professorship in a university (Columbia). In 1917 Chair of Committee to Develop National Curriculum
Lillian Wald, Ella Phillips Crandall, Mary Beard, Mary Lent, Edna Foley, Lystra Greiter, Elizabeth G. Fox	1912	Formed National Organization of Public Health Nurses. Lillian Wald, first president
Margaret Sanger	1916	Spearheaded birth control movement as a response to high maternal and child mortality. A public health nurse. Opened first birth control clinic in America
Annie W. Goodrich	1918	President of ANA. Became Chief Inspecting Nurse for Army hospitals at home and abroad. Supported formation of Army School of Nursing. Became dean of school
Mary Breckenridge	1925	Organized Frontier Nursing Service of Kentucky
Sage Memorial Hospital School of Nursing, Ganado, Arizona	1930	First school of nursing for American Indians
Lucile Petry	1943	Director of U.S. Cadet Nurses Corps
Esther Lucille Brown, Ph.D., a researcher	1948	"Brown" Study: Advocated movement of nursing education to collegiate setting
Mildred L. Montag	1952	Appointed as first Associate Degree Nursing Program Project Coordinator. Project based on Montag's doctoral thesis, "Education of Nursing Technicians." Project located at Queen's College, New York

▼▼▼ S U M M A R Y

▶ The varied and colorful evolution of practical nursing has been described with limited reference to roles played by RNs in the course of nursing history. This account is an attempt to show practical nursing students that their vocation began to develop in ancient times and is not an appendage of professional nursing. Practical nurses can be rightly proud of their own nursing "roots."

▶ The duties of practical nurses have changed according to the needs present at various times in history. Currently, practical nurses are taught basic skills during their educational program. According to some states' nurse practice acts, they are allowed to perform complex skills delegated by an RN. However, in these states, the RN must teach the complex skill involved, be satisfied with the LPN's performance, and document this for the LPN's file. Direct supervision by an RN is also required for performance of complex nursing tasks.

▶ Practical nurses play an important role in the health care system today. There is no acute shortage of nurses at this time. Unlicensed personnel are being used for patient care. The number of hospital jobs has decreased. Practical nursing employment has moved into the community.

▶ You can have a voice in the decisions affecting practical nursing. Consider the odds faced by these historical figures in nursing:

　✗ Florence Nightingale, founder of modern nursing
　✗ Clara Barton, founder of the American Red Cross
　✗ Lillian Wald, founder of public health nursing
　✗ Dorothea Dix, advocate for the mentally ill.

▶ No more frontiers, you say? Don't you believe that. You can, for example, begin by taking a stand through your vocational organization—the local and state practical nurses associations.

▶ It has been suggested by some that the history of practical nursing sounds depressing. Not so. Practical nurses have always been in the forefront of doing the real, down-to-earth nursing tasks. They have often done what no one else dared or cared to do. In the beginning most of these "nurses" had little or no training. Consider that Florence Nightingale herself left the Kaiserswerth Deaconess Institute training program after three months of training. It is with this in mind that this chapter has focused on figures in nursing history who had limited education and yet enormous courage to care for patients, most often without glamour or fanfare. What these nurses did have was the gratitude of their patients and the quiet satisfaction of a job well done. We salute you, the new practical nurses and the nurses who have paved the way for you.

▼▼▼ R E F E R E N C E S

Becker B, Fendler D. *Vocational and Personal Adjustments in Practical Nursing.* Philadelphia: J.B. Lippincott, 1990, p. 28.

Kalish P, Kalish B. *The Advance of American Nursing.* Boston: Little, Brown, 1978.

Nursing Data Source, 1994. *Focus on Practical/Vocational Nursing.* Vol. 3. New York: National League for Nursing, 1994.

Widerquist J. The spirituality of Florence Nightingale. Nurs Res. 1992; 41(1): 49–55.

▼▼▼ S U G G E S T E D   R E A D I N G

ANA Report. Trained attendants and practical nurses. Am J Nurs 1944; 44:7–8.

Brown E. *Nursing for the Future.* New York: Russell Sage Foundation, 1948.

Deming D. Practical nurses—a professional responsibility. Am J Nurs 1944; 44:36–43.

Etheridge L. National Commission on Nursing. Written testimony at public hearing, February 1981.

Goldsmith J. New York's Practical Nurse Program. Am J Nurs 1942; 42:1026–1031.

Howlett H. *History of the Entry into Practice Issue* (unpublished paper), 1990.

Kinder J. President NLN. Letter, November 1986.

Longfellow HW. *The Political Works of Longfellow,* Cambridge ed. Boston: Houghton-Mifflin, 1975.

McGuane E, Bullough B. *Proud History, Promising Future.* Practical Nurs 1992; December, 40–42.

Philips E. Practical nurses in a public agency. Am J Nurs 1944; 44:974–975.

Pillitteri A. *One Nursing Curriculum 100 Years Ago: A Retrospective View as a Prospective Necessity.* J Nurs Ed June 1994; 33(6): 286–287.

Spalding E. *Professional Adjustments in Nursing.* 3rd ed. Philadelphia: J.B. Lippincott, 1946.

Thompson M. *Cry and the Covenant.* New York: Signet Books, 1955.

The Practical Nurse's Role in the Nursing Process

CHAPTER 2

▼▼▼ O U T L I N E

▼▼▼ K E Y   T E R M S

client problem
subjective

established nursing diagnosis
NANDA

objective
strengths

▼▼▼ O B J E C T I V E S

Upon completing this chapter you will be able to:

1. Discuss what is meant by the nursing process.

2. Define your role in the nursing process according to the nurse practice act of your state.

3. Describe the four phases* of the nursing process for the practical nurse:
   ▶ Data Collection (Assessment)
   ▶ Planning
   ▶ Implementation
   ▶ Evaluation

4. Describe nursing diagnosis as the exclusive domain of the RN.

---

*As defined by the National Council of State Boards of Nursing.

The nursing process is a problem-solving method. it is a way to plan client care. It helps clients reach the goals that have been set to care for their health problems.

Currently, unlicensed persons are doing all the tasks and skills that practical nurses do. It is the nursing process that separates practical nurses from the unlicensed persons. This makes practical nurses attractive to employers because they can solve problems and think critically.

As a student you will probably develop nursing care plans. Nursing care plans are learning tools. They are traditionally used in practical nursing programs to help students learn about client needs. Using your role in the nursing process to devise a care plan is a critical thinking exercise. The exact information fitting your client is not found anywhere. You compose it. This becomes easier plan by plan. And then—presto! You graduate. You are employed. You have internalized your role in the nursing process, and you are thinking critically as a nurse.

▼▼▼
What Is the Nursing Process?

Nursing process is a method of doing the work of nursing. It is a problem-solving method. Nursing process provides the steps for client care. Nurses benefit by having a methodical way of collecting data (assessing), planning, implementing, and evaluating care. Clients benefit by participating as full partners in their personal care. See Table 2–1 for a comparison between the problem-solving process and the nursing process for the practical nurse.

▼▼▼
What Does Your State Law Say About Your Role?

It is crucial at this time that, with the assistance of your instructor, you review the nurse practice act of your state. Your role in the nursing process is spelled out in

Table 2–1
Problem-Solving versus Nursing Process

Problem-Solving Process	Nursing Process
1. Define the problem	Phase 1: Data collection (assessment)
2. Decide on the goal	Phase 2: Planning
3. Identify alternatives	
4. Choose an alternative	
5. Try out the alternative	Phase 3: Implementation
6. Evaluate the effectiveness	Phase 4: Evaluation
7. Repeat the process if the solution is not effective	

Based on Bauer and Hill, 1986, p. 188.

this law. There are variations within the state and territories. Check it out. It is the basis of your nursing practice. Table 2–2, Nursing Process and Caregiver Roles, shows one model, developed jointly by the California Nurses Association and a Union Local (Local 250). The model roles are based on the California laws and educational requirements, which define the scopes of practice of RNs and LVNs and the tasks that can be assigned to nurses' assistants (NAs) and certified nurses' assistants (CNAs). The organizations, in developing the models, stated, "We recognize that skilled, experienced NAs, CNAs, LVNs, and RNs often contribute to patient care at a level beyond what their licensure or certification requires. We believe that nursing expertise must be encouraged and respected. But we must not permit employers to exploit the fear of losing a job or the need for recognition and job satisfaction in order to force speed-ups, impose greater responsibility for lower pay, and require nursing personnel to violate their legal scope of practice."

	RN Role	LVN Role	NA/CNA Role
Table 2–2 **The Nursing Process and Caregivers' Roles**			
Assessment of Patient's Condition or Needs	• Direct observation (see, auscultate, palpate, percuss) • Data collection (measurements which require substantial scientific knowledge or technical skill) • Information gathering shaped by theory, pattern recognition or judgment • Verification/corroboration of data collected by other personnel • Synthesis or interpretation of data • Formulation of nursing diagnosis, including psychosocial and educational needs	• Direct observation (see, auscultate, palpate, percuss) • Data collection (measurements, including those requiring LVN technical skill) • Recognition of abnormal values • Collaboration with RN in nursing diagnosis	• Observation (seeing) • Data collection (basic measurements) • Reporting
Planning or Coordinating Nursing Care	• Application of theory to individual patient's findings • 3-way communication to enhance mutual respect or job satisfaction, or to promote coordination of care • Delegation, assignment, or clinical guidance for other caregivers • Partnership with patient regarding plan of care	• Collaboration with RN in planning care • 3-way communication to enhance mutual respect or job satisfaction, or to promote coordination of care	• 3-way communication to enhance mutual respect or job satisfaction, or to promote coordination of care
Implementation, Not Fragmentation	• Functions, including manual, requiring substantial scientific knowledge or technical skill • Functions requiring or closely related to patient's need for ongoing assessment • Functions requiring RN assessment • Initiate/change treatment following standardized procedures • Cooperation in implementation to promote peer support, unity, or patient or caregiver safety	• Technical or manual functions, including sterile technique or IVs within certification • Ongoing data collection while implementing care • Reporting or referral as needed • Cooperation in implementation to promote peer support, unity, or patient or caregiver safety	• Manual functions appropriate to education or skill level, or in accordance with RN and LVN regulatory rules • Reporting as needed • Cooperation in implementation to promote peer support, unity, or patient or caregiver safety

Table continued on following page

Table 2–2
The Nursing Process and Caregivers' Roles (Continued)

	RN Role	LVN Role	NA/CNA Role
Patient Education	• Ongoing integration or application of new scientific knowledge to individual patient's signs or symptoms • Assessment of educational needs and delegation of implementation as appropriate to LVN • Advice based on independent scope of RN and/or standardized procedures	• Patient education based on licensed vocational nursing curriculum • Appropriate implementation of patient education	• Basic information regarding facility environment or facility procedures • Notify licensed personnel if patient needs additional education
Evaluation	• See assessment above **The RN is responsible for evaluation of patient's overall condition or response to treatment. This is achieved by the RN's direct observation or assessment, in addition to interpretation of the LVN's physical assessment, data collection, or recognition of abnormal values, or the NA/CNA's observations and measurements.**	• See assessment role above	• Observation, data collection, or reporting as above
Patient Advocacy	• Ethical or legal obligation or responsibility for active patient advocacy, which goes beyond observing patient's rights	• Ethical obligation to use technical knowledge for patient's best interest • Ethical or legal obligation to respect patient's rights	• Ethical or legal obligation to respect patient's rights

From California Nurse, March 1995.

Developed jointly by the California Nurses Association and Union Local 250. Published in California Nurse, March 1995. Used with permission.

▼▼▼
Phases of the Nursing Process for the Practical Nurse

The four steps of the nursing process for the practical nurse as presented in the 1995 NCLEX-PN (National Council Licensure Examination for Practical Nurses) test plan are:

1. *Data Collection:* Participate in establishing a data base.

2. *Planning:* Plan to set goals for meeting clients' needs and design strategies to achieve these goals.

3. *Implementation:* Initiate and complete actions necessary to accomplish the defined goals.

4. *Evaluation:* Participate in determining the extent to which goals have been achieved and interventions have been successful.

▼▼▼
What Differentiates Your Role from the RN Role?

The RN has the major responsibility for all five steps of the nursing process. As a practical nurse, you take an active part in four steps (phases) of the nursing process according to your skill level. You assist in *data collection* (assessment), *planning, implementation,* and *evaluation* of care. You work from the established nursing diagnosis, one of the five steps of the nursing process written by the RN. You turn *nursing diagnosis* to *nursing problems.* In this way you clearly understand the nature of the problems.

Nursing diagnosis, step two of a five-step nursing process for RNs, is a summary in nursing terms of actual or risk or high-risk problems that nurses can respond to. It is considered the exclusive responsibility of the RN. Writing a nursing diagnosis is based on an established list of nursing diagnoses. This list is called the NANDA list, meaning the list developed by the North American Nursing Diagnosis Association. Registered nurses are encouraged to use the approved list to share a common language with other nurses. Nursing diagnoses are intended to create a communication bridge for all nurses, so that they can understand each other's terminology. (See Appendix II at the end of the book.)

RNs are taught assessment skills, which include client interview and physical assessment of all body systems as part of their basic education. Practical nurses may *choose* to learn complex assessment skills as part of a postgraduate course. However, practical nurses learn to collect data (assess) the client and the environment during every encounter with a client. Data collection includes taking vital signs, checking therapeutic responses to medications and treatment, assessing for symptoms of health problems, etc. The focus for data collection (assessment) is based in the unit of study for the practical nurse.

According to the NCLEX-PN test plan, effective October, 1996, the practical nurse acts in a more *dependent* role when participating in the planning and evaluation phases of the nursing process and acts in a more *independent* role when participating in the data collection and implementation phases of the nursing process.

Because of the depth of the RN's basic education, the RN functions independently in all steps of the nursing process. These actions do not need a physician's order. Both RNs and LPNs and LVNs share an *interdependent* relationship with other health team members. For example, RNs and LPNs both carry out orders for treatments and medications written by a medical doctor, podiatrist, or dentist.

▼▼▼
Data Collection (Assessment): Phase 1

Some states allow practical nurses to use the phrase "assist with assessment." Other states permit use of the phrase "data collection." A committee established by the NCLEX plans to identify the terminology appropriate to cover this process. Check with your instructor for an information update.

According to the 1995 NCLEX-PN test plan, data collection includes the following:

A. Gather information relative to the client:
   ▶ Collect information from the client, significant others, and/or health care team members; and current and prior health records.
   ▶ Recognize significant findings.
   ▶ Determine the need for more information.
B. Communicate information gained in data collection:
   ▶ Document findings thoroughly and accurately.
   ▶ Report findings to relevant members of the health care team.
C. Contribute to the formation of nursing diagnosis:
   ▶ Assist in organizing relevant health care data.
   ▶ Assist in determining a significant relationship between data and client needs and/or problems.

Your involvement in this step depends on the place of your employment and your skill level. The practical nurse usually has more responsibility in the nursing home where the client's condition is more stable. At the conclusion of your practical nursing program you have acquired strong, although incomplete, assessment (data collection) skills: "the tool box is not complete." An incomplete tool box is nothing to be ashamed of. For example, take the temperature, pulse, respiration (TPR) and blood pressure properly. Be proud of your data collection (assessment) skills. They provide valuable data. Most areas offer physical assessment as a course separate from the practical nursing program. Ask your instructor about the availability of such a course. It is an excellent way to learn interview, observation, and physical assessment skills. Whether you use part or all of these skills at work, the knowledge will improve the care you provide.

The *primary* source of information in data collection is the client. After all, she knows herself and her body better than anyone else. All questions should be directed to the client unless he or she is unable to respond. *Secondary* information is available through family members, friends, and information that accompanies the client. Clients need to be reassured that information will be considered confidential unless they give permission to share it.

Data collection begins on admission. Data collection (assessment) continues with each client encounter. The RN interviews the client to obtain his or her history and assess the body systems. The practical nurse is not taught how to interview or physically assess body systems. As part of the one-year program, learning communication skills does not include learning the formal interview process. Obtainment of initial data, including vital signs, is often assigned to the practical nurse. It is important to separate the information gathered into *subjective, objective, historical,* and *current* data.

▶ *Subjective* information is based on the client's opinion. It can include self-evaluation of pain, headache, nausea, feelings, etc. Charting starts with the words, "Client states . . . ."

▶ *Objective* information includes data that the nurse can observe and verify. Examples include vital signs, height, weight, appearance, personal hygiene, etc. Use of the senses is required: seeing, hearing, smelling, touching, and yes, sometimes even tasting. Objective information helps to support or cast doubt on subjective information. Charting states what the nurse observes and measures without judging or drawing conclusions.

▶ *Historical* information includes the health history that relates to the current condition. Charting involves being as objective as possible.

▶ *Current* information includes what is happening now. This is "where it's at" for the practical nurse who is *assisting with* data collection (assessment). Words like check, observe, monitor, weigh, measure, smell, palpate, and auscultate are clues that this is an assessment (data collection) procedure. The practical nurse develops a list of data to be collected to accompany the identified problems as a way to tell if the client is meeting the goals. Data collection (assessment) starts when you first see the client at the beginning of the shift. This is your baseline observation. It continues throughout your shifts. Florence Nightingale said that if you do not observe your client you should not be a nurse. With each contact the LPN (or LVN) must see, hear, smell, and touch the client when necessary and use all the senses to gather data about the client and the environment. Data collection is vital—the client changes throughout the day. This is why accuracy in taking vital signs, describing vomitus, bleeding, or a skin lesion, for example, is so important. "Has the client's skin lesion changed since the last time you checked the lesion? How? How much?" Sometimes LPNs do not understand that what they are assigned to do is a vital part of the total assessment (data collection). Data collection starts during admission. It continues daily at the beginning of the shift for the baseline observation, then periodically during the shift, and right before leaving.

Data collection (assessment), whether partial or total, involves courtesy. Introduce yourself to the client and explain what you are going to do. Address the client as Mr., Mrs., Miss, or other title as appropriate. Avoid using a first name unless you have the client's permission. Remind yourself that this is a professional, not a personal, relationship you are building. The most common complaints put forth by clients: "I don't know which one is the nurse," "I am treated with disrespect," "I am not their grandma," and so on. When in the client's presence, stand or sit where he or she can see you. Clients often experience fear on being hospitalized or transferred to a new facility. Confusion or lack of skills on the nurse's part serves to increase that fear. The focus of the nurse's job is to serve the client with the greatest skill possible.

Avoid asking questions that have been asked before. Be sure that you have looked at the record before entering the client's room. Explain why you are asking questions and reassure the client that he or she has the right not to answer questions that cause discomfort. Be a good listener. Encourage confidence. Request clarification rather than pretending that you understand: "I am not sure that I understand what you mean by that statement." Check out what you think you understand: "Am I correct in saying that you are worried about the kind of care you will receive here?" Avoid using reassuring promises that you cannot deliver: "Don't worry, everything will be just fine." Also avoid giving approval—for example: "That's right." This statement may make it difficult for a client to change his or her mind. Nursing responsibility does not involve judging the client's behavior, values, or decision. Finally, avoid showing or verbalizing disapproval or belittling the client: "You know you shouldn't do that." Chapter 13 elaborates on communication techniques that assist you in making the best use of the limited time you have to obtain needed data from the client.

In checking information for accuracy, it is necessary to validate it to differentiate between subjective and objective data. Subjective data is what the client feels. Sometimes it is demonstrated by objective signs. For example, the client may state that he or she feels very warm (subjective). The client has a temperature of 102°F (objective).

There are several possible barriers to data collection (assessment) to which you must be alert. They include insufficient time, poor skills in data collection (assessment), communication failure (such as a comatose client), the presence of distractions, or a client who is too sick to want to talk. What can happen, if your personal values get in the way, is labeling the client before the interview is complete instead of basing decisions on facts. Respectful distancing is necessary if the nurse is to remain objective and use all senses clearly.

Physical assessment is an important part of data collection. RNs are taught how to perform physical assessment of clients as part of their basic education. They are taught assessment of all body systems. Practical nurses in basic programs learn assessment as part of each unit of study. Additional education in assessment, acuity or severity of the client's illness, and the area of employment all determine the extent of the practical nurse's involvement in physical assessment. The practical nurse is always assessing therapeutic responses to medications for side effects, symptoms of health problems, and so on (see Table 2–3).

When all the data are gathered, you will assist the RN in looking for gaps in information that will need further checking.

Charting data collection (assessment) information varies according to the guidelines of the specific facility where you work. Maintain a separation in your own

---

Table 2–3
Examples of Practical Nurse Data Collection

Examples used can apply to acute care or the community

1. Observing results of a laxative or enema
2. Observing for signs of congestive heart failure for a client taking furosemide (Lasix) and digoxin (Lanoxin)
3. Observing an ulcer on the lower leg of a diabetic: size (measure it), location, appearance, any drainage, and so on
4. Observing No. 3 each time leg is dressed
5. Observing behavior for signs of disorientation or confusion
6. Observing NPO client drinking water
7. In acute care: observing position in bed; community: observing gait, posture
8. Observing if 76-year-old client is showing signs of ego integrity or despair. (Although the client should be at ego integrity, he is not capable of being there. Because of his cerebrovascular accident (CVA) he has to be washed, fed, and lifted everywhere. He is incontinent. His behavior reminds you of an infant. You will work at establishing trust in the client instead of ego integrity.)
9. Observing family interactions
10. Observing the environment for need for safety factors—spills, bed rails, glasses on table, and so on
11. Observing the urine for color, odor, amount, other characteristics

mind about what constitutes subjective data, objective data, historical data and current data. Remember that in a lawsuit, a nurse expert reviewing a chart may interpret sloppy charting as sloppy nursing care. Refer to Chapter 20 for tips on charting.

▼▼▼
Planning: Phase 2

Only the RN can develop the nursing plan. The practical nurse provides input into plan development. It is illegal for the practical nurse to write the plan and for the RN to initial it. According to the 1995 NCLEX-PN test plan the practical nurse's role in planning is:

A. Assist in the formation of goals of care:
   ▶ Participate in the identification of nursing interventions required to achieve goals.
   ▶ Communicate client needs that may require alteration of the goals of care.
B. Assist in the development of a plan of care:
   ▶ Involve the client and health care team members in selection of nursing interventions.
   ▶ Plan for the client's safety, comfort, and maintenance of optimal functioning.
   ▶ Select nursing interventions for delivery of the client's care.

In the planning phase, practical nurses take the nursing diagnosis and state it as a nursing problem. Practical nursing students start here, state the problem, set goals, list interventions, and then list data collection (assessments). This process seems to reverse that of the RN, but remember that practical nurses do not have primary responsibility for assessment (phase 1) and rely on the RN for the nursing diagnosis. To understand the nursing diagnosis, the practical nurse states it in objective specific terms as a nursing problem (see Table 2–4).

Whenever evidence of a new problem emerges, practical nurses collect data about the problem because of their good data collection skills. They collaborate with the RN, and the RN then formulates a new diagnosis.

For a nursing care plan to be a useful, realistic tool for the nursing staff, priorities must be established. A care plan will not include all of the clients' problems.

The most important problems, those that are potentially life threatening, must be taken care of immediately. Maslow's hierarchy of needs is commonly used by nurses to assist in prioritizing client needs. The lowest level of needs according to Maslow (1943) are the physiologic (survival) needs. This means that in prioritizing client needs, attention is paid first to problems related to food, air, water, temperature, elimination, rest, and pain.

Write an example of a problem for each survival need.

1. Food _____

   _____

2. Air _____

   _____

3. Water _____

   _____

4. Temperature _____

   _____

5. Elimination _____

   _____

6. Rest _____

   _____

7. Pain _____

   _____

Possible answers: (1) not enough or too much food intake, (2) difficulty with breathing, (3) dehydration due to vomiting, (4) temperature seriously above or below normal, (5) diarrhea, (6) sleeping too little or too much, (7) pain that interferes with functioning.

It is not uncommon when working on several problems at the same time to find that a relationship exists between problems. Priorities may also change rapidly depending on the client's condition. The nurse has to remain flexible and to recognize the need to shift priorities according to client needs. The client will be far more cooperative with the care plan if he has been

Table 2–4
Student Assignment Sheet and Patient Care Plan

Student _____

Patient _____ Room _____ Doctor _____

Age _____ Marital Status _____ Religion _____ Occupation _____

Admission Date _____ Date of Surgery _____ Diet _____

Medical Diagnosis _____ Surgical Procedure _____

Meaning in Own Words _____ Meaning in Own Words _____

Primary Nursing Problem _____

Categories of Human Function	Assessment	Nursing Problems	Goals	Nursing Intervention	Evaluation
Protective (personal care and hygiene environment, surgery)	What you will: Check, observe, monitor, weigh, measure, palpate, auscultate. (1) Assess at beginning of shift for baseline, (2) periodically during shift, and (3) right before you leave	What is the problem in your own words? Be specific and objective. May use nursing diagnosis, but . . .	The Patient Will: (Reverse the problem and state positively what client will do—realistically, measurably, time-referenced)	The Nurse Will: (Be objective and specific. Care plans in texts rarely are. What the nurse will do to help client meet goals)	What progress is client making toward goals? Results of data collection and assessment in objective terms
Sensory-perceptual					

Table continued on following page

Table 2–4
Student Assignment Sheet and Patient Care Plan (Continued)

Categories of Human Function	Assessment	Nursing Problems	Goals	Nursing Intervention	Evaluation
Comfort, rest, activity, and mobility (sleep and rest, body alignment)					
Nutrition					
Growth and development; developmental stage: Erickson's task:					
Fluid-gas transport					
Psycho-social-cultural (emotional support, spiritual support, diversion and recreation)					
Elimination					

Need for Community Resources:

included in identifying the priorities of care. Remember that regression takes place during illness. The client advances on the hierarchy as he recovers. Cooperation is much more likely when the nurse understands this and respects it.

Think back to phase 1, data collection (assessment). What did the client say on admission about what he expects, wants, or needs during the time he is a client (check the chart: important information as you assist the RN in planning the care)? Did you also remember to collect data on client strengths? (what he can do for himself)? Strengths are building blocks in developing a realistic plan.

▽▽▽
Goal Setting

Specific outcomes (goals) provide direction for individualizing the care of the client. To be useful, outcomes must be client-centered and be determined by the client and the nurse together. Goals must be (1) measurable, (2) realistic, and (3) time referenced. The focus of the outcome is on the client, not the nurse. A goal is thought of as, "The client will do this or that." To get the best results, an outcome must be set for each priority problem or need. *Reverse the problem and state it in positive terms.* Terminology will vary to some degree. Some agencies use the terms goals, behavioral objectives, or expected outcomes.

The example below shows how a client's care plan might look. Measurable, realistic, time-limited goals have been established for a *priority* problem. The goal statement specifically addresses the nursing problem. The stated time is an educated guess that becomes more accurate with experience. The examples show how the

practical nurse *changes* the nursing diagnosis into a nursing problem.

▽▽▽
Identifying the Interventions

The next step of the planning phase is to identify what nursing interventions will take place to achieve the goal. These are things the nurse will do to assist the client to reach the goals. Sometimes this means encouraging the client to do for himself. This is also called nursing approach or nursing care. Interventions focus on the "related to (R/T)" portion of the nursing diagnosis. They tell all nursing personnel who, what, where, when, and how much. Anyone should be able to carry out your interventions. Check them out. Are they objective and specific? Interventions are based on courses you have taken, additional reading, research, and so on. Interventions do not just come from the top of your head. See Chapter 8, Hints For Using Learning Resources.

Client and family strengths and weaknesses play an important part. The client and family are important partners with you in attaining the goal or goals. Building on client strengths provides a sense of contribution and some control. Maybe the client in the example given previously has the strength to feed himself but will not do so unless someone sits at the bedside. Rather than taking this strength away from the client and feeding him because it is "quicker and less messy," plan around it. The goal is to get him to take 1500 calories in 24 hours.

Sample Interventions

1. Six small ground meals at 8:00 AM, 10:00 AM, 12:00 noon, 2:00 PM, 4:00 PM and 6:00 PM. Client seated in an easy chair with minimal assistance. Encourage

Nursing Diagnosis	Goal	Nursing Problem
Altered nutrition: less than body requirements. Related to (R/T) decreased calorie intake.	The client will eat 1500 calories of ground foods and liquids during each 24-hour period. (The problem is reversed and stated positively.)	Eats only 5% of each meal. R/T loss of appetite and weakness.

self-feeding. Assist only if needed. Record time, amount, and type of food eaten.

2. Offer 240 ml of liquids at 6:00 AM, 9:00 AM, 11:00 AM, 1:00 PM, 3:00 PM, 5:00 PM, 7:00 PM, and 9:00 PM. Vary choices: likes Jello, ice-cream, 7-Up, chocolate milk, and pineapple juice. Drinks herbal tea with meals. Record time, amount, and food.

There are different kinds of care plans available. An individualized written care plan has been demonstrated. Some facilities use standardized care plans. These plans are based on research of the best possible options for a nursing diagnosis (nursing problem). To individualize a standard plan, cross out what does not apply and add appropriate interventions that apply to your client.

Computerized care plans are gaining in popularity. Individualized plans can be entered into the computer. More commonly, standardized care plans are used and then individualized to deal with the nursing problem.

Multidisciplinary care plans work well in settings in which staff from varied professions and disciplines are frequently involved with the client. An example is a long-term care or psychiatric setting. These plans are developed by a multidisciplinary team and reflect specific interventions used by each discipline, e.g., physical therapist, nutritionist, nurse, and physician. Maintaining a separate plan for each profession is often considered repetitious. The focus of a multidisciplinary plan is client problems rather than nursing diagnoses. The language used must be common to all disciplines involved.

All nursing interventions must be dated and signed.

Documenting (charting) the plan is essential. Legally, if it is not charted it is not done. Where the documentation takes place depends on the facility. It may be done on the computer or in long-hand in the nurse's notes or on flow sheets. Some agencies have special care plan kardexes or clipboards at the bedside. Eventually these become a part of the client's permanent record. Meanwhile, the plan is the recipe for meeting the client's nursing problems. Find it!

▼▼▼
Implementation: Phase 3

According to the 1995 NCLEX-PN test plan the practical nurse's role in implementation is to:

A. Assist with organizing and managing the client's care:
  ▶ Implement the established plan of care
  ▶ Participate in a client care conference
B. Provide care to achieve established goals of care:
  ▶ Use safe and appropriate techniques when administering client care
  ▶ Use precautionary and preventive interventions in providing care to clients
  ▶ Prepare client for procedures
  ▶ Institute nursing interventions to compensate for adverse responses
  ▶ Initiate life-saving interventions for emergency situations
  ▶ Provide an environment conducive to attainment of goals of care
  ▶ Provide care in accordance with client needs and/or preferences
  ▶ Encourage client to follow a treatment regime
  ▶ Assist client to maintain optimal functioning
  ▶ Reinforce teaching of principles, procedures, and techniques for maintenance and promotion of health
  ▶ Monitor client care provided by unlicensed nursing personnel
C. Communicate nursing interventions:
  ▶ Document client's response to care, therapy, or teaching
  ▶ Report client's response to care, therapy, or teaching to relevant members of the health care team

The next stage is *initiating* the nursing interventions. What were those client strengths you identified? It is time to build on them as you begin to initiate the plan. Think back to the interventions listed on page 31.

1. Can the client move from the bed to the chair

and back alone? With minimal support? With complete support?

2. Can he feed himself? Completely? With some assistance?

3. Does he eat best if someone is present? Alone? During conversation about family?

4. Are there any family members who can be instructed in how to act as partners in implementing the care plan?

5. Is the responsibility for the intervention within the LPN role?

Once again, these are samples of the many questions that may be addressed at this time.

The implementation phase includes reporting and charting the shift activities. Reporting, to be useful, should be presented in an orderly fashion.

Your responsibility will vary according to the work area in which you are involved and whether you are functioning in a beginning or expanded role. In an acute-care setting your primary responsibility will be to use the care plan as a guideline for providing direct client care, continuing data collection, making verbal reports to the RN, and charting. In nursing homes and extended care facilities, you may be functioning in the role of a charge nurse and have responsibility for managing client care under the supervision of the RN. The key for all of your activity, regardless of your position and the agency involved, is to use the care plan as the basis for your nursing actions and reporting. For example, as a student you draw information from the care plan on how to provide individualized client care. While providing care you continue to make observations based on your knowledge of the client's strengths and disease conditions. You chart on flowsheets and nurses' notes following the priorities indicated by the nursing problem, plus any new observations you have made. You use the care plan as your guideline when reporting to the RN and offer information on any changes you have noted. Specifically, you focus on the nursing interventions outlined in the care plan: Do they continue to be appropriate? What changes or lack of changes have you observed? With this information the RN can update the plan of care and needs only to validate the data.

▼▼▼
Evaluation: Phase 4

Evaluation is the fourth phase of the nursing process for the practical nurse. According to the 1995 NCLEX-PN test plan, the practical nurse's responsibility in evaluation is to:

A. Compare actual outcomes with expected outcomes of client care:
   ▶ Assist in determining the client's response to nursing care
   ▶ Assist in identifying factors that may interfere with the client's ability to implement the plan of care
   ▶ Assist in determining the extent to which identified outcomes of the care plan are achieved
B. Communicate findings:
   ▶ Document client's responses to care, therapy, or teaching to relevant members of the health care team

Have you noticed how heavily dependent each step of the care plan is on the others, and how the steps are often going on simultaneously? Evaluation begins as soon as client contact occurs. The continual data collection (assessment) helps to make daily evaluation part of the natural flow of good nursing care.

Evaluation is a way of measuring client progress toward meeting goals. You are not evaluating nursing behavior. Think of the client's goal. Look at daily data collection (assessment). If your data collection (assessment) list is complete, evaluation will be the results of your data collection. Compare this to goals. If progress is being made toward meeting goals, do nothing. If the client is not meeting goals, check the goals. Are they measurable, realistic, and time-referenced? If not, revise the portion that needs revision. Check the interventions or look for new interventions. If the goals meet the above criteria, revise nursing interventions that are not working.

Data collection (Assessment) list	Goal	Evaluation
Check intake: ▶ amount and type of liquid in milliliters ▶ amount of food taken at each meal.	The client will eat 1500 calories of chopped foods and liquids during each 24-hour period.	By day two client was able to consume 1500 calories, in ground meals and liquids, during a 24-hour period.

When the goal is written in measurable terms and an appropriate data collection (assessment) list has been developed, the evaluation is built in. If you cannot evaluate the goal, it probably was not written accurately.

▼▼▼ SUMMARY

Nursing process is the language of nursing; it is a way for all nurses to assist clients in meeting their goals. It is also a way for nurses to communicate effectively with each other whether the focus is wellness, illness, or transfer to another facility.

The RN, by virtue of a broad science-based education, has the primary legal responsibility for the four steps/phases of the nursing process. The nursing diagnosis is the RN's exclusive responsibility.

The LPN, as a full partner in providing nursing interventions, must understand his or her role in the four phases of the nursing process. The practical nurse also participates in the nursing process according to assignment and skill level.

Data collection (assessment), phase 1, includes participation in establishing a data base by (1) gathering information relative to the client, (2) communicating information gained in data collection, and (3) contrib-

uting to the formation of the nursing diagnosis. Data collection (assessment) occurs not only during admission but also during each nurse-client encounter. The client is the primary source of information.

Planning, phase 2, includes participation in setting goals for meeting the client's needs and designing strategies to achieve these goals. This is accomplished by (1) assisting in the formulation of goals of care and (2) assisting in the development of a care plan. Client problems are prioritized, realistic client-centered outcomes, and nursing interventions are established. The highest priority is always given to physiologic (survival) needs.

Implementation, phase 3, involves initiating and completing the actions necessary to accomplish the defined goals. The practical nurse accomplishes this by (1) assisting with organizing and managing the client's care, (2) providing care to achieve established goals of care, and (3) communicating nursing interventions.

Evaluation, phase 4, includes participation in determining the extent to which goals have been achieved and interventions have been successful. This involves (1) comparing the actual outcomes with the expected outcomes of client care and (2) communicating findings (NCLEX-PN Test Plan, 1995).

Critical thinking (i.e., advanced problem-solving) accompanies nursing process every step of the way.

▼▼▼ R E F E R E N C E S

Iyer P, Taptich B, Bernocchi-Losey D. *Nursing Process and Nursing Diagnosis,* 3rd ed. Philadelphia: W.B. Saunders, 1995.

Kalish R. *The Psychology of Human Behavior,* 5th ed. Monterey: Wadsworth, 1983.

Maslow A. A theory of human motivation. Psych Rev 1943; 50:370.

NCLEX-PN Test Plan for the National Council Licensure Examination. Chicago: National Council of State Boards of Nursing, 1995, (effective date, October 1996).

▼▼▼ *B I B L I O G R A P H Y*

American Nurses' Association. *Nursing, A Social Policy Statement.* Kansas City, American Nurses' Association; 1980.

American Nurses' Association. *Standards of Clinical Nursing Practice.*

Washington DC: American Nurses Association, 1991.

deWit S. *Rambo's Nursing Skills for Clinical Practice,* 4th ed. Philadelphia, W.B. Saunders, 1994.

Frisbie D. Looking at teaching through the nursing process. 1984; 23(9):401–403.

Gross J. Learning nursing process: A group project. Nursing Outlook 1994; Nov/Dec 279–283.

Ignatavicius D, Workman M, Mishler M. *Medical Surgical Nursing: A Nursing Approach Process,* 2nd ed. Philadelphia: W.B. Saunders, 1995, Chap. 3.

Linton A, Matteson M, Maebius N. *Introductory Nursing Care of Adults.* Philadelphia: W.B. Saunders, 1995, Chap. 8.

Neumann T. Speaker: representative of WI Board of Nursing, Update on legal matters in the state of Wisconsin. Fall conference of Wisconsin Association of Licensed Practical Nurses, Chula Vista Resort, Wisconsin Dells, WI, Nov. 3, 1995.

Smith C, Maurer F. *Community Health Nursing: Theory and Practice,* 3rd ed. Philadelphia: W.B. Saunders, 1995, Chap. 9.

Varcarolis E. *Foundations of Psychiatric Mental Health Nursing,* 2nd ed. Philadelphia: W.B. Saunders, 1994, Chap. 8.

The Health Care Team

▼▼▼ *O U T L I N E*

▼▼▼ *K E Y   T E R M S*

▼▼▼   O B J E C T I V E S

Upon completing this chapter you will be able to:

1. *Explain in your own words the goal of the health care team.*
2. *List ten members of the health care team (nurses count for one member).*
3. *Identify the nursing personnel that are part of the health care team according to the following criteria:*

    a. *education*
    b. *role and responsibilities*
    c. *licensing*

4. *Define nursing.*
5. *Describe in your own words the following methods used to deliver nursing service:*
    a. *case method*

    b. *functional method*
    c. *team method*
    d. *primary care*
    e. *patient-focused care*

6. *Describe the practical nurse's role in the methods used to deliver nursing services listed in Objective 5.*

▼▼▼
Who Is Responsible for Mrs. Brown's Discharge?

Mrs. Amelia Brown, aged 75, lives with her daughter on a 200-acre farm in rural Wisconsin. While working in the barn, Mrs. Brown fell and broke her right hip. She required surgery to repair the hip. While under general anesthesia during surgery, Mrs. Brown's blood pressure reached dangerously high levels, but it quickly stabilized under the anesthesiologist's interventions. Despite this setback, Mrs. Brown was discharged after six days in the hospital. She and her family agreed that she was not ready to return home at that point in her recovery, so she was discharged to an extended care facility. Here she was given physical therapy to learn how to function at home with her restrictions in ambulation. Two weeks later, Mrs. Brown was discharged from the extended care facility to her home.

Sounds like another success story for nursing, doesn't it? We will follow Mrs. Brown as she progresses through the health care system and then decide who should get credit for Mrs. Brown's discharge back to the farm.

▽▽▽
Mrs. Brown's Emergency Care

After Mrs. Brown falls, her daughter calls the emergency squad to transport her mother to the nearest hospital. This hospital is located 20 miles away in a city with a population of 98,000. The three persons manning the emergency squad are **emergency medical technicians (EMTs)**. Each EMT has taken an approximately 120-hour course in basic life support skills. Each has been certified as an EMT by means of a national test. The EMTs are currently taking a five-month paramedic course, which is preparing them to provide more advanced life support skills. On the way to the hospital, the EMTs monitor Mrs. Brown's blood pressure, pulse, respirations, and level of consciousness. They keep her right leg immobilized. The EMTs maintain contact with the hospital emergency room by means of a two-way radio.

On arriving at the emergency room (ER), the EMTs provide the **registered nurse** with verbal and written reports of Mrs. Brown's status. The **emergency room doctor** examines Mrs. Brown and orders an x-ray of her right hip. The **x-ray technician** brings the x-ray equipment to the ER and takes an x-ray film of Mrs. Brown's right hip. The x-ray technician has had a minimum of preparation in a two-year program conducted by a hospital or technical college. This technician is prepared to perform diagnostic measures involving radiant energy. The **radiologist** on duty reads the x-ray of Mrs. Brown's right hip. On the basis of the physical examination and the results of the x-ray, the ER physician diagnoses a fracture of Mrs. Brown's right proximal femur. The ER physician notifies Mrs. Brown's **family physician** and contacts the **orthopedic surgeon** she requests.

The **registered nurse (RN)** receives Mrs. Brown in the ER and assesses her and provides care until she is admitted to the hospital. The RN is a graduate of a diploma or three-year program in nursing. This nurse has passed a national examination to become an RN.

RNs who work in the ER participate regularly in continuing education courses at the hospital and at seminars given regionally and nationally for ER nurses. Mrs. Brown is prepared for surgery.

To be qualified to be in charge of the medical care of Mrs. Brown, the family physician has attended four years of college, four years of medical school, one year of internship, and approximately a three-year residency program. Medical school consists of a program that provides the basic knowledge and skills needed to be a medical doctor. Internship involves a program of clinical experiences designed to complete the requirements for licensure as a practicing physician. The residency program prepares physicians for practice in a specialty. The specialty in this situation is family practice. With some exceptions, the ER physician, the radiologist, and the orthopedic surgeon have had the same education as the family physician. The ER physician has completed a residency program in emergency or trauma medicine. The radiologist has completed a residency program in the reading and interpretation of x-rays. The orthopedic surgeon has completed a three- to five-year residency in performing surgery for problems of bones and joints. Each of these physicians has passed the board examinations, which license them as physicians and allow them to practice under the state medical practice act. Each physician in this scenario is board certified in his or her specialty area.

Laboratory studies are ordered preoperatively. **Lab personnel** draw blood for the studies. Lab personnel have varied educational backgrounds. Some have on-the-job training to obtain blood samples. A medical lab technician has two years of education. A medical technologist (MT) has four-plus years of education and can be certified by a national examination. Lab personnel are responsible for collecting the specimens needed for lab tests, performing the tests, and reporting the results to physicians and staff.

The family requests that their parish priest be contacted to give Mrs. Brown the sacrament of the sick (see Chapter 15). Because surgery is imminent, the pastoral care department is notified. A Roman Catholic **priest**, a member of the pastoral care team, anoints Mrs. Brown with holy oils, prays with her, and gives her Holy Communion. To be able to meet Mrs. Brown's spiritual needs, the priest has had four years of college and four years of theological school before being ordained.

▽▽▽
The Surgical Experience

In the ER the **anesthetist** prepares Mrs. Brown and her family for the anesthesia part of the surgical experience. This health care worker is an RN with a bachelor of science in nursing (BSN). This nurse has studied an additional two to three years in an approved school of anesthesiology after the four-year BSN program. The anesthetist provides anesthesia to patients undergoing surgery. Mrs. Brown is transferred to the surgical suite, where she undergoes a right hip pinning procedure under general anesthesia. This type of anesthesia will put Mrs. Brown in a state of unconsciousness. During surgery, the anesthetist monitors Mrs. Brown's vital signs continuously while she is unconscious. The orthopedic surgeon is assisted by the **surgical technician**. The surgical technician sets up the sterile environment. This health care worker makes sure the surgeon's instruments and supplies are available when he requests them for the pinning of Mrs. Brown's right hip. The surgical technician is a graduate of a one-year diploma program at the local technical college. The overall functioning of the surgical team is coordinated by the **professional nurse** who has a minimum qualification of a BSN.

During surgery, the anesthetist notes that Mrs. Brown's blood pressure is rising to a dangerous level. She contacts the **anesthesiologist** STAT. The anesthesiologist, a medical doctor with a residency in anesthesiology, orders antihypertensive drugs (drugs that lower the blood pressure). The situation is quickly brought under control. Surgery is completed, and Mrs. Brown is sent to the Postanesthesia Care Unit.

▽▽▽
Postanesthesia Care Unit (PACU)

The purpose of the PACU is to monitor clients' vital signs, level of consciousness, movement, and any special equipment required by the client after surgery. When the client's condition is stable, he or she is transferred to the hospital room. Mrs. Brown is assessed by a PACU **registered nurse** who is a graduate of a three-year school of nursing. After one and a half hours, Mrs. Brown is assessed as being ready to leave the PACU. Because of the episode involving high blood pressure during surgery, Mrs. Brown's surgeon orders her to go to the intensive care unit (ICU) overnight for closer observation instead of to the postoperative surgical floor. A **transport aide**, who is trained on the job, and a **staff nurse** from the PACU take Mrs. Brown to the ICU.

▽▽▽

Intensive Care—A Time of Close Observation

The ICU is staffed by RNs who went to school for either two years (Associate Degree nurses), three years (Diploma nurses), or four years (Baccalaureate nurses). Each nurse has taken the same national examination to become an RN. None of these nurses are qualified to work in the ICU immediately on graduation from their nursing programs. Most institutions prepare a nurse for the responsibilities of this unit through in-service classes after a minimum amount of experience or through a postgraduate or continuing education course. Mrs. Brown's nurse is a **two-year graduate** and is responsible for the care and observation of two clients. The family is unable to answer some additional questions about Mrs. Brown's medical history. The family physician asks the **clerk receptionist (ward clerk)** to obtain Mrs. Brown's medical records from the medical records department. The clerk receptionist assumes the responsibility for many of the clerical duties that are a necessary part of any client care area. The clerk receptionist learns these skills by taking a course that varies in length, depending on the area of the country. The course averages about one semester of theory and clinical experience. The **medical records department** is staffed by personnel who have gone to school for two to six years to learn the skills required for indexing, recording, and storing client records, which are legal documents. Thanks to Mrs. Brown's old records, which are sent to the ICU, the family physician receives answers to his medical questions. The surgeon writes postoperative orders for Mrs. Brown including an order for patient-controlled analgesia (PCA) to control postoperative pain. The hospital **pharmacist** has studied for a minimum of four to six years to become licensed to prepare, compound, and dispense drugs prescribed by a physician or dentist. The pharmacist fills the order for Mrs. Brown's drugs and intravenous solutions.

The **respiratory therapy department** is contacted to evaluate Mrs. Brown's respiratory status and suggest treatment to prevent respiratory problems. Respiratory care technicians (CRTT) are graduates of 18-month programs in respiratory therapy. Respiratory care therapists (RRT) are graduates of associate degree or collegiate programs in respiratory therapy. Within 24 hours after admission to the ICU, Mrs. Brown is judged to be in stable condition. She is transferred by a **transport aide** and an ICU **staff member** to the surgical floor.

▽▽▽

Surgical Floor—An Eye to Discharge

The **nurse manager** on the surgical floor at this hospital is an RN who has graduated from a four-year nursing program. As manager of the unit, this nurse is responsible for all the care given to clients. Mrs. Brown's **team leader** is an RN from a two-year nursing program. This nurse is responsible for formulating a plan of care for each of the assigned clients and modifying these plans as needed.

The team leader receives a verbal report and the current care plan for Mrs. Brown from the ICU personnel. The team leader begins assessment of her new admission. The **practical nurse (LPN)** helps put Mrs. Brown to bed and immediately takes her vital signs. The LPN is a graduate of a one-year vocational program in nursing. The LPN has taken a national examination to become licensed as a practical nurse. The practical nurse is assigned to give Mrs. Brown bedside care.

A referral is sent to the physical therapy department. The **physical therapist (PT)** assesses the strength of Mrs. Brown's unaffected extremities. The PT sets up a program of exercises and ambulation with no weight bearing on the right extremity. The goal of treatment is to prevent the development of complications. Physical therapy keeps up the strength of Mrs. Brown's unaffected extremities until she is able to bear weight fully on the right side. The PT has been educated in a four- or five-year college program. Some PTs have a master's degree in physical therapy. The **physical therapy assistant (PTA)** has been educated in a two-year community college or technical-school setting. The PTA carries out the plan of care developed by the PT.

Soon after being transferred to the surgical floor, the **social worker** visits Mrs. Brown and her family to discuss discharge plans. The social worker suggests that Mrs. Brown stay in an extended care facility for two weeks to participate in extensive physical therapy and then return to the farm. Social workers help clients and families solve problems with the financial concerns of hospitalization. They arrange for community agencies to provide appropriate care and services needed by clients after discharge from the hospital. Social workers also help the family communicate their health care needs more clearly. Social workers obtain a bachelor's degree in social work in four years and a master's degree in one additional year of college. Mrs. Brown's social worker talks to the PT and the family. All agree that with exercise and skills teaching, the family eventually will be able to care for Mrs. Brown at home.

As the time for discharge to the extended care facility gets closer, a **patient care technologist** (PCT) is assigned to take Mrs. Brown's vital signs. PCTs perform treatments and skills assigned to them by the RN or the LPN. PCTs are trained by the hospital for the specific duties they are to perform. Training involves classes (sometimes autotutorial or self-study classes) and a clinical component. The training a PCT gets is short and varies from facility to facility. The job titles "unlicensed assistive personnel" or "patient care assistant" are used in some facilities. The responsibilities of the licensed practical nurse in relation to PCTs are discussed in Chapter 19.

Because Mrs. Brown is 50 pounds overweight, her physician orders a weight reduction diet. The **dietician** teaches Mrs. Brown and her daughter the elements of weight reduction that will be carried out when Mrs. Brown returns to the farm. The dietician is responsible for planning the meals and supplementary feedings for patients and the cafeteria meals for staff. The dietician also supervises the preparation of food and counsels clients and their families about nutritional problems and therapeutic diets. This health professional is educated in a four- to five-year college program, followed by a year of internship in a health care agency.

Every day during Mrs. Brown's stay, the **housekeeper** cleans her room and bathroom. Maintaining cleanliness is an effort to keep up medical asepsis (absence of germs) and provide a pleasant environment. The housekeeper receives training in the needed skills by the employing institution or through a short course in a technical school.

Finally, Mrs. Brown is discharged from the hospital. She leaves by **Medi-Van** and is transported to the extended care facility.

▽▽▽
Extended Care Unit—On the Road to Rehabilitation

Mrs. Brown's roommate in the extended care facility is an 80-year-old woman who has had a stroke. She is also preparing to go home after additional physical therapy. The **PT** conducts an initial assessment of Mrs. Brown and incorporates the hospital physical therapy plan of care with her findings. The **PTA** helps Mrs. Brown daily with exercises and ambulation, using a walker and minimum weight-bearing on her right leg. A **nursing assistant** (NA) is assigned to assist Mrs. Brown with her personal care. Nursing assistants are educated to give bedside care through courses of at least 85 to 120 hours' duration. Successful completion of this course of study makes the NA eligible to be placed on the state registry of NAs.

A referral is sent to the occupational therapy department. The **occupational therapist** (OT) completes an assessment of Mrs. Brown. The **occupational therapy assistant** (OTA) carries out the plan of care. The goal for Mrs. Brown is to be as independent as possible when she returns to the farm despite her physical limitations. Occupational therapy helps clients restore body function through specific tasks and skills. Educational requirements include a four-year occupational therapy program. Some four-year graduates pursue a master's degree in their field. A two-year program prepares OTAs for their roles.

Mrs. Brown receives her newly prescribed blood pressure medication from the **practical nurse**, who also is functioning in her expanded role as charge nurse in this facility. The **day supervisor**, an RN with a bachelor of science degree in nursing, checks Mrs. Brown daily to monitor her progress. Ten days later, Mrs. Brown excitedly waits for her family to take her back to the farm. She is pleased with her progress and is confident about going back to her home. She knows that at this time she is unable to gather the eggs each day, but she is anxious to get back in the kitchen.

> *Who is responsible for Mrs. Brown's return to the farm? After reading Mrs. Brown's story, you can see that it is impossible to give any one member of the health care team credit for sending Mrs. Brown home. Everyone needs to work together!*

▼▼▼ The Health Care Team

A primary goal of health care is to restore optimal physical, emotional, and spiritual health to everyone. This goal is accomplished by promoting health, preventing illness, and restoring health when illness or accident has occurred. Health care includes a large number of specialized services. It is necessary for groups of people to work together to provide clients with all the services they need to maintain comprehensive health care. These groups of health care workers are called the health care team. For Mrs. Brown to be rehabilitated after her fall, it took a minimum of 123.5 years of education for all the health care workers in this scenario to learn how to perform their respective jobs. The x-ray technician's x-ray film confirmed the presence of a hip fracture. The narcotic pain reliever supplied by the pharmacist relieved pain after the surgical procedure, allowing Mrs. Brown to move more freely and avoid complications. The treatment by the RT helped prevent pneumonia. The PTs, OTs, and nursing staff all helped to restore Mrs. Brown's health and prevent further illness by avoiding complications. The dietician's expertise allowed Mrs. Brown to receive the basic nutrients she needed to maintain her health, heal her fracture, and lose weight. Teaching about weight reduction diets promoted health by keeping Mrs. Brown's weight within acceptable limits. As you can see, each member of the health care team, because of his or her specific preparation in a field of study, can increase the quality of health care for a client. It is impossible for one person to provide the knowledge,

expertise, and skills that the health care team as a whole can provide.

Each member of the health care team must have good communication skills. Good communication ensures that care is coordinated for the client's benefit (see Chapter 13). Fragmentation of care can be avoided. Each health care team member has to be able to anticipate problems and avoid them when possible (by using critical thinking skills). When problems do occur, the health care team needs to use problem-solving skills to find solutions in the process of delivering care. In this way, the quality of client care is continuously improved. The team must strive continually to keep their care client-oriented. The team needs to realize that a cooperative effort is needed to reach client goals.

▼▼▼ What Is Nursing?

What is nursing, and what do nurses on the health care team do? The American Nurses Association (ANA) is a national nursing organization that is recognized as being representative of professional nurses in the United States. This organization defines nursing as the "diagnosis and treatment of human responses to actual or potential health problems" (American Nurses Association, *Nursing—A Social Policy Statement,* 1980, p. 9). Another often-used definition of nursing complements this one. This definition is by Virginia Henderson. Henderson states that "the unique function of the nurse is to assist the individual, sick or well, in the performance of those activities contributing to health or its recovery (or to peaceful death) that she would perform if she had the necessary strength, will or knowledge" (Henderson, 1966, p. 15). The ANA's definition includes the diagnosis of responses to health problems. Henderson's definition includes the ill or well person. Both definitions contain important considerations for nursing. It is important for practical nurses to understand their role in Mrs. Brown's care. The direction of practical nursing has been channeled by the two definitions just given. An understanding of the education, licensure, roles, and responsibilities of the varied members of the health care team is necessary.

▼▼▼
Nursing's Place on the Health Care Team

Nursing staff on the health care team include unit managers, RNs, LPNs, student nurses, NAs, and cross-trained staff. Assisting the nursing staff are unlicensed assistive personnel (UAPs). Clerk receptionists, although not nurses, are an important part of the unit staff. The members of the health care team are generally on duty in acute or residential health care organizations 24 hours a day, seven days a week. Some members of the health care team may not be scheduled at night or on weekends or holidays, and some of these persons are available on an on-call basis. In the community, health care workers' hours vary depending on site of employment. Some sites are only open Monday through Friday during day hours. Others also offer services in the evening. And others are open seven days a week and sometimes 24 hours a day.

▽▽▽
Registered Nurses (Professional Nurses)

Education

Today there are over 2 million RNs employed in nursing. Registered nurses are the largest group of health care workers in the United States. Nursing is a female-dominated profession, although approximately 5% of RNs are male. The graduates of the three types of education programs for professional nurses—two-, three-, and four-year programs—currently take the same licensing examination. On successful completion of this examination, all of these graduates hold the title registered nurse.

▶ Associate degree nursing (ADN) programs are found in community colleges, junior colleges, and technical schools. The ADN educational program includes general education courses, including courses in the biologic, behavioral, and social sciences, as well as nursing-theory courses and clinical practice. On graduation, the two-year (associate degree) graduate receives an associate degree in nursing and is eligible to take the national licensure examination for registered nurses (NCLEX-RN) to become a registered nurse.

▶ Three-year nursing programs (diploma programs) are conducted by a hospital-based school of nursing. These nursing programs involve the same general-education courses as two-year programs as well as nursing-theory courses. Diploma programs traditionally have emphasized clinical experience. The three-year nursing graduate receives a diploma in nursing. On graduation this nurse is eligible to take the NCLEX-RN examination to become a registered nurse.

▶ Four-year (baccalaureate) nursing programs are found in colleges and universities. Baccalaureate nursing programs emphasize course work in the liberal arts, sciences, and nursing theory, including public health. On graduation, the four-year nurse receives a BSN and is eligible to take the NCLEX-RN examination to become a registered nurse.

The Role of Registered Nurses

Graduates of all three nursing programs are prepared for general-duty staff nursing in a hospital or nursing home. Nursing education programs also prepare graduates of all three programs to function in a community-based, community-focused health care system. Although you may find two- and three-year RNs in supervisory and administrative positions, only baccalaureate graduates have been prepared in their nursing education programs for advancement to these positions. Baccalaureate graduates are also prepared for beginning positions in public health agencies. Nurses with BSN degrees are the only nursing graduates that may elect to do graduate work in nursing at the master's and doctoral levels. Graduates of associate degree nursing programs outnumber BSN graduates. Starting in 1989, the number of students in BSN programs began to increase, and the trend continues. The number of diploma graduates continues to decline. This education mix is expected to continue.

All RNs function under the nurse practice act of the state in which they are working. Registered nurses use the nursing process to identify client problems, formulate nursing diagnoses, and plan and evaluate care. Standards of care are used to provide care for each client. Standards of care are used instead of care plans in many institutions. These standards include the priority nursing diagnosis for each client with appropriate assessments, nursing interventions, and expected outcomes (goals). Standards provide minimum guidelines for a consistent approach to delivering client care. Standards are used as a reference by the RN in individualizing client care.

Registered nurses assign routine care and the care of stable clients to assistive personnel. This allows RNs to carry out the roles of (1) planning care, (2) coordinating all the activities of care, (3) providing care that requires more specialized knowledge and judgment, (4) teaching clients, families, and other members of the health care team, (5) and acting as client advocate. Registered nurses function independently in nursing, initiating and carrying out nursing activities. For example, to prevent complications in the respiratory and circulatory systems, RNs assess the client on bed rest. They identify the need for a turning routine, deep breathing, leg exercises, and range-of-motion exercises. Registered nurses add these nursing interventions to planned care. Because of their level of education, RNs can identify which clients can and cannot receive these nursing interventions.

When RNs carry out the legal orders of another health professional, for example, the physician or physical therapist, they are functioning in an interdependent role. Frequently, RNs function interdependently (collaboratively) when decisions about client care are made jointly by members of the health care team. It is the independent role in decision making that distinguishes RNs from LPNs. Registered nurses have the ultimate responsibility for care given to clients.

Education Beyond the Basic Nursing Programs for Registered Nurses

Certification. After graduating from a nursing program and gaining work experience and letters of reference in their chosen field, RNs can receive certification from various professional nursing groups. The certificate that is awarded after passing a comprehensive examination indicates that the nurse has demonstrated qualifications for a select area of practice. Certification is a lengthy and costly process. The credentialing center of the ANA will require a minimum qualification of a BSN for all of its certifications by 1998.

Advanced Practice. With additional degrees or special education, RNs can pursue expanded roles, called advanced practice. **Clinical nurse specialists (CNSs)** have a master's degree in a specialty area (example, medical-surgical nursing). When employed by acute-care organizations, the CNS serves as a mentor, role model, and resource person for staff by setting standards for nursing care. The CNS also is employed by clinics, nursing homes, and other community settings. In all sites of employment, the CNS also serves as an educator, consultant, researcher, and administrator. **Nurse practitioners (NPs)** are found in the same settings as the CNS. Some NPs have their own offices. They are involved in providing primary and preventive health services. NPs diagnose and treat common minor illnesses and injuries. **Certified nurse midwives (CNMs)** provide preventive gynecologic care and low-risk prenatal and postpartum care to women at home and in hospitals and birthing centers. **Certified registered nurse anesthetists (CRNAs)** are the primary providers of anesthetics in acute care facilities. They are found in every setting where anesthesia is given. This includes operating rooms, clinics, and outpatient surgical centers. **Advanced practice nurses (APNs)** may also prepare themselves to prescribe medications, and many states have given APNs the authority to do so. Through advanced degrees or certificates, these nurses specialize in treating specific groups such as the family, adults, and children. The trend is to expect all APNs to have a minimum of a master's degree.

▽▽▽
Practical Nurses

Practical nurses are the second largest group of health care workers in the United States. The educational program for practical nurses varies in length from 9 to 12 months. The practical nursing program is found in trade, technical, and vocational schools as well as community colleges. These institutions are usually public, tax-supported institutions. Practical nursing programs are also found in private schools. Courses in the biologic and behavioral sciences as well as nursing theory are offered. Clinical experience in acute care facilities, extended care facilities, and the community is included. On graduation, the practical nurse receives a diploma in practical nursing and is eligible to take the NCLEX-PN examination to become an LPN .

Role of the Practical Nurse

Practical nurses must be aware of the content of the nurse practice act of the state in which they are employed. The practical nurse's role is found in this law, and the law differs from state to state. Regardless of the site of employment, practical nurses provide care in basic and complex client situations under the general supervision of an RN, physician, podiatrist, or dentist. In acute care facilities the increasing number of clients requiring more complex care reflects the practice of discharging clients from hospitals for continued recuperation in extended care units and nursing homes—excellent places of employment for practical nurses. Periodically, a job analysis is performed to determine the content areas for the NCLEX-PN. The findings of the latest job analysis indicate that new LPNs are continuing to provide care in acute care, long-term care, ambulatory care, and home care settings (Chornick et al, 1995, p. 1).

Practical nurses function interdependently when they offer input to the RN about the effectiveness of care or offer suggestions to improve the client's care. Because practical nurses provide actual care at the bedside in acute care situations, their collection of data while engaged in giving care is valuable in determining if progress is being made to meet client goals. A major criterion in differentiating between the roles of the registered and practical nurse is that the practical nurse never functions independently. Practical nurses must function safely and are accountable for their actions.

Table 3–1
Differences Between the RN and the LPN Using the Five Roles of the Professional Nurse (RN) as a Guide

Five Roles of RN	RN	LPN
Professional	Belongs to and is actively involved in ANA at state and local level	Belongs to and is involved in NFLPN at state and local level.
Provider of care	Independent role. Initiates all phases of nursing process; formulates nursing diagnoses	Dependent role. Assists with all phases of the nursing process; works with established nursing diagnoses; identifies nursing problems
Manager of care	Controls decisions regarding staff and care of clients	First-line manager in nursing home/ extended care. Responsible to nurse manager.
Teacher	Initiates all health teaching	Initiates health teaching for health habits (nutrition, cleanliness, health habits, etc.) Reinforces health teaching of RN in all other areas.
Researcher	Theory included in four-year program. All levels interpret and implement research findings. Participates in the research process.	Theory not included in one-year program. Assists in implementing research findings.

They should assume responsibility only for nursing actions that are within their legal role and that they feel safe in carrying out. Table 3–1 helps to identify differences between the LPN and the RN.

Practical nurses are also employed in the community. Sites of employment include physician's offices, weight loss clinics, freestanding clinics, ambulatory care centers, home health care agencies, and industry. Sites of job placement for the practical nurse in the community increase each year. These include dialysis centers, group homes, home health agencies, adult day care centers, Red Cross (as a phlebotomist), Alzheimer's disease units, companion centers, and various entrepreneurship opportunities.

Expanded Role of the Practical Nurse

In all settings, practical nurses are being used in their expanded role. Because practical nurses work under another professional's direction, the practical nurse role is called an interdependent one. Employers expect practical nurses to think critically and solve problems in client care situations. During implementation of care by the LPN, the RN is available to help in decision making when questions arise either on site (direct supervision) or by phone (general supervision). See Chapters 18 and 19 for further discussion of the expanded role of the practical nurse.

> **Refer to your state's nurse practice act to determine the circumstances under which you may function with the direct or general supervision of an RN and in your expanded role.**

▽▽▽
Student Nurses

Student professional and practical nurses come to the clinical area under the supervision of clinical instructors. The clinical area is an extension of the classroom. It provides an opportunity to apply theory to practice. When assigned to clients, students have a responsibility to give safe care and function responsibly under the supervision of the instructor. Students are in the clinical area to learn, not to give service. It is possible that a clinical instructor can remove them from the assigned unit at any time for additional learning experiences. Students are a member of the health care team. They are expected to assist other team members in addition to performing their client assignment. Examples of such assistance include passing trays, answering call lights in acute care situations, and assisting patients. These activities help students learn how to get along in a team situation. *Student nurses are responsible for giving the same safe nursing care that LPNs provide.* This is a legal matter. Therefore, the student role demands preparation and supervision.

▽▽▽
Nursing Assistants

Nursing assistants can be trained for their positions on the job by combining federally mandated classroom instruction with close supervision by RNs while in the clinical area. Vocational schools offer programs that last a minimum of 85 hours. These programs combine classroom or autotutorial instruction with clinical practice. During the course, testing for competence occurs to meet federal Omnibus Budget Reconciliation Act (OBRA) requirements. When test results are satisfactory, the names of NAs are placed on a registry. In some states NA-R (nursing assistant–registered) is placed after the names of these health care workers. Nursing assistants function under the direction of registered or practical nurses. NAs who work in hospitals, nursing homes, extended care units, or psychiatric hospitals assist in providing personal and comfort needs for stable clients. They are assigned routine tasks, sometimes involving housekeeping chores. A large number of NAs are employed by nursing homes. Currently, the supply of NAs is not meeting the high demands of employers. People in some areas of the country refer to male NAs as orderlies.

Some states offer an advanced NA course. More complex skills are taught in these courses. These skills include many of the skills performed by the practical nurse.

The demand for home health care workers continues to increase. NAs are allowed to perform a wider variety of skills in the home as home health care workers. Some states offer a postgraduate course for

NAs to prepare them for the transition to home care. The comprehensive home care program is also available to individuals without NA experience.

Unlicensed Assistive Personnel

In an effort to use health care workers more efficiently and effectively, health care organizations have added a new level of worker to the health care team. Unlicensed assistive personnel are trained by health care organizations to function in an assistive role to RNs and practical nurses. Some health care organizations require applicants for UAP positions to be registered as NAs. These workers learn selected skills, sometimes by the autotutorial method or module method combined with some clinical teaching. Actual skills learned depend on which skills are needed in specific client care units. Unlicensed assistive personnel are also known by the terms patient care technician (PCT), patient care associates, care pairs, nurse extenders, multiskilled workers, and so on. See Chapter 16 for a discussion of UAPs under What Changes in Health Care Can Tell You and Chapter 19 under Assigning Tasks in the Extended Care Unit.

Clerk Receptionists (Ward Clerks, Health Unit Clerks, Health Unit Coordinators)

The job of the clerk receptionist is mainly secretarial in nature, but the duties vary from site to site. With the clerk performing this job, nurses are freed from much of the paperwork involved in client care. Clerk receptionists are trained on the job or in programs of several months' duration in technical schools. Clerks prepare, compile, and maintain client records on a nursing unit. Duties include transcribing physician's orders, scheduling lab tests, x-ray procedures, and surgery; scheduling other appointments for services; routing charts on client transfer or discharge; compiling the client census; answering the phone; maintaining established inventories of supplies; distributing mail to clients; and generally ensuring that the unit functions smoothly.

Unit Managers

Some large health care organizations have unit managers to supervise and coordinate management functions for client units. Some college background and supervisory experience is desirable for this position. This job is combined with on-the-job training for specific duties. Responsibilities include budgeting, supervision of ward clerks, assignment and evaluation of clerical personnel, inventory of patient's valuables, coordination with housekeeping and maintenance, and clarification of hospital compliance with Medicare requirements. If a health care organization does not have unit managers, these duties are assumed by the clerk receptionist and nurse manager.

Delivery of Client Care Services in Acute Care Settings

With the goal of providing optimal care, the health care team uses different methods to assign clients to staff. The methods evolved as a response to changing needs in staffing. Each of the methods is discussed in its general form as it was intended to function. Keep in mind that health care organizations modify these methods to fit their individual needs.

Case Method

At the turn of the century, families hired nurses to meet a client's special needs in the home. By the 1920s, private duty nursing was popular. This case method of client care continued in various degrees into the 1960s. Vestiges of the case method, or a one-to-one relationship with a client, are found today in acute care situations as total care nursing (comprehensive care). In the case method one nurse is assigned to one or two clients and is responsible for the total care of these clients. Today, total care nursing occurs in intensive care or special care units, as Mrs. Brown experienced in the ICU after she left the PACU. Nursing instructors frequently use the total client care method when assigning students to the acute care clinical area.

▽▽▽
Functional Method

In the 1950s, the functional method was a popular method of client assignment. Registered and practical nurses were in scarce supply. The functional method of client care is task-oriented. The tasks that have to be done for clients are divided among the staff. For example, one person might measure all vital signs, another might do all treatments, and still another might make all the beds. This method's emphasis on efficiency and division of labor is based on the assembly line production concept found in industry.

The nursing home nearest Mrs. Brown's home schedules client assignments by the functional method. An NA helped Mrs. Brown with her physical care. A practical nurse gave her medications and did her treatments. In addition to assuming responsibility for all care given to patients, the charge nurse, a practical nurse, would be kept busy with managerial and non-nursing duties. Functional nursing can easily overlook holistic care, especially in the area of psychological needs. This results in fragmentation of care. Although this method is efficient and appears to be less costly to implement, it can discourage client and staff satisfaction. The functional method may, however, work well in times of critical shortages of personnel.

▽▽▽
Team Method

After World War II, the team method of client care was introduced because of the increasing numbers of practical nurses and NAs. The team method is more a philosophy than a method. It is based on the belief that goals can be achieved through group action. The clients on a unit are divided into small groups. Small teams are assigned to care for the clients in each group. Assignments are based on the needs of each client and the skills of the team members. The team is led by the team leader, the RN. The RN continues to have the final responsibility of planning, coordinating, and evaluating the implementation of care for each client and supervising the personnel giving the care. In this method, the capabilities of each team member are used effectively. This increases the quality of care for the client and the satisfaction of the team member. An integral part of the team method is the team conference. During this conference, which is intended to be held daily, information is shared by team members about specific clients, problems are identified and solved, and plans of care are developed and revised.

The team method is rarely carried out in this manner. When busy, the team leader may administer medications and perform treatments. Team conferences are often postponed. The team method then becomes a functional method of assigning care. Several years ago, the nurses on the medical floor where Mrs. Brown was assigned used the team method, but frequently the team leader functioned as the medication nurse.

▽▽▽
Primary Method (Primary Care)

The hospital in which Mrs. Brown was a client adopted the primary care method several years ago to replace the team method of assigning care. The intention was to increase the quality of care for clients. This method was instituted in the late 1960s as a result of the dissatisfaction of professional nurses with their lack of direct client contact and the fragmentation of care that resulted from functional and team nursing. In primary nursing RNs individualize client care and accept responsibility and accountability for total client care. Ideally, staffing for this method requires a nursing staff composed entirely of RNs. Each nurse is assigned a maximum of six clients. There are no team leaders in this method. Each primary nurse is a bedside nurse, who has received the assignment from and in turn reports to the nurse manager. The major characteristic of this method is the responsibility and accountability of the primary nurse. The primary nurse is assigned to a client on admission, develops the nursing diagnoses after the admission interview, and is responsible for the care of that client 24 hours a day until discharge. When the primary nurse is off duty, an associate RN continues care as planned by the primary nurse. If any changes are contemplated in client care, the primary nurse must be contacted.

Primary nursing facilitates continuity of care. Positive aspects of the primary method include shorter hospital stays for clients, improved communication among staff, and a more holistic focus of care. Negative aspects included the difficulty of recruiting a sufficient number of RNs when this method was first introduced. But the most negative aspect of this method is the cost of a staff composed entirely of RNs. Practical nurses are used as assistive nurses in primary care situations and have performed safely and effectively.

The severe nursing shortage of the 1980s has resolved. Around 1989, nursing journals began talking about **differentiated practice** as a system of assigning clients for care. This system recognizes that persons on the health care team with less education than RNs are important in reorganizing the delivery of client care in a more cost-effective manner. In the 1990s the **skill mix** on the health care team has changed. Acute care agencies began decreasing the percentage of RNs on staff and increasing the number of practical nurses and unlicensed personnel. Registered nurses are being used as coordinators of the health care team in these situations. These changes are regional and are continuing.

1. Investigate the skill mix of staff in acute care health agencies and health care agencies in your community.

▼▼▼
Patient-Focused Care: A New System for Delivering Client Care

Have you ever experienced the following situation in an acute care setting? Rhonda, LPN, tried to find out when her nauseated, elderly client was scheduled to have his chest x-ray, physical therapy session, and special lab studies. The radiology department, physical therapy department and laboratory were unable to give even a ballpark time frame when Rhonda called. Instead, they answered, "We'll come when we can." So Rhonda started the bath. After she finished washing the client's face, a transport aide appeared at the door to take the client to the radiology department. Rhonda cautioned the transport aide that the client was nauseated, but the aide said she wasn't trained to take care of things like that.

After 40 minutes, the client returned to his room. Fortunately, he did not have to vomit while he was in the x-ray department. After Rhonda started the bath again, lab personnel came to take the client to the laboratory for the special blood test that had to be done in that department. The lab personnel looked shocked when Rhonda included the emesis basin with the client with instructions that they might need to assist him. Forty-five minutes later, the patient returned to his room.

Rhonda continued the client's bath from where she thought she left off. Then the physical therapy transport aide came to take the client to his physical therapy session. Thirty-five minutes later the client was back, but he had not had his physical therapy session. The client was waiting in line for his turn for therapy when he had to go to the bathroom, but nobody was available to help him get to the bathroom. The client could not have his physical therapy because he had been incontinent.

Identify two ways of doing things differently in this acute care situation that could help make the situation more patient-focused and efficient and would make more sense.
    The client would benefit if:

1. _____

   _____

2. _____

   _____

The following are innovations created by management people to apply to acute care situations similar to the one just described:

1. Move the separate departments to the client instead of making the client go to them.

2. Cross-train health care workers so that each has the skills and can perform the tasks of other health care workers.

▽▽▽
What Is Patient-Focused Care?

Patient-focused care is an attempt to improve the quality of care by using hospital resources more efficiently to better meet the needs of clients. It is a consolidation and change of inpatient services that affects all departments found in hospitals. The major change in patient-focused care is "decentralizing" centralized service departments within hospitals and locating them in each client unit. For example, in this system of delivering care, the radiology department would cease to be a department of its own. Each client care area would have its own radiology suite, and an x-ray technician would be assigned to this area. Each unit could also have its own pharmacy and lab areas and even an admitting desk. These health care workers would also be cross-trained to perform specific skills on the unit when needed by clients. Examples of cross-trained skills would be drawing blood, giving baths, feeding clients, taking x-rays, assisting patients with basic needs, providing health teaching about medications, and so on. As coordinator of the team, the RN would assign care duties to this team of health care workers. Patient-focused care can build a stronger team delivering higher quality care because the resources of the health care organization are focused on the client.

Patient-Focused Care
One of the authors recently had an outpatient mammogram at a hospital she has been using for years. The hospital recently went through a major renovation and restructuring. In the past, the author had to fight for a parking space, walk one block to the outpatient admission desk, walk one block to an elevator, another one-half block to the x-ray department and then retrace her steps to find her car. After the restructuring, the author walked a total of 70 steps from valet parking to the registration desk and then to the mammogram room and back to the valet for her car.

▼▼▼ S U M M A R Y

▶ Health care organizations include a large number of specialized services and health care workers to provide these services. As a result, clients in the United States have some of the best and most expensive health care services in the world. Each member of the health care team provides a valuable service to the client. All members of the health care team are equal in importance to each other. Nurses on the health care team include registered nurses, practical nurses, student nurses, and cross-trained staff. Unlicensed assistive personnel, clerk receptionists, and managerial personnel round out the nursing team. To understand where you as a practical nurse fit into the picture, it is important for you to be aware of the educational background, role, responsibilities, and possible licensing requirements of all levels of personnel on the health care team. To understand your position on the health care team, it is necessary for you to keep up to date about new levels of health care workers and the different methods of delivering client care. As we approach the year 2000, practical nurses are recognized as important members of the health care team in acute care facilities and the community.

▼▼▼ R E F E R E N C E S

American Nurses Association. *Nursing—A Social Policy Statement.* Kansas City: American Nurses Association, 1980, pp. 9–13.

Chornick N, Yocum C, Jacobsen J. *Job Analysis Newly Licensed Practical/Vocational Nurses 1994.* Chicago: National Council of State Boards of Nursing, 1995.

Henderson V. *The Nature of Nursing: A Definition and Its Implications for Practice, Research and Education.* New York: Macmillan, 1966.

▼▼▼ *B I B L I O G R A P H Y*

Barnum B. On differentiated practice. *Nurs Health Care* 1991; 14(4):171.

Enrollments surging in BSN schools; New men's movement into nursing seen. *AJN* 1993; 93(3):99, 100.

Hurley ML. The push for specialty certification. *RN* 1994; 57(6):36–44.

Manuel P, Sorensen L. Changing trends in healthcare: Implications for baccalaureate education, practice and employment. *J Nurs Ed* 1995; 34(6):248–253.

Mason D, et al. *Policy and Politics for Nurses.* Philadelphia: W.B. Saunders, 1993.

Multiskilling and the Allied Health Workforce. A seminar sponsored by the Health Resources and Services Administration, Bureau of Health Professions, Washington DC and the Connelly Allied Health Education Center of Methodist Hospital of Indianapolis, Indiana, Nov. 30–Dec. 1, 1994, Washington, DC.

Nursing Data Source; 1994. Focus on Practical/Vocational Nursing. Vol. 3. New York: National League for Nursing, 1994.

Porter-O'Grady T. Working with consultants on a redesign. *AJN* 1994; 9(4): pp. 33–37.

Prism: NLN Research and Policy. Louden D, PhD, Zemokhol R [eds.] 1994; 2(4):1–8.

Smith C, Maurer F. *Community Health Nursing: Theory and Practice.* Philadelphia: W. B. Saunders, 1995.

Swanson J, Albrecht M. *Community Health Nursing: Promoting the Health of Aggregates.* Philadelphia: W. B. Saunders, 1993.

Wesorick B. *Standards of Nursing Care: A Model for Clinical Practice.* Philadelphia: J.B. Lippincott, 1990.

The Adult Learner

CHAPTER 4

▼▼▼ O U T L I N E

▼▼▼ . K E Y   T E R M S

▼▼▼ *O B J E C T I V E S*

Upon completing this chapter you will be able to:

1. *Identify yourself as a traditional adult learner, returning adult learner, or recycled adult learner.*

2. *Identify personal areas of strength that will help you ensure success in the practical nursing program.*

3. *Identify personal areas that could interfere with your success in the practical nursing program.*

4. *Explain in your own words three rights of learners.*

5. *Discuss personal responsibility for learning and active participation in the learning process as learner responsibilities.*

6. *Identify the purpose of evaluation in the practical nursing program.*

7. *Discuss 10 learner responsibilities.*

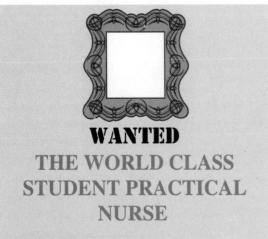

WANTED
THE WORLD CLASS STUDENT PRACTICAL NURSE

Age: Late teens up to the sixties and beyond.

Gender: Male and female

Personal characteristics:

• Married, single, looking, not looking.

• Has had work experience in a variety of settings and/or may have been through another program of study.

• Needs more knowledge and skills.

• Has clear, specific goals.

• Motivated and responsible.

• Serious about education.

• Seeking to have mind opened to the world of practical nursing.

• Would like to change practical nursing for the better.

• Willing to make considerable sacrifice of time, money, family, and personal pleasures.

• Wants to master practical nursing skills for the twenty-first century.

Does this describe you? Put your picture in the frame.

Welcome! You are one of thousands of adult learners in the United States who have decided to pursue a formal program in education this year. Every year adults enroll full-time and part-time in educational activities and programs. These programs and activities help them achieve job skills, increase self-esteem, and generally improve their quality of life. You are not alone.

You are entering school at an excellent time. Because of a decrease in the number of 18-year-olds, schools have put full effort into attracting and keeping adult learners in their programs. The adult learner is a very serious and capable learner. These learners help to increase standards in our schools. Schools have looked seriously at the special needs of adult learners. To enable the adult learner to succeed, schools have taken these needs into consideration when setting up educational programs. And to think, over the years you might have been saying, "I was born too soon," or "I was born too late." It turns out you were born at just the right time.

▼▼▼
The Adult Learner Defined

Who is the adult learner? Adult learners perceive themselves as adults and have adult responsibilities. The traditional adult learner comes to an educational program directly from high school or from another program of study. Many traditional adult students are in their late teens and early 20s. Traditional adult learners are in transition from late adolescence to young adulthood. In addition to their own developmental tasks, these students are being propelled into situations of responsibility for others. The returning adult learner has been out of school for several years. Many have not taken any courses since high school. Although returning adult learners can be any age, most are in the mid to late 20s. Returning adult students are experiencing many different life transitions. Because of life experiences, returning adult learners have built a strong foundation for the personal commitment and transitions needed in nursing school and practical nursing.

Another type of adult learner has emerged on the scene in practical nursing. This student shares some of the characteristics of both the traditional and the returning adult learner. But this adult learner might have technical school or college experience or an undergraduate or a graduate degree in a discipline other than nursing. Because these adult learners are starting a new cycle in their lives, we call them recycled learners. Reasons for choosing to enroll in the practical nursing program include:

1. Lack of jobs in the field for which the person has a degree. The outlook for a job with benefits may be more promising in practical nursing.
2. Desire to change careers.
3. Desire to acquire new job skills.

Regardless of the reason for enrolling in the one-year practical nursing program, recycled learners find that the practical nursing program meets their needs both in time and cost. In addition to characteristics of returning adult learners, the recycled learner brings experience in tackling a challenging educational program and valued life and work experience. Just as recycling is good for America, recycled learners are good for practical nursing programs. Nursing in general and practical nursing in particular are benefiting from the maturity and experience of this new type of nursing student.

Which type of adult learner are you? Survey your classmates. Determine who considers themselves to be traditional, returning, or recycled adult learners.

▼▼▼
Formal and Informal Educational Experiences

Generalizations can be made about each type of learner. Keep in mind that generalizations are broad sweeping statements. The characteristics of each type of adult learner are not found in each individual. The traditional adult learner is accustomed to planned, organized learning. This type of learning is called formal education. The practical nursing program in a vocational–technical school or junior college is an example of a program of formal education. Frequently, returning adult learners say they are rusty and have not been to school since high school. Only the latter part of this statement is true. They might not have been in a classroom for some time. But they have been learning. They have had informal educational experiences every day of their lives. Some examples of their informal educational experiences are learning to make a new recipe, using a new tool, programming the VCR, filling out a new income tax form, driving a new car, and handling a new family problem.

List at least five informal educational experiences you have had since high school.

_____

_____

_____

_____

_____

Returning adult learners tend to put more emphasis on formal educational experiences. They underemphasize the value of informal learning experiences. As you read your nursing texts, you will find that these experiences can be helpful when you are learning new material. Recycled learners may have recently graduated from college. Some may have entered practical nursing after a career in another field of work. Recycled learners have many formal and informal educational experiences that help them in a practical nursing program.

▼▼▼
Geared for Success

All adult learners have things going for them that allow them to succeed in school. Traditional adult learners are generally experts at educational routine. They know how to get through registration as painlessly as possible, find the fastest way to get from one class to another, and the best time to get through the cafeteria line, and how to take a test using a computerized answer sheet. In comparison, some returning adult learners may feel they have used up the last bit of their energy in trying to find a parking space, and once they do, they may be puzzled about how to find their way to their assigned classroom. Traditional adult learners have been given the opportunity to develop reading, writing, studying, and test-taking skills. They are at their prime physically, are filled with energy and stamina, and often have fewer out-of-school responsibilities to distract them from their studies. The returning adult learner is a serious learner who is ready to work. Returning adult learners have had many responsibilities and life experiences that help them relate well to new learning, make sense out of it, and get the point quickly. They are mature, motivated, and self-directed and have set a goal for themselves. Many have made economic, personal, and family sacrifices to go back to school. Recycled learners are also experts in educational routine, and they too have had the opportunity to develop reading, writing, studying, and test-taking skills. They are serious, motivated, and self-directed students. All adult learners are geared for success, and each group has their own strong points. But each group also has some liabilities—things that could stand in the way of success.

▼▼▼
Liabilities, Pitfalls, and Hidden Dangers

▽▽▽
Hidden Danger Shared by All Adult Learners

One of the greatest liabilities shared by all adult learners is the fear of failure. Fear of anything is a very strong motivator but in a negative sense. Fear of failure in school is a feeling that usually develops as a result of past negative experiences with learning situations. Perhaps you did not do well in some high school or college classes. Maybe you did not study, studied the wrong way, or allowed yourself to be put down by teachers or professors in the past. Maybe you allowed yourself to underachieve because of peer pressure. Regardless of the cause, you may look at school in a negative, threatening way.

A surprise is in store for you. Your past is history. You have a clean slate ahead of you! Many adult learners with the same history and fears as you may experience have succeeded in their educational programs. You are not a child in grade school. You are an adult in an adult educational experience. You will do yourself a favor if you begin to picture in your mind the rewards of succeeding in the practical nursing program. Forget the failures and setbacks you may have suffered in high school and other educational experiences. Replace your fear of failure with the desire for success. Keep your thoughts positive. Practice these positive thoughts continuously. Watch the content and tone of your thoughts and words. Negative thoughts and words can play like a tape. As surely as you learned this negative script, you can learn a positive script. But it takes time. Replace all your "I can'ts" and "I never coulds" with "I want to," "I can," "I will," and "I'm going to." Do not dwell on the past but look to the future. Dominate your thoughts with positive ones. You know, go all the way with PMA—positive mental attitude. If you consistently expect to succeed and combine this expectation with hard work in your studies, you will succeed. Did you know that your brain believes anything you tell it? Well, if it believes you can fail, it can learn to believe you can succeed. Start today to engage in positive self-talk.

Sometimes students who have not succeeded in other nursing programs enroll during mid-term in the practical nursing program. Reasons for not making it in prior nursing programs are varied, personal, and confidential. These students may feel the need to be on their guard. They may behave in a defensive manner, especially if there were teacher-student conflicts in the prior nursing program. It is good for these students to remember that the past is history. All that counts is their performance in the present. For them, it is possible to start over with a clean slate.

▽▽▽

Dangers for the Traditional Adult Learner

Although traditional adult learners have fewer outside responsibilities to distract them from their studies, they may allow social events to compete with school and study time. A serious interference with school responsibilities is a party mentality. Parties and "hanging out" used to be special occasions for celebrating and getting together. They were a well-earned and much-needed break from work and everyday routine responsibilities. Today, sometimes work and everyday responsibilities in life and at school get in the way of the traditional adult learner's party habit. Another interference is the amount of time occupied by employment outside of school hours. Ask yourself, "How much of the time I am employed outside of school is necessary for food, shelter, and other realistic expenses?" Many explanations can be given for these behaviors. Some traditional adult learners may still be working at developing an awareness of who they are and what life is all about for them. They may lack a sense of direction and have no clear goal or idea of what they really want to do in life. These examples of pitfalls for traditional adult learners are good examples of generalizations. They may or may not apply to the traditional adult learners you know.

▽▽▽

Dangers for the Returning Adult Learner

Returning adult learners may experience difficulties with academic behavior. Their reading, writing, test-taking, and study skills may be rusty. Physical changes occur as adults age and can affect learning. The senses of vision and hearing are at their peak in the adolescent years and decline very gradually through the adult years. As the decades go by these adults may notice the need for more illumination when they read. They also may experience problems with reading small print. Some returning adults note that they are not as energetic as they once were. Socially, returning adult learners have many roles to play outside of school. They may be husbands, wives, daughters, sons, grandparents, employees, or volunteers, and generally they are very busy people. Returning back to school may result in

feelings of guilt because they know it will affect their relationships and routines outside of school.

Because of their many roles, more demands are placed on returning adult learners. Some families may not support mom's or dad's choice to continue their formal education. Spouses may object to the extra demands placed on them. In many cases, the returning adult learner must struggle with learning how to juggle the worlds of learner and head of the family.

Despite these demands, returning adult learners, like traditional and recycled adult learners, need to learn how to manage their time. They need to learn how to concentrate when time for concentration is made available. Sometimes returning adult learners set unrealistic goals for themselves and have to readjust their game plan. Although past experience can be an asset, returning adult learners may have to rethink and possibly unlearn some things they have learned in the past. They might have allowed some of these things to become habits.

> When faced with obstacles, some adults may decide to throw in the towel and write off school as a bad idea. This book can help you to avoid this negative way of thinking and to go on to succeed.

▽▽▽

Dangers for the Recycled Adult Learner

The recycled adult learner shares the same pitfalls as the traditional and returning adult learner. Depending on their age and personal responsibilities, recycled adult learners may feel an energy crisis as they pursue their academic life. An additional danger for recycled adult learners may be an attitude that because they have earned a degree or have some college experience, the practical nursing program will be a breeze to get through. It is good to remember the difference between obtaining a college degree and obtaining a technical college education. In college, a student might have no practical experience with his or her major subject until junior or senior year or after graduation when hired for the first job in the chosen field. In the practical nursing program in a technical college, application of current learning is stressed continuously. Students need to apply theory continuously to the clinical area. What you learn on a Monday will be used on a clinical basis on Tuesday. And you will be expected to apply learning from past nursing classes consistently. Cramming for exams will be useless with this consistent expectation of application of theory to the clinical area.

▼▼▼
Special Challenges for Practical Nursing Students

No matter what type of adult learner you are, some students have special challenges to success in practical nursing. Students with a spouse at home may be extremely busy with school and family affairs. Single parents may feel overwhelmed when the student role is assumed in addition to all their other roles. It may be good for students with spouses to imagine what it would be like to be a student without a spouse to offer support.

Occasionally, practical nursing students with English as their first language complain about the difficulty of schoolwork and the amount of time it takes to complete assignments. It may be good for these students to imagine being responsible for the same amount of schoolwork when English is the second language. Students who speak English as a second language need to strive continually to understand content presented in a language different from their native tongue. This is comparable to presenting English-speaking students with textbooks written in Spanish or Russian.

The authors have met many students facing such challenges and commend them for the good job they have done, against great odds, in the practical nursing program. They are a testimonial that success is within your reach even if you are faced with these special challenges.

▼▼▼
Learners Have Rights

You must start thinking about some fundamental rights that you have been granted as an American citizen through the U.S. Constitution that will affect you as a learner. The First Amendment gives you freedom of expression as long as what you want to express does not disrupt class nor infringe on the rights of your peers. So, when your instructor asks you to join in a discussion, do not be afraid to do so. Instructors want your input in a class session. They have no intention of holding your comments against you. The Fourteenth Amendment assures you due process. Due process means that if you are charged with a violation of policies or rules, you will be presented with evidence of your misconduct and will be entitled to state your position. So relax. The institution in which you are enrolled cannot terminate you at whim, nor do they want to. They exist to help you succeed. A more detailed account of these two rights can probably be found in your school's student handbook. You did not get one? You lost yours? Hurry to Student Services and get a copy today.

An important learner's right is the right to have an organized curriculum and a responsible instructor who is prepared to teach it. Although your tuition and fees do not pay for all the services you receive at school, you are the most important person on campus. You are the reason the instructor was hired. You do not interfere with the instructor's work—you are the focus of it. You have the right to know the requirements of each course and how you will be graded for each course.

▼▼▼
Responsibilities of Learners

The first responsibility of learners is to learn. The authors want you to test your knowledge about the process of learning before you read any further. Read the following four statements and answer "true" or "false" to them. As the chapter continues, these statements will be discussed. You will be expected to check the accuracy of your responses. *Remember, your answers are for your eyes only.*

_____ 1. The instructor has the responsibility for my learning.

_____ 2. If I fail, it is the responsibility of the instructor.

_____ 3. If I succeed, the credit for my success should go to the instructor.

_____ 4. My instructor has the responsibility to pass on to me all the information I will need to know in my career as a practical nurse.

▽▽▽
Teaching Versus Learning

Many years ago, a wonderful thing happened in the area of adult education. Teachers were exposed to the difference between teaching and learning. Great emphasis was placed on the role of the learner. The authors think learners need to be aware of the exciting world of learning and the roles of teaching and learning in that process. In doing so you will know what is expected of you as an adult learner.

Many of you (and this includes the authors and some of your instructors), have had educational experiences in the past that encouraged dependency and passivity on the part of the learner. Think back to the educational experiences you have had. Did they involve sitting in classes in which the teacher did most of the talking and you just took notes? Did you view the teacher as someone who possessed knowledge and somehow was going to pass it on to you? And if you did not pass, did you say, "The teacher flunked me"? When you think about it, these situations are characterized by the adjectives _dependent_ and _passive_.

The last time you were dependent from necessity was when you were an infant. Even then you were far from passive. When you became a toddler, you became very independent and began to learn about the world in earnest. You very actively pursued your learning—that is, the acquiring of new knowledge and skills. And you did it with gusto! Now, here you are an adult learner. How unfair of an instructor to expect you to become dependent and passive in your learning. This is especially true because studies have proved that people learn best when they are actively involved in their own learning and have an interdependent relationship with the instructor. Today, instructors are viewed as facilitators of learning. You have already learned that it is the instructor's responsibility to set up a curriculum. Your state's Board of Nursing dictates the content of the curriculum in a school of nursing. It is then up to the faculty of your school to decide how that content will be included in the nursing program. Instructors have the responsibility to create a learning environment in which learning can take place. They do this by arranging for a variety of activities and experiences. Part of that learning environment involves being available to learners when they encounter questions and problems they cannot solve themselves. Instructors also have the responsibility to evaluate learning. They do so by testing and observing learners.

To learn is to acquire knowledge and skills. The verb _acquire_ means to obtain or gain by one's own effort. Learners must open themselves up, reach out, and stretch to gain their knowledge and skills. They are agents of their own knowledge and skill acquisition. Learning is a very active activity, not a passive one. Learners have the personal responsibility to acquire knowledge and skills. It is impossible for instructors to pour knowledge and skills into the heads of learners. Learners must become self-directed in their learning. Instructors will not hover over you and guide your every step. Instructors are there to help you along when needed. Do not expect the teacher to assume your skill for you, be your medical dictionary, or replace Chapter 2 in _Body Structure_ because you did not have time to study. Instead, expect your instructor to observe you while you are trying to work through a difficult skill. The instructor will make suggestions and demonstrate a point here and there to help you along. If you are having trouble, expect your instructor to help you put a definition of a medical term in your own words. Expect the instructor to answer specific questions you may have on Chapter 2 in _Body Structure_. These are the roles of teacher and learner and examples of their interdependency.

If you are to learn and succeed, you must become actively involved in your own learning. You say you are too old to learn? You say you cannot teach an old dog new tricks? Much study has been done in this area. To date, studies of adult learning clearly indicate that the basic ability to learn remains essentially unimpaired throughout the lifespan. Now review the answers to your true/false questions on page 56. Are there any answers you want to change before looking at the key?

1. _False._ You have the responsibility for your own learning. You must become actively involved in the learning process.

2. *False.* If you fail, it is your own fault. Adult educational programs are geared for success. You are geared for success. Although you could list many reasons why you might not succeed, the teacher's flunking you is not one of them. Learners sometimes allow themselves to flunk.

3. *False.* When you succeed (and you are perfectly capable of doing so), only you can take credit for the success. You were the person who assumed responsibility for your own learning. You became actively involved in the learning process.

4. *False.* Instructors have had much experience in nursing. They do not know all the experiences *you* will have in your career as a practical nurse. Even if they did, there would be no time or way to transfer this knowledge to you. Instructors help learners learn how to learn. This is important in an ever-changing field like nursing. Your instructors will encourage you to develop critical thinking and problem-solving skills. These skills will enable you to handle new situations as they arise in your nursing career.

If you had no wrong answers, you should be an expert on learning. Now put your expertise to work for you. If you had one wrong answer or more, the authors suggest you reread the section, Teaching versus Learning.

▽▽▽
The Role of Evaluation

The second responsibility of learners is to receive and participate in an evaluation of self. Evaluation plays an important role in your education in the practical nursing program and throughout your career. You have set a goal to become a practical nurse. As the year goes on you will be evaluated by your instructors in several different ways as a means of determining whether or not you are progressing in the achievement of that goal. When you graduate, you will be evaluated periodically while on the job, sometimes as a means of determining whether you are to receive a salary increase. At other times you will be evaluated to see if you are functioning well enough to keep your job. Evaluation generally occurs in two areas: written tests that measure your knowledge of theory and performance evaluations that

measure your progress in the clinical area. Evaluation in these areas is a learning experience in itself.

Theory Tests

Learners and instructors look at test results very differently. Learners focus on the number of items they answered correctly. Learners need to identify what they did right on a test so they can apply the process of getting the right answer to future tests. Instructors focus on the specific items the learner had wrong. Wrong items indicate critical knowledge the learner does not have. Do not just ask for your grades. Try to arrange time with your instructors to review your tests. It is impossible to say grades do not count. You must earn the minimum grade established by your nursing program. But consider this. If you got 80% on a test, that means you failed to answer 20% of the questions correctly. Now place yourself in the client's slippers. What about the 20% your nurse got wrong? Was it something the nurse should have known to care for you safely? For this reason, try to look at tests as learning experiences. Be as interested in your wrong answers as you are in your correct answers. Take time to look at your test with the goal of understanding why the correct answers are correct and why the wrong answers you gave are wrong.

Clinical Performance Evaluations

The most meaningful evaluations you will receive during the year will be the performance evaluations given while you are in the clinical area. Because these evaluations give you an opportunity for career and personal growth, it is important to understand this form of evaluation and the responsibilities you have with regard to it.

In the clinical area, instructors will be observing you as you go about caring for patients. They are observing you to discover the positive things you are doing to reach your goal of becoming a practical nurse. These behaviors are to be encouraged. They indicate that learning has taken place and you are growing and progressing toward your goal. Instructors are also observing you to discover behaviors that stand in the way of reaching your goal. These behaviors are to be discouraged. Your instructor will update you daily on your progress in a verbal or written manner. At the end of a clinical rotation, you will receive a written performance evaluation during a conference with your clinical instructor.

From the start, you need to look at performance evaluations as a two-sided coin. The instructor is on one side and you are on the other. As part of their job, instructors have the responsibility of evaluating your performance. As a learner, you have the responsibility of being aware of your clinical behaviors. You are responsible for self-evaluation. The National League for Nursing has indicated that practical nursing students, at the time of graduation, should be able to look at their nursing actions and be aware of their strong behaviors and behaviors that need improvement. Development of the ability to be aware of one's behaviors begins with day one in the practical nursing program, including the skills laboratory. Objective awareness of one's own behaviors is an important skill to have as an employee. A learner does not automatically have this skill when he or she graduates. Learners must consistently work at viewing themselves objectively. Instructors will help in this area. For example, when learning how to make a bed, ask yourself, "Is the finished product as good as I had intended it to be when I started?" *Do not wait for the instructor to identify areas of success or areas of needed improvement.*

Think back to when you received comments from your teachers and parents about your behavior in grade school and high school. How did you feel when you received these comments? Many people grow up with bad feelings about these episodes of criticism and even about the word itself. Criticism means evaluation. Many persons attach a negative meaning to criticism and view it as a put-down.

> *The phrase constructive criticism may evoke negative feelings. The phrase constructive evaluation is frequently used instead. This choice of words may help you look at evaluation of your behaviors in a positive way. It is important to distinguish what is being evaluated. You must separate your behaviors or actions from yourself, the person.*

Constructive evaluation directed toward your behaviors has no bearing on your value as a person. Look at your behaviors as being either positive and helping you to reach your goal or as needing improvement. Behaviors needing improvement must be modified so that you can reach your goal.

As you progress in the nursing program, you will learn about a systematic way of conducting client care called the nursing process (see Chapter 2). An important part of the nursing process is evaluation of client goals while giving client care. If your actions are not helping clients to reach their goals, they must be modified. Knowledge of the nursing process will help you develop your ability to look at your actions and evaluate them. Comments from instructors will help your self-awareness. Remain open with yourself. The comments you receive are directed toward your behaviors and not you as a person.

A good way to start learning self-evaluation is to look at yourself in everyday life. Ask yourself how you look through the eyes of others:

How would you like to be your own spouse?
How would you like to have yourself as a learner?
How would you like to be your own mother or father?
How would you like to be your own nurse?

If you would not like to be any of these people, identify the reasons why. Another good exercise is to make two lists. On one list note your assets or strong points. On the other list note your liabilities or areas that need improvement. When asked to evaluate themselves, learners traditionally rate themselves more negatively. They tend to neglect their strong points. Identifying strong points is not proud or vain behavior. It is dealing with yourself honestly and openly. After you have identified assets and liabilities, review your assets periodically. Make an effort to continue these strong points while modifying your liabilities. Pick one liability at a time to work on. If you do so, your assets list will grow and your liabilities list will shrink.

A good place to start self-evaluation in nursing is in the skills lab of your basic nursing course. Practice becoming very observant of the results of your actions. Are the top sheets centered when you are making an unoccupied bed? Are you using the bath blanket as a drape to avoid chilling and invading the client's privacy? Are you aware of the effect of the tone of your voice on your instructors and peers?

Evaluation is an ever-present reality in any career. Getting into the practice of self-evaluation early in your program of study will help you to develop a skill you will use daily in your career and personal life.

> List one of your strong areas that you have identified as a new practical nursing student.
>
> _____
>
> List one area needing improvement that you have identified as a practical nursing student.
>
> _____

▽▽▽
Dealing with Referrals

If you are assessed by your instructor as having areas that need improvement, the instructor will refer you to the counselor for your division at school. Examples of areas that require referral are a grade below passing in a major test and frequent absences from class. Counselors at technical colleges and junior colleges are academic counselors who have expertise in helping students identify reasons for academic problem areas. A referral to a counselor is an attempt to help you succeed. These counselors can help students set up a plan of action to remedy the problem. We have seen some students resist "going to the counselor." Some students think this is a waste of time.

> **What could be one reason for thinking that an appointment with the counselor is a waste of time?**

▽▽▽
Other Responsibilities of Learners

In addition to assuming responsibility for your own learning, becoming actively involved in the learning process, and receiving and participating in evaluation, it is necessary to be aware of some other responsibilities you have as a learner.

1. Be aware of the rules and policies of your school and the practical nursing program. Abide by them.

2. When problems do develop, follow the recognized channels of communication both at school and in the clinical area. The rule is, go to the source. Avoid "saving up" gripes. Pursue them as they come up.

3. Be prepared in advance for classes and clinical experiences. You expect teachers to be prepared. They expect the same of you. When you are unprepared for classes, you waste the time of the instructor and your peers. When you are unprepared for clinical experiences, you are violating an important safety factor in patient care. When you are scheduled for the clinical area, your state board of nursing expects you to function as a licensed person would function under your state's nurse practice act.

4. Prepare your own assignments. Use your peers and the experiences and knowledge they have and learn from each other.

5. Seek out learning experiences at school and in the clinical area. Set your goals higher than the minimum.

6. Seek out resources beyond the required readings. Examples of these resources can be the library and information from past classes.

7. Assume responsibility for your own thoughts, communication, and behavior. Do not give in to pressure from your peers. BYOB: Be Your Own Boss.

8. Be present and on time for classes and clinical experiences. Follow school and program policies for reporting absences. Getting into this habit will prepare you to be a favored employee.

9. Enter into discussion when asked to do so in class.

10. Treat those with whom you come into daily contact with respect. Be mindful of their rights as individuals.

11. *Seek out your instructor when you are having difficulties in class or in the clinical area.* Often instructors can tell when students are having problems. More important are the times when they cannot tell and only

the student knows a problem exists. Do not be afraid to approach your instructors. They are there to help you.

12. Keep a record of your grades as a course proceeds. At the beginning of a class, the instructor will explain the method of calculating your final grade. You are responsible for knowing how you stand gradewise in a course at any point in time.

▼▼▼ *S U M M A R Y*

▶ Adult learners are numerous today on campuses throughout the United States. Adult learners can be classified as traditional adult learners, returning adult learners, and recycled adult learners. Each category of learner possesses characteristics that can help them to succeed in the practical nursing program. Each group also possesses characteristics that can prevent success. Liabilities occur in areas where learners have control over their solutions. They are not concrete barriers to success. Although learners have rights, they also have responsibilities. The most important of their responsibilities are the personal responsibility for learning, taking an active part in the process, and participating in the evaluation of their learning and growth.

▼▼▼ *B I B L I O G R A P H Y*

Apps J. *Mastering the Teaching of Adults.* Malabar, FL: Krieger, 1991.

Brookfield S. *Understanding and Facilitating Adult Learning.* San Francisco: Jossey-Bass, 1990.

Chenevert M. *Mosby's Tour Guide to Nursing School.* St. Louis: Mosby Year-Book, 1991.

Cross KP. *Adults as Learners: Increasing Participation and Facilitating Learning.* San Francisco: Jossey-Bass, 1992.

Davidhizar R. The changing face of nursing students. J Pract Nurs 1994; 44:8–11.

Galbraith M. *Facilitating Adult Learning: A Transactional Process.* Malabar, FL: Krieger, 1991.

Knowles M. *Andragogy and Pedagogy.* New York: Associated Press, 1970.

Knowles M. *The Modern Practice of Adult Education: From Pedagogy to Andragogy.* New York: Cambridge Books, 1980.

Knowles M. *The Adult Learner: A Neglected Species,* 4th ed. Houston: Gulf Publishers, 1990.

Kurz J. The adult ESL baccalaureate nursing student. J Nurs Edu 1993; 32(5):227–229.

Polson C. Teaching adult students. Idea Paper No. 29. Sept. Center for Faculty Evaluation and Development, Division of Continuing Education, Kansas State University, 1993.

The Class of Dr. Lisa Miller, We're ready . . . are you? Teaching for Success 1995; 7(5):4.

How To Begin

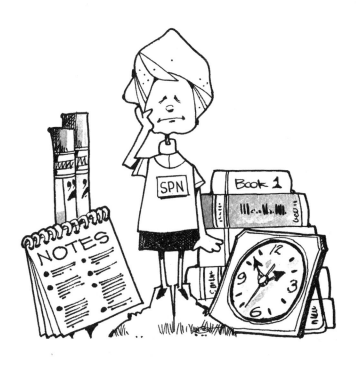

For the Organizationally Challenged

▼▼▼ O U T L I N E

▼▼▼ K E Y   T E R M S

assessment
daily schedule
delegating
effectiveness
efficiency
evaluation
gathering data

habit
high-priority task
implementation
long-term goal
low-priority task
mini-task
planning

priorities
procrastination
semester schedule
short-term goal
support system
weekly schedule

▼▼▼ O B J E C T I V E S

After reading this chapter you will be able to:

1. *Discuss three benefits of time management for an adult student.*

2. *List the activities of the various roles you fill in daily life.*

3. *Arrange the list in two columns according to whether they are high-priority or low-priority items.*

4. *Keep at least a one-day activity log to determine the present use of your time.*

5. *Devise a semester schedule and a weekly schedule to reflect present time commitments.*

6. *Make a daily "to do" list.*

7. *Carry out weekly and daily schedules for two weeks.*

8. *Evaluate the effectiveness of a personal time management plan and modify it if necessary.*

Becky, a full-time student in the practical nursing program, consistently scores As and Bs on her tests and quizzes. She always hands assignments in on time. She is always prepared to demonstrate nursing procedures in the skills lab. On Thursday evenings, she bowls with her husband in a couples' league. It is hard to believe she is the mother of six children, aged 3 to 17.

Have you noticed at school and in your personal life that some people seem to get more done than others? Worse yet, some of the busiest people are the ones getting the most done. To add insult to injury, all of us are given the same amount of time, 168 hours a week, in which to get the job done. How can some individuals get the job done and some not? The answer does not lie in the fact that some people have fewer responsibilities and less to do in a week's time. The answer lies in their ability to manage their own time.

There are several explanations for being disorganized and managing time poorly. These traits can be related to a trauma in your personal life. Organizing may be the last thing on the mind of a person who has been through a divorce or a death in the family. A state of disorganization may be the result of a disorganized upbringing. Disorganization can be the style you grew up with. You might continue this style as a source of comfort. Other disorganized persons may not have committed themselves to something they really want to do. They may use disorganization

as a symptom of their discontent. Regardless of the reason for disorganization, millions of dollars are spent annually to hire time management experts to help people get organized. This chapter contains information and tips that can help you get organized and manage your time more efficiently and effectively. If you follow the suggestions, they will help make a challenging year more tolerable for you.

▼▼▼ Self-Test of Time Management

Time management is a major skill that contributes to learner success. It is also a necessary skill for practical nurses so they can better manage their time in the clinical area to meet client goals. To start this chapter, it is necessary for you to take a self-test of time management so you will know how you stand with regard to this important skill. If you are going to be responsible for managing clinical time, you must be able to manage personal time. Answer yes or no as you read each of the statements in the Self-Test of Time Management and apply them to your personal use of time.

The answers to the self-test are the ones suggested by time-management experts. Although different time-management techniques work for different people, these suggested answers reflect basic time-management techniques that could help you succeed in the practical nursing program.

Self-Test of Time Management

_____ 1. I keep a semester or course calendar to reflect requirements and due dates of work for all my classes.

_____ 2. I keep a written weekly schedule of everything that must be done at school and in my personal life.

_____ 3. I keep a written daily list of things I must do at school and in my personal life.

_____ 4. Daily I list and rank in importance my priorities for using school and personal time.

_____ 5. After listing and ranking my daily priorities for school and personal life, I stick to the list I have made.

_____ 6. I use my best working time during the day for doing my high-priority work for school.

_____ 7. I plan to do lower-priority schoolwork before higher-priority schoolwork.

_____ 8. I start school tasks before thinking them through.

_____ 9. I stop a school task before I have completed it.

_____10. I spend the few minutes before class talking to my classmates about anything other than the class.

_____11. I have trouble starting a major task for school.

_____12. I become bored with the subject I am studying.

_____13. I have a hard time getting started when I sit down to study.

_____14. Sometimes I avoid important school tasks.

_____15. I find myself easily distracted when I study.

_____16. I always try to get everything done in my personal life that must be done.

_____17. I frequently watch television instead of doing schoolwork.

_____18. I manage to turn a short coffee break into a long coffee break.

_____19. I study nightly for my classes.

_____20. I frequently have to cram for exams.

Suggested Answers to Self-Test

1. Yes	6. Yes	11. No	16. No
2. Yes	7. No	12. No	17. No
3. Yes	8. No	13. No	18. No
4. Yes	9. No	14. No	19. Yes
5. Yes	10. No	15. No	20. No

Count the number you disagree with and plug yourself into one of the following categories:

1–5 Disagree with   You deserve the *Alan Lakein** award.

5–10 Disagree with   Hang in there! With a little guidance you will get on the right track.

11–20 Disagree with   We know you must be exhausted, but keep on reading, fast!

*Alan Lakein is a famous time-management expert. In 1973 he first published a very readable book entitled *How to Get Control of Your Time and Your Life.* The key to using time wisely has not changed since his first edition was published.

▼▼▼
Benefits of Time Management

Time management is a technique designed to help you do not only the things you have to get done but also the things you want to finish in a definite time period. Time management can put you in control of your life rather than making you a slave to it. You will have to give up some of the things you were accustomed to doing before you became a practical nursing student. Time-management techniques can help you gain some personal time for your family and yourself so you will not feel that there is time only for school. Time management can help you work smarter, not harder. It will not give you more hours in the week but will help you use what hours you do have more efficiently and effectively. *Efficiency* will help you get things done as quickly as possible. Time management does not deal solely with efficiency, as did the efficiency experts of the 1950s. The efficiency of the 1950s can bring images of robotlike individuals working to get *every* task done in the shortest time possible in a machine-like manner. Efficiency needs to be balanced with effectiveness. *Effectiveness* involves setting priorities among the tasks that need to be done and doing them the best way possible. Efficiency involves doing things as quickly as possible. Effectiveness involves choosing the most important task to do and doing it the right way.

▼▼▼
Review of Personal Goals

How did you score on the self-test? If you are a typical adult, you are probably reading quickly right now to find out what to do to improve. Take heart. Very few of us get the Alan Lakein award. Most of us could stand to learn how to use our time more efficiently and effectively. Ineffective use of personal time is learned behavior, better known as a habit. Any behavior that is learned can be unlearned if you work at it, and new habits can be acquired.

If you have set a goal to be a practical nurse, you are already on the right track in time management, no

matter what you scored. This is the bullseye to which you will direct your efforts for the next year. It would be beneficial to write that goal on a recipe card and place it where you will see it frequently. Some suggestions are your car visor, the bathroom mirror, and the refrigerator door. Be sure to include the date of your graduation. There will be some tough days in the months ahead, and the visibility of your long-term goal can keep you going. To realize this long-term goal, you must break it down into smaller, more manageable goals. These are called your short-term goals. Examples of short-term goals are passing each of the courses you must take to graduate from the practical nursing program. These short-term goals can be broken down even further to include the individual requirements for each of the courses you must take. For example, for your professional issues course you might have to meet the following requirements to pass the course:

1. Earn a minimum grade on each of a certain number of major tests.
2. Give two oral reports.
3. Write a four-page paper on a selected topic.

Fulfilling each of the requirements will eventually lead to passing the course. When each of the courses you are required to take is passed you will graduate from the program. While keeping your eye on your long-term goal, you will fulfill requirement after requirement until that goal is reached. Now, let us start learning how to manage your time.

▼▼▼
Getting Organized with the Nursing Process

At all levels, nursing has a special way of getting organized called the nursing process. You have studied the nursing process and how it relates to you as a practical nurse. The nursing process and its four components—data collection (assessment), planning, implementation, and evaluation—will be used to help you get organized as a student and in your personal life.

▽▽▽
Data Collection (Assessment)

According to *Webster's,* assessment is the act of placing a value on something. To do this, the element of judgment must be brought into the picture. **Data collection (assessment)** in time management involves two important areas: (1) *collecting data* on how you actually *spend your time* and (2) *discovering* what *roles* you fill in your daily life.

Enrollment in a vocational–technical program, whether you are single, divorced, widowed, or married, requires some degree of change in the activities in which you were involved before entering the program. Regardless of your state in life, all the roles you fill can be classified in any of five general categories: school, job, family, community, and recreation. The activities involved in going to school are very structured. You must get there, attend classes, and get home. When you are enrolled in a vocational–technical program such as practical nursing, your school day is chock full. Seldom do you even have the choice of when you will take a specific course. The same structure is not evident in the other four roles. In your other roles, you might be involved in activities that you either did not plan to do, do not enjoy doing, do not have time to do, or do not feel need to be done. You are encouraged to complete the activity on page 364 of Appendix B in order to collect data about your *personal roles and activities* for the data collection (assessment) portion of time management. A sample exercise and explanation is on page 363 of Appendix B. You are now ready to document how you actually use your personal time. Ideally, a time log should be kept for about one week to document how you use your personal time. Because time is marching on, a one-day time log can give you a general idea of how you use your time at present. Page 365 of Appendix B explains the exercise entitled Use of Personal Time. On page 366 of the Appendix, you will find a blank page on which to record your Personal Time and Activity Log. Now, supply only one more piece of information and your assessment will be complete. After this paragraph, list one activity you wish you had time for. The activity could have been listed under your roles, but maybe it was not listed at all. Re-

member, the sky's the limit as long as your wish is something that is really important to you.

My special wish is _____

_____

_____

▽▽▽
Planning

When you have completed the assessment (data collection) exercises in Appendix B, you will be ready to proceed to the planning stage. The planning phase of time management will result in a blueprint for action. In this phase you will learn how to plan use of your precious 168 hours a week. **Planning** involves thinking about setting priorities (most important tasks), but to be successful, these thoughts must be written down. You need to devise written schedules for yourself so that you can program your time on a monthly, weekly, and daily basis. The schedules should include the activities that are part of all the roles you fill and not just your role as a student. Your schedules should reflect the total of your activities.

Schedules help keep you honest. They reflect the classes you must attend and the studying you must do to reach your long-term goal. With a schedule you will avoid the roller-coaster phenomenon all too familiar to students—falling behind in school and then trying to catch up. Schedules help you include time for friends and family. Schedules help you avoid overlooking an important part of your well-being: recreation. And schedules help you avoid the pitfall of allowing extracurricular activities to come before schoolwork. Allowing extracurricular activities to come before schoolwork is the major reason for failure in post-secondary educational programs.

Arguments Against Planning

At this point some individuals will say they do not have time to plan and will pass off the suggestion about scheduling. Individuals who are too busy to plan are the very persons that should be planning. They cannot afford not to plan. If you do not plan, you will overlook priorities and possibly miss some available free time. For the small amount of time planning takes, the benefits are great. Some persons who say they do not have time to plan really do not want to find time to get priority work done. They may use lack of time as an excuse. Some individuals look at planning and scheduling as leading to inflexibility and loss of freedom. They want to "hang loose" and go in different directions as the opportunity arises. Flexibility of this sort can result in disorganization and the accomplishment of few, if any, important tasks. As imposed deadlines near, guilt, frustration, and anxiety appear. These individuals wind up being a slave to time instead of being its master. A schedule written in accordance with the principles of time management will help you be a master of time and not a slave to it. The schedule will be written with flexibility in mind, and you will be able to trade time with yourself when unexpected events come up.

Unlearning old habits and learning new habits is not an easy task. It takes work in the form of self-discipline and determination to drop old, comfortable ways. But it is possible. Be sure to practice the new habit whenever the opportunity to do so presents itself. In doing this, the new habit will eventually become a part of you. Ah! You say you slipped up and reverted to old habits. Do not give up! Start from where you left off and try again.

Scheduling Time

The only special equipment you need for scheduling is a calendar. Ideally, you need one that has blank space for each date so that you can list activities. These calendars should be available at the bookstore. Some school bookstores provide a semester calendar for students. You can also make your own monthly calendar by copying a current calendar. To schedule your time, you should be able to set priorities and delegate activities.

Setting Priorities

In Appendix B on page 367 there is an exercise entitled Setting Personal Priorities to help you decide which of your activities are most important or which activities need to come first.

In order to have a successful year in the practical nursing program, teamwork is important. Identify the persons in your life who make up your team. This is your support system. Inform them of the goals and priorities you have set for yourself for this school year.

List the persons in your personal support system.

_____   _____

_____   _____

_____   _____

Delegating Activities

Some of your activities can be delegated to specific persons on your team. On pages 71 and 72 is a chart of activities with examples of tasks that can be delegated in this manner. Taking growth and development into consideration, the tasks listed for children are excellent ways for them to learn responsibility.

As in the study of growth and development, these suggested activities apply to the typical child of each age group. The suggestions may or may not apply to your children. But do not underestimate your children. You will be able to come up with some ideas that do fit your children and add to the list. At first it may take some time to instruct your children, but in the long run it will be worthwhile. Have you ever heard of the saying "You have to spend money to make money"? Well, in time management, sometimes it takes time initially to teach the people near you what is expected of them. In the long run it will pay off handsomely in time saved. Plus you get the added bonus of encouraging independence. The same principle will be used in client care. It may take time to teach clients how to master a skill for themselves. In the long run it will save you time once they learn, and as a bonus the clients gain independence. These suggestions are a wonderful way to help a child become independent and develop lifelong skills.

Are you having trouble getting your spouse to cooperate? Do not interpret stubbornness as lack of love or laziness. Chances are that your spouse grew up in an environment in which household chores were divided by sex. The spouse may feel that his masculinity or her femininity is jeopardized by assuming new tasks. Gather your thoughts and decide on the areas in which you think your spouse could be most helpful during this hectic time of your life. The answer lies in communication. Talk to your spouse (and only you know the best time and situation for this). Hopefully, you both agree that you should be going to school and have identified the positive features of this endeavor for both of you. Review these positive features. If you have not identified them, do so together. Then collaborate on solutions to ease your lack of time. While you are at it, establish some precious "spouse-only" time to be honored during your hectic year at school. You do not want to create in your spouse the feeling of being left out during this whole experience.

Page 367 in Appendix B has an exercise entitled Delegating Activities to help you decide which personal roles and activities can be delegated.

Chart of Shared Tasks That May Be Delegated

Significant Other	Preschool and Early School Age (4–8 years)	School Age (9–12 years)
Pay bills	Fold laundry	Cook simple meals
Help clean	Make laundry piles	Wash dishes
Take charge of car maintenance	Deliver laundry to correct room	Dry dishes
Mow the lawn	Clear dishes from table (not best china)	Put dishes away
Paint		Start laundry
Do small repairs		Shop for a few food items as indicated on list
Sort laundry		Dust
Transfer laundry to dryer		Run vacuum
Shovel snow		Sew patches on own shirts
		Plant garden
		Weed
		Shovel snow
		Make own bed

Rationale for activities chosen for:

Preschool and early school age. Children in these age groups are experiencing muscle development, and notice their psychomotor development; they want to try new things. Make-believe rides high with these kids and they love to play house. Capitalize on this.

School age. These children are adults-in-training. Muscles continue to develop and psychomotor skills are increasing. They need tasks of the real world to engage in and should be encouraged to carry them through to completion.

ADOLESCENTS (13-18 YEARS)	FRIENDS	RELATIVES
Run errands with family car if they have a license; use bike if no license	Replace you at bowling the night before a big exam	Substitute for mom or dad at scout meetings, PTA meetings, or school activities

Box continued on next page

Chart of Shared Tasks That May Be Delegated (Continued)

ADOLESCENTS (13-18 YEARS)	FRIENDS	RELATIVES
Plan menus	Replace you in car pool (or substitute)	Spend time with children
Prepare grocery list within budget	Feed you occasionally	Holiday baking or shopping
Mow the lawn		
Paint		
Make own bed		

Rationale for activities chosen for:

Adolescents. Sometime during adolescence, the ability to think as an adult will develop, allowing this age group to budget, apply principles of basic nutrition, etc., to everyday life. One of the tasks of adolescence is to become independent. Help its development by delegating meaningful activity to this age group.

School-age children and adolescents can also do activities in the column to the left of their column but would probably prefer the specific activities listed for their age group.

▼▼▼
Learning Exercise

Semester Scheduling

Time Involved: Approximately 10 minutes

On your planning calendar, list the things that must be done during this time frame. Examples of activities to include here are

▶ Your class schedule
▶ Dates of major exams
▶ Dates papers are due
▶ Dates of doctors' appointments
▶ Dates of club meetings
▶ Dates for haircuts, and so on

Include activities that are delegated. Indicate them by circling the activity on the calendar. Write the name of the person who is responsible for it. Post these sheets, one month at a time on your refrigerator for you, your family, or your roommate or significant other to see. The semester schedule is done only once, in pencil. Additions or corrections are made as needed. This is also a way of communicating your new life to those with whom you live. Keep in mind, if you do live with other people, that your new schedule is something to which they must get accustomed.

Weekly Schedules

Time Involved: Approximately 10 minutes

The weekly schedule is for your peace of mind. A blank form can be found on page 368 of Appendix B. You can copy this sheet on looseleaf paper. Fill in all your classes and other fixed activities for the week. Photocopy as many sheets as there are weeks in the semester or time period of your current classes. Use some time each weekend to plan your week. Be sure to include in your planning the time you spend before and after classes. As assignments are made, add them to your weekly schedule. Your weekly schedule will not only reflect study time but also will specify what should be studied when. The following are some suggestions to keep in mind when planning your week.

1. Schedule studying for your prime time. Prime time is the time you are most effective in doing a task. High-priority courses should be studied for during prime time.

2. Schedule blocks of time for studying by identifying your personal attention span for various school activities. For example, when reading, note the time you start reading and when you begin to lose your concentration. Note the amount of time that has passed. Do this for several sessions of studying. You will begin to see patterns in your attention span. Take a three- to five-minute break at this point in your studying. Vary your activity.

Some people may find they have a 20-minute attention span. Others may have an attention span of one hour. The important thing is not to let your break extend beyond a few minutes. Condition yourself to get right back to work, without the need for start-up time.

It is impossible to tell you exactly how much time you will need for studying for each of your classes. This will vary from student to student and from class to class. Does the class meet daily? If so, you will have a daily assignment. The old suggestion of two hours of study for each hour of class will be just right for some classes, too much for others, and not enough for the rest.

3. Identify small blocks of time. Make them work for you. They are important sources of time. These minutes can add up quickly to large time losses. These small blocks of time usually occur between classes. Get up. Stretch. Take deep breaths if staying in the same classroom. Walk briskly while taking deep breaths to get to your next class. Review in your mind the class you just attended. These activities will force more oxygen into your bloodstream and help it circulate to your brain. This results in better thinking and a fresher state of mind. One of the worst things to do is to grab a soda or a cigarette. The soda, if nondiet, will quickly elevate your blood sugar level and encourage insulin to be deposited in the blood. The insulin will quickly lower the sugar content of your blood, leaving you with a tired, dragged-out feeling. Smoking constricts your blood vessels and decreases the amount of oxygen carried to your brain. Your brain needs oxygen to help you think and to keep you alert. While waiting for your next class, select one of the following activities.

   ▶ Review your notes from the class you just finished. This will allow you to fill in any gaps you may have in your notes. You will aid your retention and understanding of the material by reviewing it in this way.

   ▶ Mentally prepare for your next class. If it is a lecture or discussion class, review your assignment. If it is an autotutorial class, review your plan of activities for the class. School is a social activity, but do not waste time by fooling around during all of your small blocks of free time. The more you get done at school, the less you will have to do at home.

   ▶ Discuss an assignment with a peer.

4. Write only what is essential on your schedule. Details take too much time to write down and are a real turnoff.

5. Plan for three meals a day with appropriate snacks, based on the food pyramid. Eating properly will help avoid tiredness and irritability. With a busy schedule, you need to avoid being tired and irritable at all costs.

6. Plan for adequate sleep. Individuals have personal sleep patterns. Try to get in tune with yours. Do you ever wake up before your alarm? Next time you do, calculate how many hours sleep you have had. Odds are your hours of sleep are some multiple of 1½ hours. Brain research has shown that you will function

better if you get up after 6 hours or after 7½ hours of sleep rather than after 7 or 8 hours. Apparently, we repeat a sleep cycle every 1½ hours. If you get up one-half hour into your next cycle, you could be very sluggish. Think of this when you set your alarm. And when the alarm goes off, resist the temptation to reset the alarm on snooze.

7. Remember, although some sacrifices must be made, your life is more than just school. Review your sky's-the-limit wish on page 69 of this chapter and include it on your weekly schedule.

Daily Schedule

Time Involved: Approximately 5 minutes

This schedule could prove to be the most important one as far as getting things done. Alan Lakein, the time-management expert, calls the daily schedule a "to do" list. He states that both successful and unsuccessful persons know about "to do" lists. Successful persons use such a list every day to make better use of their time. Unsuccessful people do not (Lakein, 1989, p. 64). This is the simplest schedule to make. Use a 3-by-5-inch card and head it *To Do.* List the items you want to accomplish. Be sure to include the high-priority activities for school and your personal life that you identified on pages 364 and 367 of Appendix B. Refer to your weekly calendar to refresh your memory about your assignments and their due dates. Rank your activities so that you can handle first things first.

Decide for yourself the best time of day for writing your "to do" list. Some persons like to make up this list while eating breakfast as a way to get into the activities of the day. Some people like to make up the list right before they go to bed. These persons may be getting an extra benefit that they are not aware of. Their subconscious will be able to go over the to do list while they peacefully sleep and renew themselves. Carry your list with you. Stick to the activities and priorities you have listed. Cross off the activities when you have completed them. Ah, what a feeling!

Planning takes so little time. It can be fun and not a chore. Just think of all the benefits that come out of taking 10 minutes to plan each month, 10 minutes to plan each week, and 5 minutes to plan each day. What great returns for so little effort! And, by writing your schedules and lists, you have freed your brain from one more source of clutter and saved it for all the learning you must do.

▽▽▽
Implementation

This is the part of your time-management program in which your plans become action. The only value of a plan lies in its being used. Thanks to the planning you have done, you now have an incentive to get started because you already know exactly where you have to be and what you have to do. Now for some hints on how to follow that plan.

General Hints

As you begin to follow your personal plan, you may notice that some of your peers at school are not planning their time. They may even give you static for attempting to plan yours. Even if it means leaving some peers in the shuffle, have the intestinal fortitude to follow your schedule. You paid your tuition and have your own personal-time problems to contend with to get full mileage out of that tuition. There may be some students who put their efforts into games instead of scholastic pursuits. They think they will look better if others do not succeed. You will recognize these students when they tell you straight out that your efforts will make them look bad. Whose problem is that, anyhow? Make sure you never miss a class, regardless of peer pressure or any reason other than an emergency. When you miss a class, you spend more time than the class would have taken trying to obtain the information from the class. You may never capture all of it.

In actually carrying out your schedule, be aware of

a pitfall that can happen when you assign a specific time to a task. Sometimes the time it takes to do a task, whether for home or school, can stretch out to fill whatever time you have assigned to it. So practice setting realistic time limits in which to complete tasks so you do not fall into this trap.

Procrastination

You know what you have to do and when it must be done, but do you ever find yourself putting off high-priority tasks to some time in the future? Take time now and list one task that you have put off this week.

_____

_____

_____

_____

How did you feel about postponing this task? Such action usually leads to tension. What is causing your reluctance? Reevaluate the task you have been avoiding. Is it really a high-priority task? Remember, your planning should be flexible. The priority status of tasks can realistically change. But be careful if you find yourself using this explanation too frequently. Other causes for putting off what is important are ill health (you do not have the energy), laziness (you do not have the motivation), and past successful episodes of procrastination (if you did not do it, someone else did or nobody cared). Regardless of the cause, we all procrastinate to some degree. Some persons make more of a habit of it than others.

If you look truthfully at the tasks you keep postponing, odds are they are unpleasant, difficult, or time consuming. It seems we never postpone things that are fun or simple to do. In fact, sometimes we avoid high-priority tasks and do a bunch of low-priority ones. This action gives us an immediate yet false feeling of accomplishment. For others, fear of failure causes them to put off things to the last minute. This provides the individual with an excuse for not doing well.

A sure way to finish those unpleasant, difficult, and time-consuming tasks you have been putting off is to reduce the entire task to a series of mini-tasks. There are

two rules for doing this. First, the mini-task must be simple to do and take no more than five minutes of your time. Second, for best results, the mini-tasks should be written and carried in your pocket for quick reference. Many students fear upcoming major tests and put off studying for them. Some examples of mini-tasks for this situation could be:

1. Before and after each class, review your current notes and related material covered previously.

2. Write the more difficult information you must know for the test on index cards. For example, write a term on one side of the card and its definition on the other. List causes of, consequences of, prevention of, and differences between items of class content and have these cards handy for quick reference whenever you have a spare minute. One of your authors studied vocabulary for a German final in this way while having a root canal procedure done.

3. Follow the same procedure as in mini-task 2 for items you got wrong on quizzes.

4. Talk to a peer about course content.

Refer to Chapter 6 for information on identifying your personal learning styles.

Now, write some mini-tasks for the high-priority task you identified as having put off.

1. _____

2. _____

3. _____

These mini-tasks will get you involved in starting the task in a less painful way. Just starting a task, even in a minimal way, is a positive force. Getting started takes more effort than keeping going.

Whatever the cause of your procrastination, to be behind in work is to be behind in success. Most times it takes more time and energy to escape the task than to do it in the first place. Start today to keep life in the present. Avoid deferring life and all its opportunities to the future.

Hints for Handling the Home or Apartment

No matter how much you delegate, if you are a spouse and parent, a single parent, or a single adult, you must realize that your house or apartment is not going to be as spic and span while you are a student. A few hints may help ease the transition. Some of these hints are also helpful for spouses who are helping out while the other goes to school and for single adults who are living on their own for the first time.

▶ Grandma always said tidy up to make it look like you really cleaned. Pick up papers and magazines as you pass through a room. If you don't have time to wash dishes, rinse and stack them to be done later rather than just collecting them on the counter in the kitchen. Make your bed each morning when you first get up. It only takes a minute and improves the appearance of the bedroom dramatically. In fact, you can teach yourself to smooth out the top covers before you get out of bed and then slither out. Place dirty clothes in a laundry basket in your bedroom or bathroom instead of just heaping them on the floor. Hang up other clothing instead of just draping it over furniture. Clean the tub after using it by soaping up your washcloth and washing the sides of the tub while it is still warm. The soap and dirt ring will not have to be scoured. (Be sure to put your washcloth in the laundry and get out a clean one.) Put hair dryer, cool curling iron, and so on away after use or collect them in a basket to reduce clutter. These suggestions take hardly any time and really help things look straightened up.

▶ If you live in a two-story home, put a box at the top of the stairs and another one at the bottom for objects that need to go upstairs or come down. There is always something coming or going, and this will save extra trips.

▶ Having trouble with the family remembering their assigned chores? Draw the shape of a house on cardboard, draw 31 windows on the house and number them in sequence. Cut three of the four sides of each window so that it opens up.

Place the cardboard over a piece of shelf paper and write in names and chores for each day on the paper. Paste this chore sheet in place and tape up the windows. The first month takes the most time, but the chore list is a snap after that. Be sure to include a surprise or treat occasionally.

▶ A fun and fast way for an adult or child to dust is to wear a washed garden glove, spray the glove with furniture polish, and go to it.

The sky's the limit as far as creative ideas for saving time at school and in your personal life. You will come up with some ideas out of sheer necessity as the year goes by. When you do, be sure to share them with your peers.

▽▽▽
Evaluation

Evaluation of your time-management program will take place continuously from the minute you start implementing your plan. Evaluation involves determining how well your plan is working and how you are progressing toward meeting your long-term goal. It is a crucial part of time management. Why continue with a plan if it is not helping you reach your goal?

If the plan is not working, modify it. Ask yourself, "What changes should I make in my plan so that it will help me reach my long-term goal?" The best gauge you have for evaluating your plan is your test grades. They will tell you if you are devoting as much time as you need to make the grade in a course.

And how is your daily participation in class? Do you have assignments completed when they are due? Are you even aware that you had an assignment? Did you forget the test was on Thursday because you didn't mark it on your weekly calendar? Are you lapsing into the habit of procrastination? Not only will evaluation help you see how well you are progressing toward your goal, it will also help you develop the evaluation and modification skills you will need as a practical nurse.

▼▼▼ S U M M A R Y

▶ Time management is the efficient and effective use of personal time to meet long-term goals. Techniques of time management can help you gain control over your life rather than being a slave to it, and can help you work smarter, not harder. By using elements of the nursing process, you can set up time-management techniques to fit your personal life. Assessment includes collecting data about present personal-time use and the activities included in the various roles you fill. Planning involves writing semester, weekly, and daily schedules to include high-priority activities. Implementation involves carrying out your plan. Evaluation involves deciding whether your plan is helping you meet your long-term goal and modifying it accordingly.

▼▼▼ R E F E R E N C E S

Lakein A. *How to Get Control of Your Time and Your Life.* New York: New American Library–Dutton, 1989.

▼▼▼ B I B L I O G R A P H Y

Chenevert M. *Mosby's Tour Guide to Nursing School.* St. Louis: Mosby–Year Book, 1991.
Mayer J. *Time Management for Dummies.* Foster City, CA: IDG Books, 1995.
Meltzer M, Palau M. *Reading and Study: Strategies for Nursing Students.* Philadelphia: W.B. Saunders, 1993.
Pauk W. *How to Study in College,* 5th ed. Boston: Houghton-Mifflin, 1993.
Shepherd J. *College Study Skills.* Boston: Houghton-Mifflin, 1990.
The great Alan Lakein on time management . . . 20 years later. Bottom Line/Personal. 1993; 14(18):11–12.

Discovering Your Learning Style

CHAPTER **6**

▼▼▼ *K E Y   T E R M S*

adult ADD
auditory learner
critical thinking
left brain

linguistic learner
logical learner
musical learner
right brain

spatial learner
tactual learner
visual learner

▼▼▼ O B J E C T I V E S

Upon completing this chapter you will be able to:

1. *Define critical thinking in your own words.*

2. *Explain what is meant by learning style.*

3. *Discuss three major learning styles.*

4. *Describe four secondary learning categories.*

5. *Identify your personal learning styles.*

6. *List five characteristics of the right and left sides of the brain.*

7. *Describe five characteristics of an undependable memory and learning system.*

▼▼▼
Introduction to Critical Thinking

Critical thinking is an advanced way of thinking. It is the problem-solving method plus more. Critical thinking is used to resolve problems and to find ways to improve even when no problems exist.

Critical thinking changes according to where you are and what is going on. For example, critical thinking in the classroom and nursing lab is quite different from critical thinking in the clinical area. This represents the difference between simulated practice and real life.

Critical thinking is an essential part of nursing. The overall purpose of nursing is to assist people to (1) stay well or (2) regain their maximum state of health as quickly as possible, in a cost-effective manner, and in a way that fits with their belief system. Decisions nurses make affect both. Nursing decisions must be accurate and must be based on sound thinking and data. As a nurse, your critical thinking skill will vary according to your education and clinical experience. Challenge yourself critically by:

1. Anticipating questions that the client or instructor might ask.

2. Asking for clarification for what you do not understand.

3. Asking yourself if there is more you can do.

4. Rewording what you have read or been told in your own words (for example, stating the nursing diagnosis as a nursing problem).

5. Making comparisons to something similar to help you understand.

6. Organizing information in more than one way to see if you have missed anything important. This is to avoid being impressed when the "facts" fall into place but you have missed the obvious.

7. Asking your instructor to check out your conclusions.

8. Striving for objectivity. Keep an open mind and avoid drawing conclusions in advance.

9. Reviewing all your data again, especially after a period of time. It may look different.

10. Getting used to saying "I do not know but I will find out."

11. Learning from mistakes. Fix them if you can, and for goodness sake, do not hide an error. Someone's life may be at stake, plus others can learn from your error.

12. Thinking about what you are reading about while you are reading it.

Ask your instructor to challenge you to think critically while you are on the clinical unit.

▼▼▼
Discovering Your Learning Style

Most individuals have wondered why one classmate takes voluminous notes while another just listens, and another equally successful student says, "I'll understand this better when I practice it." Everyone learns differently. Some of you may have attempted to emulate a classmate's learning style because of his or her success. Perhaps you continue to practice a learning method that has never been as successful for you as you would like it to be. The authors are here to say that if a learning style is not working for you, change it. After completing this chapter, you are encouraged to review what you have learned about learning styles and to support or change your present learning styles accordingly. Before reading any further take time to complete the self-evaluation quiz given here.

Self-Evaluation of Major Personal Learning Style

Identify Your Major Learning Style

Directions: Underline the answer that is most accurate for each statement.

	Yes	Sometimes	No
Prefers to talk rather than read.	○	△	□
Likes to touch, hug, shake hands.	△	□	○
Prefers verbal directions.	○	△	□
Uses finger spelling as a way of learning words.	△	□	○
Likes written directions better than verbal directions.	□	○	△
Reads to self by moving lips.	○	△	□
Likes to take notes for studying.	□	○	△
Remembers best by doing.	△	□	○
Likes or makes charts and graphs.	□	○	△
Learns from listening to lectures and tapes.	○	△	□
Likes to work with tools.	△	□	○
Might say, "I don't see what you mean."	□	○	△
Good at jigsaw puzzles.	□	○	△
Has good listening skills.	○	△	□
Presses pencil down hard when writing.	△	□	○
Learns theory best by reading the textbook.	□	○	△
Asks to have printed directions explained.	○	△	□
Chews gum or smokes almost continuously.	△	□	○

Scoring

Count all of the ○ △ □.
The highest number indicates the major learning style(s).

Key

□ = visual
○ = auditory
△ = tactual

Adapted from and used with the permission of Jeffrey Barsch, Ed.D. Complete copies of the test may be obtained by writing directly to Jeffrey Barsch, Ed.D., Ventura College, 4667 Telegraph Rd., Ventura, CA 93003.

Congratulations! You have taken the time to identify your major learning styles. There are specific categories that further define your learning style.

▶ Logical learner (organized, consistent)
▶ Musical learner (hums, sings, plays instruments)
▶ Linguistic learner (enjoys words and new vocabulary)
▶ Spatial learner (likes more boxes and diagrams: less words)

Now to find out what it all means.

▼▼▼ Major Learning Styles

Different people think differently. They think in the system corresponding to the sense of vision, hearing, or touch. Those who think in terms of vision (visual learners) generate visual images—that is, they think primarily in pictures. People who think in terms of hearing (auditory learners) talk to themselves or hear sounds. Individuals who think in terms of touch (kinesthetic or tactual learners) experience feelings in regard to what is being thought about. This does not mean that a learner thinks exclusively in any one of these overall systems. What it does mean is that most people think more in one system than another. There are ways to enhance learning by supporting the overall system.

No learning style is better than another. It is usually easier to feel connected to someone who shares a similar learning style: "we think in the same language." It is easy to label a peer with a different learning style as either smart or dumb. A similar implication is there for an instructor.

A learning style just is. There are ways to make it work for you.

▽▽▽ Visual Learner

If you are a visual learner, you learn best by watching a demonstration first. You learn something by seeing it. Make this style work for you by:

1. Sitting in front of the class.
2. Staying focused on the teacher's facial expression and body language.
3. Making notes in class, and highlighting important points.
4. Rewriting notes in your own words as a form of studying. Writing notes in the margin of your book.
5. Using index cards for review or memorization.
6. Reviewing films or video tapes.
7. Looking for reference books with pictures, graphs, or charts or drawing your own.
8. Requesting demonstrations and observational experiences prior to demonstrating a new skill.
9. "Picturing" a procedure rather than memorizing steps.

▽▽▽ Auditory Learner

If you are an auditory learner you learn best by hearing. Make this style work for you by:

1. Reading aloud or mouthing the words. Concentrate on hearing the words, especially when reading test questions.
2. Reading important information into a tape recorder and then playing it back.
3. Listening to the teacher's words instead of taking notes during class. Tape presentations and discussions if permission is granted by the instructor and students. Play the tapes back several times.
4. Finding a "study buddy" with whom to discuss class content. Verbalizing the information aids in learning the material.
5. Requesting permission to make audio tapes or oral reports for credit instead of written reports.
6. Making up rhymes or songs to remember key points.
7. Requesting verbal explanations of illustrations, graphs, or diagrams.

▽▽▽ Tactual Learner

If you are a tactual learner you learn best by doing. You have difficulty in processing both visual and auditory input. You follow directions best by watching and doing. Make this style work for you by:

1. Handling the equipment before you practice a nursing procedure.

2. Moving while reading or reciting facts; rocking, pacing, using a stairmaster or stationary bike, and so on.

3. Changing study positions often.

4. Using background music: your choice.

5. Taking short breaks and doing something active during that time.

6. Offering to do a project as a way of enhancing a required classroom presentation. For example, you have been asked to explain how oxygen gets out of the capillary and carbon dioxide gets in. You develop a project to use as the basis of your explanation.

▽▽▽
Specific Categories of Learning Styles

Logical Learner

If you are a logical learner as well, you learn best by using an organized method of study. Make this style work for you by:

1. Taking the time to organize a method of study that fits you personally.

2. Redoing your notes to fit your study method; categorizing the material under titles.

3. Studying in an area that is orderly.

Musical Learner

If you are a musical learner, you learn best by humming, singing, or playing an instrument. Make this style work for you by:

1. Playing your favorite music or humming when studying. Remind yourself what music relates to the content you are studying.

2. Playing an instrument while reviewing information in your head.

Linguistic Learner

If you are a linguistic learner you learn best by reducing the number of words you have included in your notes. Make this style work for you by:

1. Taking notes when you read this text. Use those notes as your study source. Your love of words and vocabulary may cause you to become distracted from the key points.

2. Reviewing all written work before handing it in. Delete extra words and phrases that are not directly related to the topic.

Spatial Learner

If you are a spatial learner you learn best by studying diagrams, boxes, and special lists in the text. Make this learning style work for you by:

1. Making your own diagrams, boxes, or lists when they are not available in the book.

2. Redoing your notes using key concepts only.

3. Boxing key information in the text.

Choose ideas from those suggested to fit the combination of learning styles that defines you; add or subtract as needed.

▼▼▼
One Brain: Two Different Ways of Thinking

In most people, the left side of the brain is associated with academic activities and the right side of the brain is associated with creative intuition. One side of the brain is no more or less important than the other. You need each side to make sense out of the world. Table 6–1 compares the different functions of the right and left sides of the brain.

The two sides of the brain are designed to form a partnership and are complementary to each other. In the activity of speech, for example, the left side of the brain, being very verbal and fluent, would

Table 6–1
Comparison of the Two Sides of the Brain

Left Brain	Right Brain
Thinks in words	Thinks in images
Looks at the parts that make up the picture or entire situation	Looks at the whole picture or entire situation
Logical side	Emotional side
Breaks down the whole to individual parts and takes them one at a time, step by step (analyzer)	Combines parts to make a whole (holistic, a synthesizer)
Works like a digital computer	Works like a kaleidoscope
Speech, word center	Visual center
Slower working	Faster working
Special activities: 　Reasoning 　Numbers (mathematics) 　Expression of thoughts in words 　Verbal awareness 　Verifies ideas	Special activities: 　Music 　Rhythm 　Insight 　Imagination 　Intuition 　Nonverbal memory 　Generates ideas 　Daydreams 　Visualize in three dimensions 　Visualizes in color

cause us to talk in computerlike patterns if the right side were not available to add tone and inflection to our voice. The right side of the brain helps us to recognize a face in the crowd quickly, even if the person had shaved off his beard, whereas the left side would puzzle over this missing part. In school, the left side helps us break down new information into bits and pieces so we can master it. The right side gives us the total picture of our learning. In nursing, the right side generates new ideas to use in improving client care, the left side verifies the safety of these new methods.

This brain partnership can be encouraged or dis-couraged in an individual. We have been accused of living in a left-brained world. Education in the United States has typically encouraged activity of the left side of the brain and ignored that of the right side. Individually, we have allowed the left sides of our brain to be more active. This bad habit helps make our brain partnership a lopsided one. We can learn to be more aware of both sides of our brain. From the standpoint of learning it would benefit each of us to do so.

When the full power of both sides of the brain is used, humans can achieve great things. To overlook one side or the other in everyday life, including learning situations, is to function with only half of our potential.

This situation has occurred throughout the history of humans when one side or the other is favored.

▼▼▼
Undependable Memory and Learning System

There are average and above average individuals with potential and talent who embrace failure messages and low self-esteem. Some of these individuals are part of a population who continue to live with an untreated attention deficit disorder (ADD) as adults. Among the characteristics of adult ADD is an undependable memory and learning system.

Signs of Possible Adult ADD

Check the statements that apply.

_____ 1. Trouble hanging on to a steady job.

_____ 2. Difficulty getting assignments in on time; late in filing taxes or renewing driver's license.

_____ 3. Supervisor or instructor complains that you do not do your share of the work.

_____ 4. Feel others are responsible for what happens to you.

_____ 5. Impulse buyer: I need, I want, I must have. Credit cards frequently maxed out.

_____ 6. Thrill-seeking impulsive behavior: live for the moment without considering consequences.

_____ 7. Use alcohol, tobacco, and caffeine to pick you up or calm you down.

_____ 8. Overreact to everyday situations: very happy, very sad, very angry or irritable, grumpy, pessimistic.

_____ 9. Short attention span: easily distracted.

_____ 10. Superfocused: Difficulty detaching from task at hand.

_____ 11. Normal noise, sight, or sound causes feelings of intense anxiety or irritation.

_____ 12. Protective of own physical space but will invade others' space without forethought.

_____ 13. Experiences shame after unexplained explosive outbursts.

_____ 14. Fatigued: seen as a night person but often stays up until exhausted because of nightmares and disturbed sleep patterns.

_____ 15. Problems with organizing activities of daily living.

_____ 16. Uses charm and humor to manipulate.

_____ 17. More comfortable with monologue than with dialogue.

If you recognize several of these traits check with your school counselor for further information. The authors also recommend the book *You Mean I'm Not Lazy, Stupid or Crazy?!* (Kelly and Ramundo, 1993).

▽▽▽
Some Suggestions for the Student with Adult ADD

1. Identify your learning style from the categories presented in this chapter. Practice the suggestions offered.

2. Use relaxation exercises to quiet your mind and reduce anxiety.

3. Use background music (not TV) to shut off background noises.

4. Schedule study time for when you feel most alert and fresh.

5. Use color to help focus your attention. A col-

ored transparency over the page you are reading or a large colored poster board on the desk where you work help to draw your attention.

6. Use physical activity to enhance study: Play study tapes while walking, or ride a stationary bike while reviewing notes.

7. Invent your own comfortable ways of studying.

▼▼▼
Putting It Together

It is not unusual to read information but then say, "But of course this doesn't apply to me." This information does apply. You have had an opportunity to (1) identify your main learning style and (2) receive hints on how to enhance your learning style.

To become a self-directed learner:

1. Behave in a successful manner. Successes reinforce this attitude.

2. Set realistic goals and evaluate the results to see if these goals are being met. **It is an obstacle to learning to think that learning can take place without effort.**

3. A personal point of view affects learning. Do not let established styles harden into such fixed beliefs that new styles cannot be tolerated; at that point, education ends.

4. Tie in new learning to previous lessons and experiences. This gives the material meaning and makes it easier to remember.

5. Seek help when needed; sometimes being alone is best. Sometimes it is best to study with others. Beginning studies, problems with studies, or the need to be with someone are reasons for seeking out others.

6. Learn beyond the point necessary for doing or performing the skill. Keep reviewing and practicing the skills learned.

▼▼▼ S U M M A R Y

▶ Critical thinking is an advanced form of thinking. It is used to solve problems and to find ways to improve even when no problems exist. It is an essential part of nursing.

▶ People think in different representational systems; the way they think determines their major learning style. Some think in pictures (visual learners). Some hear sounds or talk to themselves (auditory learners). Some experience a feeling in regard to what they are thinking about and learn best by doing (tactual learners). Each learning style can be enhanced through specific techniques.

▶ There are secondary learning categories as well. Identifying whether you are a logical learner (organized, consistent), a musical learner (like to hum, sing, or play instruments), a linguistic learner (love words and new vocabulary), or a spatial learner (likes boxes and diagrams rather than words) further enhances your learning ability.

▶ The right and left sides of the brain have separate and distinct functions. Thinking and learning are affected by the more active or dominant side. Students in whom the left brain is more active tend to read and write well, solve problems logically, and enjoy learning details and facts. Those who have a dominant right brain are more creative, express their feelings freely, use an intuitive approach to problem solving, and prefer an overview of the subject. Learning to use the less active side enhances functioning of both sides of the brain.

▶ One's personal attitude toward learning also influences the learning process. Attitude is closely related to whether you are a reactive learner who expects to be taught or an active learner who takes charge of his own education.

▼▼▼ *R E F E R E N C E S*

Alfaro-LeFevre R. *Critical Thinking in Nursing: A Practical Approach.* Philadelphia: W.B. Saunders, 1995.

Barsch J. *Understanding Your Learning Style.* Ventura, CA: Ventura College Learning Disability Clinic.

Iyer P, Taptich B, Bernocchi-Losey D. *Nursing Process and Nursing Diagnosis,* 3rd ed. Philadelphia: W.B. Saunders, 1995.

Kelly K, Ramundo P. *You Mean I'm Not Lazy, Stupid or Crazy?!* New York: Scribner, 1993.

▼▼▼ *B I B L I O G R A P H Y*

Bandler R, Grinder J, Stevens J (eds). *Frogs into Princes.* Moab, UT: Real People Press, 1979.

Buzan T. *Use Both Sides of Your Brain,* 3rd ed. New York: New American Library, Dutton, 1991.

Griggs D, Griggs S, Dunn R, Ingham J. Accommodating nursing student's diverse learning styles. Nurse Educator 1994; 19(6).

Learning How to Learn

CHAPTER 7

▼▼▼ KEY TERMS

active listener
application
external distractions
idea sketches
internal distractions

knowledge
mapping
mental imagery
mnemonic devices
outlining

passive listener
study groups
tutoring
understanding
vocalization

▼▼▼ OBJECTIVES

Upon completion of this chapter you will be able to:

1. Identify techniques that increase your degree of concentration in learning situations.

2. Identify techniques that improve your listening skills in learning situations.

3. Describe techniques that enhance understanding of information needed to be a practical nurse.

4. Evaluate your personal need for help with reading skills to increase speed of reading and degree of comprehension.

Of all the reasons for not succeeding in school, lack of study skills is high on the list of causes. From our teaching experience, we have seen students fail owing to lack of study skills more often than lack of time to devote to school. In fact, when failure is attributed to "I don't have the time," it really is often due to lack of knowledge about how to study and to use time to advantage. Many vocational schools and junior colleges offer courses in how to study before the student enters a program and have departments that offer study skill services after a student is enrolled. Not everyone who needs these services is aware that they need them. Many learners think they will succeed because they have succeeded in high school or college courses. Learners cannot assume they have the study skills necessary to succeed in the practical nursing program because they have attended high school or college. Students who have developed study skills will be surprised at how much more effectively they can learn after reviewing their study habits.

Before going on, you must be aware of two things. First, you must get yourself organized into a study habit. Some people dislike the thought of being organized. Many times this feeling arises out of habit. The feeling can be overcome by keeping your educational goals in front of you and developing some organizational skills for studying. Second, you must realize that it is hard work to acquire the knowledge and skills needed for your chosen career. We cannot say it will be easy. Learning is hard work. It takes time and effort. Study skills are like any other skill. They are developed by practice and hard work.

▼▼▼
General Hints for Learners

▽▽▽
Concentration

Concentration is the ability to keep your mind completely on the task at hand. The major enemy of concentration is distraction. There are many distractions in a learner's life that compete with the need to buckle down to school assignments. These distractions can be summarized as two types: (1) those that come from outside yourself (external distractions) and (2) those that come from inside yourself (internal distractions).

External Distractions

External distractions occur in your physical and social environment.

Personal Study Area.   Your physical environment is a potential enemy of concentration. Locate one or two realistic areas for studying. The chosen areas should be associated with learning and not daydreaming or napping. The learning resource center at your school, if your school has this resource, can be used between classes and after school. Another area can be a place in your home or apartment. This could be the kitchen, a corner of your bedroom, or part of the basement. The place you choose should be away from family or roommates. The area should have a writing surface, a lamp, and a chair. Have a supply of pens, sharpened pencils, a highlighter felt marker, loose-leaf paper, scrap paper, index cards, a calendar, an English dictionary, thesaurus, and a medical or nursing dictionary at hand and add additional tools you have identified that help you learn. Keep these items organized and at hand. You will save time and aggravation by not having to look for your study tools each time you sit down to study. Choose a chair you feel comfortable in but not one that you associate with snoozing. Avoid studying in bed.

Lighting.   The light you choose for studying is almost more important than your chair. Many students have a table lamp. This is fine as long as the bulb is shaded and your writing surface is light colored to reflect light. It is important to eliminate glare. The shade and light surface will help in this matter. Try using a "soft white" light bulb to reduce glare further. Be sure that the bulb is screwed into its socket to ensure a tight connection to reduce flicker. If a ceiling light is also available, turn this on in addition to your table lamp to reduce shadows. Eyestrain can occur if lighting allows glare, shadows, or flicker to exist in your study area. If you have tried to eliminate these three unwanted lighting conditions and you still experience symptoms of eyestrain, such as headaches, dizziness, tiredness, or blurred vision while reading, it is time to have an eye examination to rule out the need for corrective lenses. Some students discover that they need glasses only after they enroll in an educational program demanding much reading, such as the practical nursing program.

Background Sounds.   Keep in mind that research studies on learning styles show that some students concentrate better with background sounds (music, voices). Other students require quiet surroundings. Honestly identify the type of environment that allows you to get the most out of your study time. Your grades will be the criteria by which you can judge whether your environment is helping or hurting. Strive for a study environment that meets your learning style preference (see Chapter 6). If you require a quiet environment, sometimes home does not provide this. Past students have told us they were successful in disciplining themselves to ignore noise and concentrate on studying. Television, stereos, radios, and CD players are considered background noise. Frequently, despite learning style preferences, students state that they study best in the presence of these external distractions. If these habits are a carryover from high school and are interfering with your concentration, establish new habits to help you with your more difficult subjects. High school and college study habits do not automatically guarantee success in the practical nursing program.

List any external distractions that are affecting your concentration. _____

_____

_____

_____

What can you do to eliminate these

distractions? _____

_____

_____

Your Peers.   Are the persons you associate with at school encouraging your progress in the practical nursing program? Do you support and encourage each other? Do you pick a special person to sit with in class so you can privately chat while others are talking? Do you seek out other students who have negative attitudes? If so, what are the conversations you engage in during a supposedly relaxing coffee break? Do the persons you associate with love to belittle, complain, and tear down the instructor, the course, and various students in your group? Does your anxiety level increase when you carpool with certain students on test days? The energy devoted to any of these activities can seriously deplete the energy needed to achieve success with less stress and frustration.

Answer the questions asked under Your Peers above.

_____

_____

_____

_____

_____

_____

Internal Distractions

You can have the perfect desk, lighting, chair, noise level, equipment, and peers for studying but still not be able to keep your mind on the task at hand. The culprit may be distractions arising from inside yourself. Here are some common examples of internal distractions and suggestions for overcoming them.

Complaints of Mental Fatigue.   Most students confuse boredom with fatigue. In setting up a study schedule, make sure you do not study one subject so long that you get bored with it (see Chapter 5). Keep up your physical self with proper food, sleep, and exercise. At the first sign of "getting tired," take a short break (not a snooze) and come back to new material so that you can get your mental second wind.

Daydreaming. Daydreaming can be a creative adventure or wasted time. Every time you find your mind wandering from the topic at hand, put a check mark on a piece of paper that you keep at your side. This will remind you that you are drifting off and need to get back to work. Students who use this technique find that the number of check marks decreases dramatically as the days go on.

List four topics that you daydream about when studying. _____

_____

_____

_____

_____

List internal and external distractions that encourage you to daydream. _____

_____

_____

_____

_____

List suggestions for reducing or eliminating these distractions. _____

_____

_____

_____

_____

Another Technique for Improving Concentration

The following technique has been used successfully by students to improve their concentration. Try it out to see if it can help you.

Simple tools such as a pencil or highlighter will keep you active in your learning. Underlining or highlighting *main* ideas, writing in the margins, and so on, will keep you active and your concentration at its peak. Remember the hints related to your personal learning style (see Chapter 6).

▽▽▽
Listening

The human voice takes up much of class time. Whether you are involved in a mini-lecture class or a discussion or activity, or are viewing videotapes as part of a course, you are going to miss a lot if your mind wanders. Listening is much more than the mechanical process of hearing. There are two kinds of listeners. Which type are you?

▶ The **passive** listener receives sounds with little recognition or personal involvement. This "listener" may be doodling, staring out the window, or even staring at the instructor but thinking about having to change the oil in the car or deciding what to cook for dinner.

▶ The **active** listener listens with full attention, is open-minded and curious. This listener is searching for relevant information and strives to understand it. Active listeners realize that listening is an important method of gathering information and work at developing this skill. The active listener looks for ways that the speaker's words can be put to practical use regardless of the student's level of interest or degree of fondness for the instructor or the instructor's dress or mannerisms.

▶ Are you an active or a passive listener? Hints for effective listening include:

1. Be well rested for class.
2. Have assignments, including extra readings, completed.
3. Ask questions before, during, and after class.
4. Listen for key information and central ideas, not specific facts.
5. Make eye contact with the speaker.
6. Listen when other students are speaking.
7. Seek help when a difficult concept is not understood.

▽▽▽
Notemaking

An important part of listening is remembering what you have listened to. Some students say that taking notes interferes with their listening skills. They are correct if they are in the business of *taking notes. Research has shown that a student remembers only 50% of a 10-minute lecture when tested immediately afterward and only 25% of that lecture when tested two days later.* The secret to improving those percentages to as much as 80% to 90% is to engage in **notemaking** whenever you are listening. Because teachers derive test questions from mini-lectures, discussions, activities, videotapes, and readings, that 80% to 90% could translate into a comparable test score. Notemaking will help you to pay attention, concentrate, and organize your ideas.

Hints for Notemaking

Never try to capture every word the speaker says. This is **notetaking** and is impossible. A speaker can put out about 100 to 125 words per minute or more. Time yourself to find how many words you can write per minute. Have a peer time one minute and another peer read for the same time while you try to write everything down. The number will shock you. Besides not being able to get every word down, you will also not be able to capture the meaning of what was said. Instead, strive for **notemaking**, forming condensations of what is said in a telegramlike manner. Actively listen for the main ideas. Capture them in a way that reflects your personal learning style or styles. You are recording ideas or key concepts that you will later add to, correct, and study.

Have One 8 $\frac{1}{2}$- × 11-inch Loose-leaf Notebook with Dividers for Each Class.
Spiral notebooks have the disadvantage of not allowing handouts to be easily included with daily notes. With the loose-leaf system, the notebook can be left at home and a supply of paper taken to school daily. Make sure your name, address, and telephone number are in the notebook in case you misplace it.

Do Not Take Notes in Shorthand.
Shorthand notes have to be transcribed after class, another poor time-management technique. Develop your own personal symbols, abbreviations, and shorthand of sorts to help you capture the main ideas yet retain readability without having to transcribe the notes. Use your medical abbreviations as presented in your charting classes. Make your notes in pen so that they don't smudge. When a mistake is made, cross out the error, but do so neatly. Erasing is time consuming. Avoid typing or rewriting your class notes word-for-word. Instead, use this time to think about what is important in the notes and condense them as you rewrite. This is especially helpful for visual learners. At first your notes may seem to be a disaster, but remember that you are not competing for a penmanship award. With practice, they will improve. Your goal is a set of notes you can use today, next week, and at the end of the program for review for the NCLEX-PN.

Two Methods for Making and Reviewing Notes

Outlining Method. The first method is the *outlining method,* which has been used for ages. It involves adapting normal loose-leaf paper so that you have room to take notes and summarize content, and can test yourself on your notes. This method can be used to prepare you continually for testing of the material. This method is useful for taking notes when reading textbooks. Figure 7–1 is an example of traditional **notemaking,** used to summarize this chapter so far. Use the margin at the top of the page to write the date and course number and any assignments that are given. Extend the left margin another inch. Take your notes in your personal learning style to the right of this line. After class, in the area at the left of the page, record key words or phrases that serve as cues for the lecture notes on the right. Also, use this area as a space for questions or comments. These will be useful in testing yourself. The bottom inch of each page should be left blank. A summary of the content of the notes on that page can be made in this section. This summary forces you to think about and come to grips with the ideas in your notes. Some students think that writing material in note form alone will help them retain the material. Active and

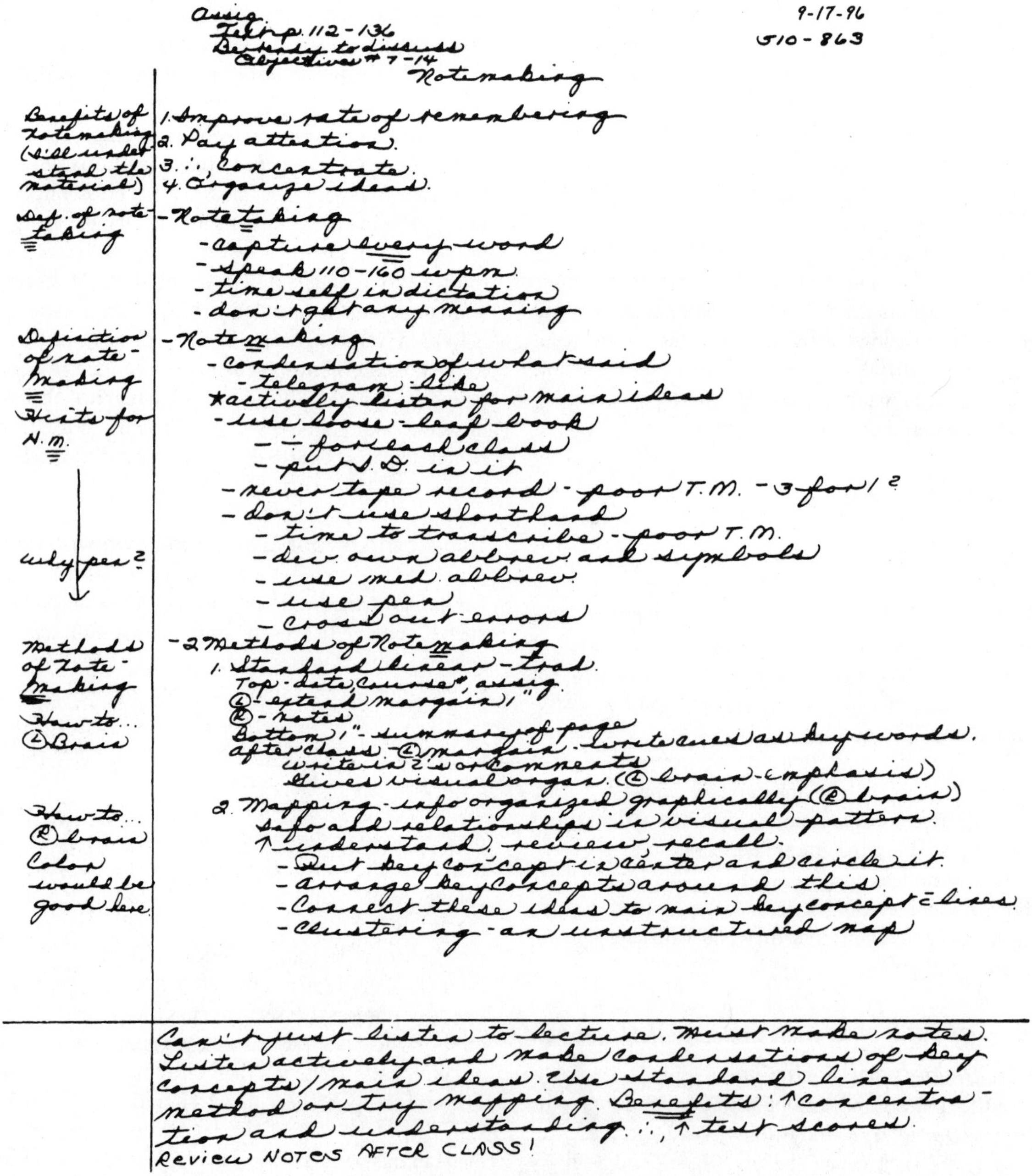

Assig
Jextrp. 112-136
Be ready to discuss
Objectives # 7-14

9-17-96
510-863

Notemaking

Benefits of notemaking (will understand the material)
1. Improve rate of remembering
2. Pay attention.
3. ∴, concentrate.
4. Organize ideas.

Def. of note taking
—Notetaking
  —capture every word
  —speak 110-160 wpm
  —time self in dictation
  —don't get any meaning

Definition of note-making ≡ Hints for N.M.
—Notemaking
  —condensation of what said
    —telegram: like
  *actively listen for main ideas
  —use loose-leaf book
    —∴ for each class
    —put I.D. in it
  —never tape record - poor T.M. -3 for 1?
  —don't use shorthand
    —time to transcribe - poor T.M.
  —dev. own abbrev. and symbols
  —use med. abbrev.
  —use pen
  —cross out errors

why pen?

Methods of note-making
—2 Methods of Notemaking
  1. Standard linear - Trad.
  Top - date, course #, assig.
    (a) extend margain 1"
    (b) - notes
  Bottom 1" - summary of page
  after class (a) margain: write cues as key words.
    criteria? or comments
    gives visual organ. (b) brain-emphasis)

How to... (1) Brain

How to... (2) brain
Color would be good here

  2. Mapping- info organized graphically. (②brain)
  info and relationships in visual pattern.
  ↑ understand, review, recall.
    —Put key concept in center and circle it.
    —arrange key concepts around this.
    —Connect these ideas to main key concept ⊂ lines.
    —clustering - an unstructured map

Can't just listen to lecture. Must make notes.
Listen actively and make condensations of key
concepts/main ideas. Use standard linear
method or try mapping. Benefits: ↑concentra-
tion and understanding ∴, ↑ test scores.
REVIEW NOTES AFTER CLASS!

Figure 7–1

Traditional notemaking.

frequent review of your notes is an important step in retention of material.

Mapping. An alternative to the linear method of notemaking has been suggested by brain researchers. It encourages using the right side of the brain with its emphasis on images. Information presented in a linear manner, as in traditional notemaking, is not as easily understood as information presented by key concepts. The use of key concepts is the primary way in which the brain processes information. The brain takes these key concepts and integrates them in relationships. So, if the brain does not work in lines or lists, the method of notemaking called **mapping** can enhance your ability to understand, review, and recall this information. Mapping is a method in which information is organized graphically so that it is seen in a visual pattern of relationships. Figure 7–2 summarizes the information presented in this chapter so far in an unstructured mapping form called clustering.

▼▼▼
Remembering and Forgetting

We all can recall things from the past, indicating that our brains have the ability to store information. But how many times have you said "I forgot," or "I can't remember"? Possible causes of forgetting include:

1. A *negative attitude* toward the subject, which interferes with the motivation to remember.
2. *New knowledge,* which interferes with the recall of old learning.
3. *Old knowledge,* which interferes with the recall of new learning.

Valid as these causes of forgetting may be, perhaps the most common reason why students cannot remember is that *they never grasped the information in the first place.* They really did not internalize the information and understand it to begin with. Perhaps they did not listen actively, or they just read words and created a mental blur. To store information in your long-term memory, a neural trace or a record of the information must be laid down. Psychologists have found that it takes four to five seconds for information to move from the temporary, or short-term, memory to the permanent, or long-term, memory. To form a long-term memory of information, you must strive to understand that information. In doing so, you will give your brain the chance to lay down a neural trace. Presto! You have created a memory of that information. Short but frequent study periods will help you to understand information and store it in your long-term memory.

▼▼▼
How to Understand (Comprehend) Information

You will be exposed to much new knowledge during your year in the practical nursing program. You will gain knowledge as stated in the course objectives. Your real test as a practical nurse will be your ability to understand that information and use it as the basis for critical thinking in the clinical area. The national licensing examination for practical nurses tests at the level of knowledge, understanding, and application. The following definitions will help you comprehend the meaning of the words knowledge (knowing), understanding, and application.

1. *Knowing* means the ability to repeat information you have memorized. This is the lowest level of learning. Defining a concept *as stated in a dictionary* is an example of knowledge.
2. *Understanding* (comprehension) means to grasp the meaning of the material. This is the lowest level of understanding. Repeating information *in your own words* indicates that you understand the concept.
3. *Application* means being able to use learned material in new situations. For example, you apply what is learned in class to your clinical work. Application is a higher level of understanding, which helps you retain what you are learning.

Understanding and application are what employers expect of a practical nurse on the job. Your instructors will also expect this level of competence in the clinical area as you continue to practice your critical thinking skills. Past students with college degrees have told us that the consistent need to apply both prior and newly learned information is the area

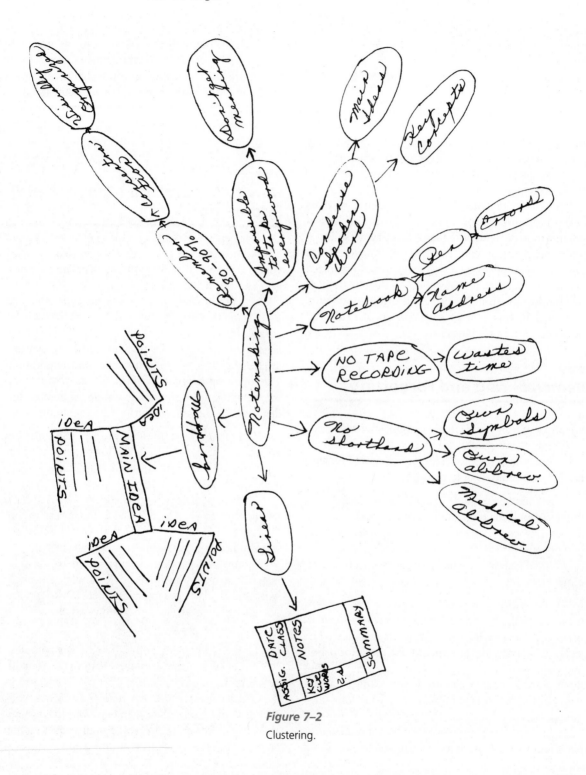

Figure 7–2
Clustering.

about practical nursing that differs most from their college experience.

▽▽▽
Visual Strategies to Enhance Understanding

Your scholastic world is bombarded with words, sentences, and paragraphs. One of the most beneficial techniques used to understand and remember all the new information is to balance this verbal mixture with visual strategies. Each of the following visual strategies will help you to understand and ultimately remember information better. They deal with the right side of the brain. You will be tapping a resource that perhaps you have not used before. If you have right brain dominance, your understanding will be improved by adopting left brain strategies of organizing information, as discussed in Chapter 6. These strategies include improving the general organization of material and writing and restating new information in your own words.

Draw Idea Sketches

These drawings will probably be comprehensible only to you. The emphasis is not on the quality of the drawing but on the process you must go through to take a verbal concept and represent it graphically, without words. To go through this process you must understand the verbal concept. You can even set it up as a cartoon. Use stick figures and describe the concept verbally. Figure 7–3 is an idea sketch illustrating the function of

the drug Lanoxin (digoxin), which is used to slow and strengthen the heartbeat.

> Choose a concept you are having trouble with in one of your classes. Draw an idea sketch to help you increase your understanding of that concept.

Use Color in Whatever Form of Notemaking You Use

Use highlighters, crayons, colored pencils, or felt-tip pens. Avoid merely underlining the page. Use the different colors to help capture and direct your attention to information that fits in different categories. The different colors will help your brain organize and retrieve information.

Make Your Own Diagrams as You Read

If you commit ideas to memory only by using words, you are using only half of your brain's resources, those of the left side. If you also produce a sketch of that idea, you will have brought the right side of your brain into use. The use of both sides of the brain is a powerful tool that encourages the storage and retrieval of information.

Engage in Mental Imagery

This technique will really help you to remember because it demands that you understand the information.

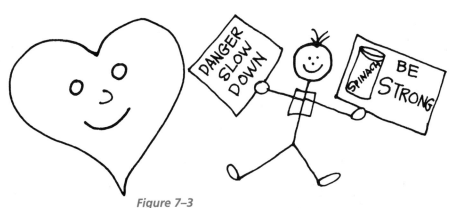

Figure 7–3
Idea sketch. Action of Lanoxin (digoxin).

When you use mental imagery, you become the idea that you are having difficulty understanding. The right side of your brain generates pictures of the idea, and the left side supplies the script to explain what is going on in the pictures (and always in your own words).

The following is an example of a mental image developed by a practical nursing student to give herself a simple understanding of the function of insulin, a hypoglycemic agent that increases glucose transport across muscle and fat-cell membranes. Notice how she used the senses of hearing and feeling and also body movement to help achieve understanding. She also uses a metaphor, equating something she knows about with something she is trying to learn. The student recites this image to herself while she closes her eyes and visualizes it. At first, she had her roommate read the story while she visualized the scenario.

I Am Insulin—A Job Description.   I am insulin and I am shaped like a canoe. In fact, I am a canoe, a green one. My job is to make the sugar or glucose in the blood available to most of the cells of the body for energy. I like my job. I like things that are sweet but not too sweet, so blood sugar is just my thing. Sometime after the person who owns the pancreas where I am stored in my canoe rack eats a meal, a whistle blows, and I know this is a signal for me to launch myself into the bloodstream. As I ride the currents of the blood, I rock gently back and forth and the sugar in the bloodstream jumps right in to be passengers. Blood sugar likes me. I think this is because I am green, but I might be wrong. When I am pretty full, but not full enough to swamp, I pass through the blood vessels, paddle through the sea of tissue fluid (boy, it smells salty) around the cells, pass through the cell membrane, and deposit the sugar by making these molecules jump out of the canoe and into the fluid inside the cell. I feel pretty important in my job. Without me, the blood sugar molecules would be unable to pass through the cell membranes. Because of this, I am given the official job title of hypoglycemic agent, because I lower the level of sugar in the blood. Excuse me, there goes the whistle.

Perhaps a physiologist would wince at this description. But it is nothing to be ashamed of if it helps you understand a concept. Plus, mental imagery can be fun!

▽▽▽
Other Methods of Increasing Understanding

Form a Neural Trace.   Positive mental attitude is a factor in allowing you to understand and remember. Remind yourself that all the basic courses in which you are now enrolled are essential. They are the building blocks for all the remaining courses you will take in the practical nursing program. You have already started your career. Most of the following techniques help increase understanding of your work by allowing neural traces to be recorded in your brain.

1. **As you listen or read, seek out key concepts, basic principles, and key ideas.** Be selective and learn to sift out and reject unnecessary details. You cannot memorize everything. If you could, you would not have an understanding of anything. The student who memorizes has difficulty in applying course information and solving problems in the clinical area. The activity of being selective helps you lay down neural traces. Emphasize accuracy, not speed. You want correct information to make a clear neural trace. It is difficult to unlearn wrong information and replace it with correct information.

2. **Short study periods followed by short rest periods are better than long study marathons.** This type of study will reenergize you and allow neural learning to continue during rest periods. Those seemingly wasted 10 minutes between classes or standing in the cafeteria line can be used to your advantage.

3. **Use as many body senses and as much body movement as possible when trying to learn new information.** Recite the information aloud as you read, using your own words. If you can explain it, you must understand it and will know it. Hearing yourself say the information aloud is an additional channel that allows neural traces to be recorded. Write down the information in your own words. *Do not copy word-by-word from a book.* This muscle action will help you clarify ideas and improve thinking. Vary your body position while studying. Lean against a wall. Sit on the floor. Pace. You will keep alert and awake. Using your muscles by gesturing can help to improve memory of information by matching a gesture to information that needs to be remem-

bered. When the gesture and word are associated in your mind, the word can be retrieved by performing the gesture. Physical motion can jog memory and promote recall. You should see some of the motions students go through during an exam. If it works, don't knock it. These techniques of using body senses and body movement are all elements of tactual learning. They all help lay down the neural trace. Try them . . . they may work for you. Adopt the suggestions that help you understand the material in your classes. They will increase your long-term memory of that information.

▽▽▽
Study Groups

Do you have a desire to achieve better grades? Do you need to study more efficiently? Do you need a little support? Joining a study group could be the strategy for you. Students usually form their own study groups out of need. Studies have shown that despite each person's preferred learning style, actively participating in a study group can improve academic performance. Notice we said *actively* participate. Sometimes students join a study group thinking that the group will help them pass, and they avoid active participation. Kind of like a freeloader. Study groups work when students use them to become actively involved in their own learning. The group provides an outlet for oral rehearsal of material, which promotes retention. Active study group members usually develop questioning and reasoning skills on a higher level.

▽▽▽
Tutoring

Tutoring is a very select study group. For best results, tutoring is arranged through a special department through instructor referral or self-referral by the student. The purpose of tutoring is to help a student understand the material better and pass the course. We guarantee one thing in tutoring. The person doing the tutoring will probably get an A. Students who need tutoring *sometimes* have learning disabilities. In these situations, because of an excellent attitude on the part of these students and their active participation in the tutoring process, tutoring can be beneficial. Students

without learning disabilities who actively participate in the tutoring process also are successful in passing courses.

We are concerned about students at risk for failure who expect the tutor "to learn for them." These students do not actively participate in the tutoring process. We have also seen some privately arranged tutoring situations fail because the tutor felt that the student at risk needed to "be saved." *Please note: Students cannot be saved. Nothing can replace active participation on the part of the learner. If you want to pass a course, you must become actively involved in your own learning.* There are also students who need tutoring but say they do not have time for it. Comment on this response.

▼▼▼
Memory Aids

Mnemonic devices are examples of memory aids. You know what they are. Some examples:

▶ Rhymes
  Thirty days hath September . . .
  I before *e* except after *c* . . .
  In fourteen hundred and ninety-two . . .
▶ Acronyms
  Every good boy does fine . . . (to remember the line notes of the treble clef.)

There are also devices in nursing that can help you remember information. For example,

▶ CMTSP (for assessment of the nerve and blood supply to an extremity)
  C = color
  M = motion
  T = temperature
  S = sensation
  P = pulse
▶ PERL (for assessment of the pupils)
  P = pupils
  E = equal
      and
  R = react
  L = to light

Memorizing these acronyms can help the practical nurse remember series of information. They do not take the place of understanding the information.

▼▼▼ Reading

To think critically, you must have information. To acquire information you must be able to read with understanding. Because you are responsible for large amounts of reading in a practical nursing program, the ability to read with understanding (comprehension) is a necessary skill. Most of us are able to read the printed words on a page. But the reading demanded of a learner and future employee involves much more than this. Reading to learn and understand involves a rate of speed and a degree of understanding that are effective. You probably had to take a reading test as part of your pre-entrance tests for the practical nursing program. Generally, these tests are brief. If you scored low, you were referred for help with this skill. Perhaps you are one of those who achieved an acceptable score on these short reading tests but could use some hints on how to increase your reading efficiency. Evaluate your reading habits by answering yes or no to the following questions.

1. Do you ever reread a sentence before you come to its end?
2. Do you ever have trouble figuring out the main point of an author?
3. Do you stop your reading every time you come across a word you cannot define and look up the word immediately?
4. Do you read novels, popular magazines, newspapers, and textbooks at the same speed?
5. Do you ever have trouble remembering what you read?
6. Do you ever have trouble understanding what you have read?
7. Do you ever think of other things while you read?
8. Do you ever read every word of a sentence individually?

If you answered yes to any of the above questions, you could benefit from some help with your reading efficiency. We suggest a visit to your school's study skill center for assistance with reading your textbooks with more organization and efficiency.

▽▽▽ Hints to Increase Reading Efficiency

1. **Read in phrases, a few words at a time, rather than word by word.** Although the brain can only view one word at a time, it only understands when words are in phrases. For better understanding, you should read as you speak, in phrases.
2. **Move your lips while reading.** Vocalization, whether out loud or to yourself, is a tool used by the auditory learner to increase understanding. For some students, reading aloud word by word can decrease speed and comprehension.
3. **Put expression into your reading.** You do not speak in a monotone, so why read that way? Musical learners can benefit by singing what they are reading. Try it. It may work for you.
4. **Be aware of your reading assignments that are technical or scientific in nature and vary your reading speed accordingly.** The more recreational your reading material (novel, newspaper, and so on), the faster you can read. For more technical or scientific material, you must slow down. As you become accustomed to this type of reading, you will find yourself increasing your speed.
5. **Underline unfamiliar words as you read.** When you are finished reading, copy the words on an index card and look them up in an appropriate dictionary. Most of the unfamiliar words you come across will be medical terms and can be found in your medical dictionary. At first you will think these words are Greek, and you are right. Quite a few of them are derived from the Greek language. The rest are derived from Latin. Write the definition on the other side of the card. Break the word down with vertical slashes into its prefix (the word beginning), root (core word), and suffix (word ending), so that you can begin making associations with other words with the same prefix, root, or suffix. If your medical dictionary does not include this information

with each word, the information can be found in medical terminology texts in your learning resource center.

Nursing involves learning a whole new language. If possible, include your own drawing to represent the definitions of these words with the verbal definition. This can help you recall the meaning of the word. Using index cards allows your language development to progress because you can take the cards with you wherever you go. Learning can occur whenever you have a few minutes to spare.

6. **Underline key phrases and write in the margin.** We assume you own your textbooks. Underlining will keep you active and result in the identification of key concepts for study and review.

▼▼▼ S U M M A R Y

▶ Learning how to learn is important because the theory and skills needed by the practical nurse can be understood and stored in the long-term memory and used as the basis for critical thinking. When theory and skills are stored in long-term memory, they can be retrieved or recalled when needed. There is no easy way to learn information. There are some techniques that have been proven effective in increasing your level of concentration, improving your listening skills, and enhancing your ability to understand information. Perhaps your most important skills for success in the practical nursing program are your reading skills.

▼▼▼ B I B L I O G R A P H Y

Alfaro-LeFevre R. *Critical-Thinking in Nursing: A Practical Approach.* Philadelphia: W.B. Saunders, 1995.

Buzan T. *Speed Reading.* New York: New American Library-Dutton, 1991.

Buzan T. *Use Both Sides of Your Brain.* New York: New American Library-Dutton, 1991.

Griggs D, et al. Accommodating nursing students' diverse learning styles. Nurse Educator 1994; 19(6):41–45.

Hancock O. *Reading Skills for College Students.* Englewood Cliffs, NJ: Prentice Hall, 1995.

Kay G. How to help students develop better notetaking skills. Teaching for Success 1995; 7(3):8.

Meltzer M, Palau S. *Reading and Study Strategies for Nursing Students.* Philadelphia: W.B. Saunders, 1993.

Pauk W. *How to Study in College,* 5th ed. Boston: Houghton-Mifflin, 1993.

Williams LV. *Teaching for the Two-Sided Mind: A Guide to Right Brain/Left Brain Education.* New York: Touchstone, 1986.

Hints for Using Learning Resources

▼▼▼ *O U T L I N E*

▼▼▼ *K E Y   T E R M S*

audiovisual materials
bucket theory
call numbers
CD-ROM
community resources
compare and contrast

computer-aided instruction
computer simulation
cooperative learning
copyright laws
course outline
discussion buddy

guest speakers
interlibrary loan service
learning resource center
lecture-discussion
librarian
microfiche

microfilm

nursing organizations

nursing skills lab

online catalog

periodical indexes

periodicals

PQRST

reference materials

stacks

study skills lab

syllabus

▼▼▼   *O B J E C T I V E S*

Upon completing this chapter you will be able to:

1. *Describe each step in the PQRST method of textbook study.*

2. *Discuss the value of reading assigned periodicals.*

3. *Locate an article related to nursing by using:*
   a. *Cumulative Index to Nursing and Allied Health Literature*
   b. *one CD-ROM database (if available)*

4. *Discuss six hints used to gain full value from lectures.*

5. *Discuss your responsibilities for each of the following classroom learning strategies:*
   a. *mini-lecture—discussion, activities*
   b. *cooperative learning*

6. *Discuss the value of these learning resources to your personal learning:*
   a. *syllabus or course outline*
   b. *nursing skills lab*
   c. *study skills lab*

   d. *audiovisual materials*
   e. *computer-assisted instruction (CAI) and computer simulations*
   f. *learning resource center (LRC)*

7. *Describe how the following resources help you stay current in practical nursing:*
   a. *periodical indexes*
   b. *CD-ROMs*
   c. *nursing organizations*
   d. *community resources*
   e. *guest speakers*

There are three basic methods of obtaining theoretical information to prepare yourself to become a practical nurse: textbooks, professional journals, and classroom learning strategies. The purpose of this chapter is to provide suggestions to help you get full mileage out of these methods. In addition, other learning resources used by schools of practical nursing are discussed. How to stay up-to-date is also included. Even if you have past experience in an educational program of study, you will find the information in this chapter helpful. The information will help you adjust to and succeed in the practical nursing program with less stress and frustration.

▼▼▼
Textbooks

"I read the material four times and got a D. My friend read the material once and got an A. It isn't fair." The learner speaking is correct. It takes a lot of time to read material four times for a test. The missing ingredient is critical thinking. To think critically in nursing, you must have information. To acquire information, you

must be able to read with understanding. Earning only a D is a poor return on your time investment. The experts in study skills have come up with a variety of study systems for using textbooks and related reading materials. These systems are basically the same in that they present a method of reading that will increase comprehension by ensuring that the information is stored in long-term memory. We have chosen the PQRST method as described by Staton in *How to Study,* which was first published in 1959 and is still available today. It is the method we used in nursing school, but do not ask which edition we used. Believe us, this method has stood the test of time.

▽▽▽
The PQRST Method of Textbook Study

Each letter stands for a step in the study method. *Regardless of the length of time available for studying, studies have shown that learners who use each step of this method consistently scored higher on tests.* But each of the five steps in the method must be used. Learners have reported that the system is easier to use than they thought it would be. Each of the five steps will be discussed by identifying the meaning and benefits of each step and then describing how to carry it out and why it works.

P = Preview

What It Means.   Preview is an overview or survey of what the material is all about. It gives you the general big picture of what the author wants to accomplish, not the fine details.

Benefits.   Previewing helps you look for and recognize important points or main ideas of the reading material.

Why It Works.   The Preview step makes you reflect or think about the material. It also increases your concentration level. These are important elements in the storage of information in long-term memory.

How To Do It

1. When you first buy your textbooks, look at the table of contents. This will give you a general sense of the organization of the book.

2. Read the Preface to find out the author's purpose for writing the book, the organization of the material, and suggestions for reading the book.

3. Preview the method of the author of each of your textbooks. Before reading each assignment,

▶ Read each of the topics and headings.
▶ Read the summary.
▶ Read the first and last sentences of each paragraph.
▶ Using the general hints listed for reading, read the assignment.

Q = Question

What It Means.   As you preview the reading material, ask yourself **questions** that may be answered when you read.

Benefits.   Formulating your own questions as well as using the author's questions will give you pointers about what details to look for in your reading. These questions will help you prepare for exams.

Why It Works.   By providing you with clues, this step points out what to look for in your reading. The Question step will also make you reflect on your reading and increase your concentration level.

How To Do It.   Look at the chapter title and each heading. Turn them into questions. Some authors include questions at the end of a chapter. If so, read these before going on to the next step. Most authors include learning objectives at the beginning of each chapter. Use these to keep your mind inquisitive and to seek ends to these objectives.

R = Read

What It Means.   In this stage you actually **read** the material. You are now gathering information to be stored. Look carefully at pictures and charts. They may contain new information or clarify what you have read.

Benefits.   You will accumulate information and facts and be able to store them in long-term memory.

Why It Works.   Being an active reader by seeking answers to the questions you have formulated will keep up your level of concentration and allow you to store information in your brain.

How To Do It.   Review the general hints under Reading in Chapter 7 and practice them so you can remain active during this step. You are seeking the answers to the questions you formulated. Remember to underline key phrases and to write notes in the margin.

S = State

What It Means.   To state means to repeat in your own words what you have read.

Benefits.   You will understand the organization of the material you are reading and the relationship of the facts to each other. By increasing understanding, you will be able to apply the information in the clinical area. *Rote memory fails when it comes time to apply information.* Stating will help you evaluate whether you did indeed store the information.

Why It Works.   Stating something out loud involves another sense (hearing) and provides an additional channel for information to be stored. Stating facts in your own words indicates knowledge and understanding of the material.

How To Do It.   At the end of each paragraph, look away from your book. Ask yourself the main ideas that were covered in the paragraph. State the ideas out loud and in your own words. This is the key to the success of this step. As you become more proficient in this step, you will find that you are able to read more than one paragraph and still state the main ideas and the answers to the questions you have formulated. Look at your marginal notes. Try to elaborate on them.

T = Test

What It Means.   This final step occurs some time after your first study session and involves **testing** yourself on what you remember.

Benefits.   Because the testing step is ongoing, it will indicate your weak areas and give you time to remedy them before an exam. Better grades are sure to follow.

Why It Works.   This stage settles once and for all whether the information is in your long-term memory. It also indicates your comprehension of the material. When you identify your weak spots, you can review them and make sure they are retained in your long-term memory. You will be covering the information in small doses but more frequently. This activity is the best way to encourage the brain to remember.

How To Do It.   This testing stage is really a review stage. Review your marginal notes. Restate the main ideas presented in the chapter. Review your class notes. Relate them to the information in the textbook. Write down the information you are having trouble with on index cards to be carried with you so you can test yourself while on the run.

To be effective, your authors suggest that about half of your study time be devoted to the Preview and Read steps. The other half should be devoted to Question, State, and Test. These steps require critical thinking (reflective thinking), use of your memory, and organi-

zation of ideas through your own efforts. The strength of this system lies in the State step. The reflective thinking required in this step takes work. Resist the temptation to skip over State.

An important part of any textbook is the index found in the back of the book. The subject index includes a list of topics that can be found in alphabetical order. Page numbers are included for information discussed. This index will help you locate information quickly.

▼▼▼
Professional Journals

Practical nurses need to be aware of sources that will provide up-to-date information on nursing topics. Professional journal articles give you the opportunity to stay on top of the latest research in nursing and its application. In addition to articles that are assigned reading, practical nurses need to find and use articles that pertain to selected nursing topics and nursing problems in the clinical area. Student practical nurses need to be self-directed in looking up articles that apply to their current learning needs. Professional journals of interest to practical nurses include but are not limited to the following:

1. The Journal of Practical Nursing
2. RN
3. Nursing 97 (the year in the title changes each year)
4. The American Journal of Nursing

Identify these nursing journals in the learning resource center. Determine which of them help you to keep up-to-date in nursing.

▽▽▽
Articles

Learners are all looking for the perfect textbook, the one that is complete and self-contained. But it does not exist! Specific articles may be assigned to give you up-to-date information to supplement the readings in your textbooks. Use the PQRST method and hints for reading textbooks to read these articles. Copyright laws prohibit the instructor from copying an article for each of you. For this reason, the required reading articles are available on a reserve basis in the learning resource center. You can make notes from these articles. Because copyright laws allow you to have one copy of an article, photocopy the article for your own use. Underline, highlight, and write in its margins. Remember, the instructor knows you are busy. Articles are not busy work but are a necessary part of any career education to keep current in your discipline.

▼▼▼
Magazines and Newspapers

Include newspapers and popular magazines as sources of information on health-related topics. Magazine articles never replace professional journal reading, but they do provide information that your clients read. As one practical nursing student said, "I better be up-to-date and understand what my clients are reading." Be aware of the author's expertise. This will help you to evaluate the accuracy of the information on the topic.

> **List two newspapers or popular magazines that you read.**
>
> _____
>
> _____

▼▼▼
Classroom Learning Strategies

▽▽▽
Lectures

Some of your teachers may have been taught using the "bucket theory" of education. The bucket theory suggests that merely by lecturing, a teacher can transfer knowledge from the teacher's mind to the mind of the student. This teaching method evolved from the time of Aristotle. The teacher was considered the source and the vehicle of transmission of information. Of course, the printing press had yet to be invented! Although traditional lecturing is an outmoded form of instruction, **brief lectures** (mini-lectures) can be valuable as a

means of enhancing your assigned readings. However, they are passive learning experiences that do not actively involve you in the learning process. Research has shown that "most students learn best from methods other than lecture" (Jerit and Taylor, 1991). A mini-lecture situation should be a brief episode, taking no more than 30% of class time. Mini-lectures should enhance your reading assignment, not replace it. A mini-lecture should reflect the fact that the teacher spent time searching, reading, selecting, and organizing information for your benefit. The instructor has done all the work and has become smarter in the process. You need to remain especially alert and actively involved during the mini-lecture to be able to benefit from this method of teaching.

The instructor may introduce various techniques to keep you actively involved during the mini-lecture.

1. You will be assigned to a **discussion buddy** before the class starts.
2. The two of you will be given a discussion task.
3. Focus carefully on the mini-lecture so you will be able to formulate an answer to the discussion task.
4. After the mini-lecture, discussion buddies share their answers with each other. A new answer is formulated from both of your responses. The instructor will choose students at random to share their newly composed answers with the class.

What goes on in the classroom is just as important as what goes on in a reading assignment. There is, however, one great difference between the two. *You can repeat a reading assignment but you can never repeat a missed class.* Here are some hints to help you learn from a mini-lecture or any class situation.

1. *Never skip a class unless you are faced with an emergency.* Some students skip class to get another hour's sleep, use the time to prepare for another class or an exam, or get in their legal number of cuts. When an emergency does make it necessary for you to miss class, photocopying notes is not the answer to catch up on what you missed. Ask a peer to go over his notes and tell you about the class. Recall what you learned in Chapter 6 about your personal learning styles.

2. *Come to class prepared.* By having the assignment completed, key terms and concepts will be familiar to

you. You will be ready to participate in learning activities. You will save yourself embarrassment by avoiding questions that are answered easily by the readings. Come to class in time to get a seat close to the instructor and the blackboard. Heading for the last row is heading for distractions and lower grades. Have a pen and papers pertaining to the assignment ready to go.

3. *Listen for verbal cues that will inform you of key points during mini-lectures.* Some examples can be found in Table 8–1. Keep vigilant for nonverbal cues given by the instructor that will also inform you of key ideas. Examples are raising the hands, a long dramatic pause, raising or lowering the voice, and leaning toward the class. Be sure to copy everything that is written on the blackboard.

4. *The instructor speaks at a much slower rate than you are capable of thinking.* The fact that you can think faster than the instructor can speak allows you to relate this new information to information you have learned in the past and formulate questions when you do not understand. Ask these questions in class or seek out the instructor after class. It is your responsibility to question what you do not understand.

5. *Look over your notes as soon after class as possible.* Use the hints given in Chapter 6 about your personal learning styles. It is essential that you follow these techniques to place the information you learned in class into your long-term memory.

6. *Be present while in class.* Avoid using class time to work on other projects.

Table 8–1
Verbal Cues for Key Ideas in Mini-Lectures and Discussion Activities

"The most important difference is. . . ."
"The major principle in this situation is. . . ."
"To sum up. . . ."
"The main point is. . . ."
"Finally. . . ."
"In conclusion. . . ."
"Moreover. . . ."
"To repeat. . . ."

▽▽▽ Lecture-Discussions

In the **lecture-discussion** strategy, the instructor shares several ideas with the class and then stops so that the class can discuss the ideas. Sometimes the instructor may say that the next class will be nothing but discussion of the assignment. The instructor then acts as a discussion leader. The instructor has developed several learning strategies to help keep your discussion focused on course objectives. Here are some hints for participating in discussions and related activities.

1. Be prepared to participate in the discussion by completing your assignment. This will allow you to be an active participant.

2. Be sure to have made a list of questions about the assignment. Discussions are the perfect time to clear up questions.

3. While other learners are speaking, listen to what they have to say. Some learners make the mistake of using other learners' speaking time to formulate their own comments.

4. You may disagree with others during a discussion. Do so assertively and firmly. Avoid yelling matches at all costs. It enriches your world to listen to another's point of view before responding.

▼▼▼ Cooperative Learning

Cooperative learning is a technique that emphasizes individual accountability for learning a specific academic task while working in small groups. Cooperative learning encourages you to: (1) be actively involved in your learning, (2) develop critical thinking skills, and (3) develop positive relationships with your peers. Besides helping you learn the course content, cooperative learning will help you encourage traits you will need in your future job. Cooperative learning encourages the development of teamwork. The ability to work in a team situation is what an employer is looking for in an employee. Use the suggestions listed under Lecture-Discussions to help you get full mileage out of this learning strategy.

▼▼▼
Other Learning Resources

▽▽▽
Syllabus and Course Outlines

A **syllabus** is an up-to-date course document given to you at the beginning of a course. It includes, at a minimum, a course description, course objectives, course requirements for a passing grade, required textbooks, grading scale, instructor information (office location, office phone number, office hours), course policies, and testing policies.

Some schools of practical nursing also use **course outlines** for each course. These outlines are a great help to an adult learner. They contain unit-by-unit course objectives and content areas, which indicate what the learner must know. Each objective begins with a verb. Watch the verb carefully. The verb tells you the level of understanding you must achieve to meet the objective. If an objective states you must *list* something, that task is quite different from having to **compare and contrast** the same information. Instructors develop their test questions from the course objectives and course content. The course outline will include a list of resources indicating where the information to answer the objectives is found. Supplementary material in the form of worksheets, charts, activities, and additional reading may be included to round out your learning.

▽▽▽
Nursing Skills Lab

The nursing skills lab is a resource that will allow you to practice and develop your physical bedside skills. It is to be used throughout your program of study. This lab contains the physical items needed to make the practice area as similar to the workplace as possible. *Skills must be practiced.* Reading about them, watching a film, and watching other students practice are only the first steps in developing a physical skill. *Practice until you are proficient in each skill, so that you will feel comfortable performing these tasks in the clinical area.* Remember that you recall 10% of what you hear, 20% of what you see,

50% of what you read, and 90% of what you do, so *do* all you can.

You will be required to make appointments to give a return demonstration of skills. This routine will give you an opportunity to organize your time. This is what is expected of the practical nurse as part of client care. When you make an appointment with the skills lab, you are entering into an agreement with the lab personnel. Your responsibility is to practice the skill until you can perform it in the time frame of your appointment. If you are unable to keep your appointment, inform the lab personnel. This will allow them to schedule other students into lab time for skills testing.

▽▽▽
Study Skills Lab

The **study skills lab** is available to help you with academic problem areas. Examples of areas in which help is available are: study skills, time management, reading (including vocabulary and comprehension), listening skills, math skills, test-taking skills (especially situation tests), notemaking, writing, and any other academic problem you may have. You can go to the skills lab on your own or by referral of your instructor or the counselor.

> *Some students who need the study skills center state they do not have time to go for help. Comment about this response.*

▽▽▽
Audiovisual Materials

In addition to lectures, discussion/activities, textbooks, and articles, the instructor may have included films and videotapes as part of your assignment. **Audiovisual (AV) materials** are not considered extra or additional assignments. They are a significant part of all areas of learning. These learning resources give faith to the saying, "One picture is worth a thousand words." AV materials provide an additional sensory channel for learning compared to reading. In some nursing courses, especially autotutorial skills courses, the AV medium *is* the course. The student progresses independently, attending periodic lecture–discussion classes and seeking out the instructor when questions arise. Approach the AV material as you do a class. Realize that you have the option of repeating all or part of the presentation when you do not understand it. Remember, television is a source of information for nursing and related topics.

▽▽▽
Computer-Aided Instruction

No segment of society has been left untouched by the computer. **Computer-aided instruction** (CAI) is an increasingly used teaching strategy in nursing education. It has the following benefits:

▶ It allows learners to be actively involved in their own learning.
▶ It encourages problem solving, a skill employers expect in practical nurses.
▶ It provides immediate feedback by quickly evaluating answers and decision-making strategies.
▶ It provides an opportunity to develop the ability to follow directions.

Learning by CAI is enhanced for students in whom the right side of the brain is dominant. CAI can also be used effectively by any student to master new material. It simplifies concepts and reinforces skills that have been presented previously. If CAI is used in your practical-nursing program, you will be taught the skills necessary to use the computer. The process is simple even if you do not have any computer experience. Many of you will also be using the computer in the clinical area to store and retrieve patient information. And in less than one year, all of you will be taking the NCLEX-PN examination by computer.

Computer Simulation

Computer simulation is a learning activity that makes use of an imaginary patient situation. The student is required to gather data, set priorities, plan, and evaluate care as in an actual clinical situation.

The computer patient simulation continually changes, as it would in the clinical area. This requires the student to evaluate the situation and plan new nursing interventions. Computer simulations may be used when the patient census is inadequate for patient assignments, when a desired patient situation is unavailable, or when enhanced learning of specific concepts is desirable. A review of the available software reveals that few computer simulations are intended specifically for practical nursing students. Your instructors can suggest modifications of existing simulations for your use.

▼▼▼
Learning Resource Center

If you are over 30, you know this resource as the library. Its new name, often abbreviated LRC, merely reflects the increased scope of the library as we approach the year 2000. It consists of a lot more than books. How do you feel when you find out you must use the **learning resource center**? If you have some negative feelings, perhaps it is because you are unfamiliar with the sources of information contained in this resource, their location, and how to use them. If you investigate your school library you will find that it contains a wealth of services that will help make your time in the practical nursing program much easier. Ask the librarian for a tour. Some libraries have self-guided tours on audiotape. An hour spent touring can save you many wasted hours and much frustration later in the school year. Ask for a library brochure so that you have an idea of the library's general hours of operation and its physical layout. Identify the special study areas available to you and groups of learners. Because the library is a learning area, you should help keep it a quiet environment.

▽▽▽
Resources of the Library

Librarian

This is perhaps the best resource in the whole school. The **librarian** is a college-educated specialist in what the library has to offer in the area of information and where that information can be found. Look at the librarian as a professional educator about information for learning and as a person who is always ready to assist you. When you do go for assistance, be sure to watch the process the librarian uses to obtain the information you need. Next time, you will be able to help yourself.

Interlibrary Loan Services

Interlibrary loan services allow your LRC to borrow materials you need that are not in your library's holdings. Books and audiovisual materials are available through this service. If your LRC does not have the periodical in which an article you need is located, a photocopy of the article, free of charge, can be obtained from a library that does have the periodical. Allow yourself about one week to receive articles obtained in this manner.

Vertical File (Pamphlet File)

The **vertical file** contains pamphlets of various subjects arranged in alphabetical order by topic.

Circulation Desk

The **circulation desk** is the area where library materials are checked out and returned. Materials reserved by your instructor will probably be found here and can be checked out for short periods, along with audiovisual equipment to use with the material, if needed.

Online Catalog

There is a lot of information you can obtain in a library by yourself once you understand the cataloging system. Most libraries have converted their card catalogs to an **online (computerized) catalog**. All books found in your LRC, except magazines and newspapers, are indexed in this computerized system. Cataloged materials also include audiotapes and videotapes. You can search for desired materials by subject, title, or author. Sometimes you know an author's name but not the title of the material you need. Select "author" on the initial computer screen. Type in the author's last name and first name. All the materials in the LRC by that author will appear on the screen with their call numbers (location in the library). If you know the title but not the author, information will appear on where to locate the material. Sometimes you are investigating a topic but have no information about authors or titles of material on that topic. Type one or two words describing the topic you are investigating. Authors and titles relating to that topic will be displayed on the screen. Some systems will indicate if the material is on the shelf or checked out. If the LRC does not have the material you are seaching for, but another library on the system does, this information might be included also. This system of cataloging can save students valuable time and energy.

Directions and brochures for how to use the online catalog are located next to the computer terminals. It is impossible to give you a step-by-step guide to using the online catalog because different libraries use different computer systems to organize this information. However, a few hints might help you keep body and soul together at the computer terminal.

1. Read the directions on the screen, top to bottom.
2. Locate the keys with arrows up ($\uparrow$), down ($\downarrow$), left side ($\leftarrow$), and right side ($\rightarrow$). Up and down arrows move the blinking cursor up a line or down a line. These arrows can also be used to scroll through lists quickly (the information appears on the screen and rolls by). The side to side arrows can move the blinking cursor left or right.
3. When you press the enter ($\leftarrow\!\shortmid$) key, do so firmly, but do not hold it down. Press it and remove your finger quickly.
4. If your system tells you to press a letter and a number (for example, F1), look for keys that have the letter and the number on one key. These are located at the top of the keyboard. Do not type an F and then a separate 1.
5. If you are unsuccessful in finding information, ask an LRC staff member.
6. YOU WILL NOT CAUSE THE SYSTEM TO BREAK DOWN.

▽▽▽

Locating Your Material

Now to locate your material in the LRC. Libraries may choose to use either of two systems to classify materials so they are easy to locate: (1) the Dewey decimal system and (2) the Library of Congress classification system. Regardless of the system your library uses, the **call number** shown on the author, title, or subject screens is the same number as that on the material itself. Get in the habit of copying, in order, *all* the letters and the numbers in the call number.

The Stacks

Armed with the call number, you can proceed to the stacks—the place where the majority of materials that can be checked out is located. When you do find the material you are looking for, note that materials covering the same subject are shelved in the same area. You might find additional useful material on the same shelf.

Reference Material

Reference materials include dictionaries, including medical and nursing dictionaries, encyclopedias, almanacs, yearbooks, atlases, handbooks, and other similar categories of books. You will find up-to-date information on any subject in this area. Reference material generally does not circulate. It cannot be checked out. Some libraries allow certain reference books to circulate for brief periods. Information from reference materials may be copied on a copy machine.

▼▼▼
Staying Current in Practical Nursing

▽▽▽
Periodicals

Because magazines are published weekly, monthly, and quarterly, that is, periodically, they are often called **periodicals**. They are also referred to as journals—publications that contain news or material of current interest to a particular discipline. Professional journals contain articles that include the most recent information available on a specific subject and subjects that are too new to be included in books. This is the reason periodicals are important resources for a learner in a

field changing as quickly as nursing and health care. The titles and authors of various articles cannot possibly be included in the online catalog. These can be found instead in two sources: bound books called periodical indexes and CD-ROM databases.

Periodical Indexes

Entries in periodical indexes are listed by author, title, and subject. There are two periodical indexes of special value to practical nursing students.

Reader's Guide to Periodical Literature. This comprehensive index to more than 160 **popular American nontechnical magazines** includes articles published between the dates printed on its cover. This guide is useful for recreational reading on specific topics, such as setting up a workshop, decorating with stenciling, and learning about the Internet. The **Reader's Guide**, or green book, is valuable for practical nursing students because technical data on health topics are presented in understandable language for the general public.

Cumulative Index to Nursing and Allied Health Literature (CINAHL). This comprehensive and authoritative periodical index contains current listings for nursing and 17 allied health fields and for others interested in health care issues. Six hundred and fifty nursing, allied health, and related journals are reviewed, indexed, and included in five bimonthly issues and cumulative (arranged by year) bound volumes of past issues. Figure 8–1 illustrates the information found in a typical entry in the *Cumulative Index to Nursing and Allied Health Literature*.

Near the indexes is found a **periodical listing**. The listing includes the professional journals and magazines and the dates of the issues that are found in your library. If the article you need is in a journal or magazine that is not held in your library, see the librarian. The librarian will track down the article in another library and arrange for you to receive a photocopy by interlibrary loan. If your library has the date and issue you need, go to the section of the library that contains the periodicals. If the issue you need is not there, it may be on **microform**. To conserve space, back issues of maga-

---

1-ANTIBIOTICS
  2-Bugs and drugs: antibiotic resistance in the
    1990s **3-** (Rickman LS) **4-** (tables/charts)
    5- TODAYS OR NURSE 6- 1994 Sept-Oct; **7-** 16(5):
    8- 7-12 **9-** (12 ref)

    Key: 1. Subject. 2. Title of the article. 3. Author of the article. 4. Additional
information found in article. 5. Periodical in which the article appears. If the
periodical is abbreviated, the periodical index will have in the front of the book
a list of periodical abbreviations and the full name of the journal for which
those abbreviations stand. 6. Date of publication. 7. Volume and number of
periodical. 8. Pages of the article. 9. Article has a bibliography with 12
references.

Figure 8–1
An entry from the *Cumulative Index to Nursing and Allied Health Literature.*

zines are microphotographically produced. Two commonly used microforms are **microfilm** and **microfiche** (mī-crō-feesh).

    1. Microfilm. Using microfilm, a whole year's issues of magazines can be reproduced on 16-mm or 35-mm film that threads on a wheel about 3½ inches in diameter with room to spare.

    2. Microfiche. Microfiche involves a 4- by 6-inch film card that carries reduced images placed on the card in rows. One microfiche can contain up to 98 pages of text.

    Both of these microforms must be read with a device that enlarges the very small image. Many libraries have reader–printers that will print the image seen on the screen on a sheet of paper you can take with you. See the librarian for help with microforms.

CD-ROM

Public and school libraries have these valuable sources of information. The audio CDs you use at home play music. The CD-ROM in the library plays "information." This information, via disk, may already be loaded into the computer so you do not have to insert a disk. CD-ROM systems differ in the subjects and the level of coverage they offer. See CD-ROM Databases for examples of specific CD-ROMs that would benefit practical nursing students.

CD-ROM Databases

Nursing and Allied Health on CD-ROM

This is the *Cumulative Guide to Nursing and Allied Health Literature* discussed under Periodical Indexes but in CD-ROM form and with some additional information. The library receives monthly updates of information from all vendors. Information can only be retrieved back to 1982. Summaries of important points in the texts of articles in over 200 journals are presented and can be printed out for student use. CINAHL CD-ROM also includes access to information from selected journals on consumer health, health care books, nursing dissertations, selected conference proceedings, standards of practice, audiovisual materials, and educational software in nursing.

Health Reference Center on CD-ROM

This CD-ROM service provides an extensive database of all aspects of health, fitness, diseases, drugs, and nutrition. Coverage includes the full text of approximately 100 health care consumer-oriented magazines, newsletters, and professional journals, over 500 medical education pamphlets, and the full text of Mosby's Medical Dictionary plus four other reference books. You can view or print the full text of journal summaries, articles, pamphlets, and definitions. This database is also updated monthly.

NewsBank Comprehensive Search

NewsBank contains full-text newspaper articles of current issues and events selected from over 100 newspapers from across the United States and Canada. Articles that provide the most current, up-to-date information are selected. Practical nursing students will find valuable information for nursing courses under Health and Science and Social Issues.

SIRS Researcher (Social Issues Resources Series)

This database contains full-text articles selected from more than 800 domestic and foreign magazines, newspapers, journals, and U.S. government documents. Practical nursing students can search subject headings, title-browse articles under broad topics, and do keyword searches to find current information for class, clinical applications, and everyday life. The text of each article published in this database can be printed out by the student. Articles that do not have copyright clearance are presented in summary form.

CD-ROMs are also a source of textbook-type information for practical nursing students. Check your LRC to see if any encyclopedias are available on CD-ROM. Examples of other helpful sources are *Time Almanac* and *Five a Day Adventure* (child's nutrition game that can reinforce vitamin information gained from your nutrition class in a fun way). *The Family Doctor* answers questions about 280 medical conditions and 1600 prescription drugs, provides information on 900 diseases, and includes a full-motion video covering the anatomy of all body systems.

Because of computer technology, the process of "keeping up to date" has been simplified as far as finding information is concerned. All you need is time! CD-ROM databases are expensive sources of information. If your LRC has this technology available for student use, be sure to use it. The systems are user friendly. Combined with a helpful LRC staff, you cannot lose! Here are some hints when using these systems.

1. Read the directions that appear on the screen and are posted around the terminal.

2. When doing subject searches, be sure to narrow the topic. Provide the computer with key words so it can make a search that fills your needs.

Using CD-ROM Databases
Identify one nursing problem or topic area to research on a CD-ROM database. Print out one article or newspaper story about this problem or topic. Suggestions: Write an objective sentence describing the problem or topic. Then pick key words from the sentence and type these for the subject search. Example: You have been assigned to do a report for Personal Vocational Issues class. You need information about health and illness beliefs of various ethnic groups, and you chose Korean-Americans (problem statement). Key words that apply to this statement would be ethnic groups, Korean-Americans, health beliefs, and illness beliefs.

3. Review suggestions for accessing the online catalog.

4. Avoid confusing the online catalog terminals (holdings ·of the library) with the CD-ROM database terminals (contains summaries and full text of articles, newspaper stories, and so on).

Citing CINAHL

Despite the popularity of CD-ROM databases, they are costly and may not yet be in your school's LRC budget. Some schools of practical nursing may share a computer system with other health care institutions. Student use of these databases may be restricted. Understanding how to use a periodical index is still a necessary skill. How well do you understand the information found in a periodical index entry? The beginning of each CINAHL book contains directions for using the source. Ask the LRC staff if they have the 12-minute videotape See the Cites with CINAHL. The video teaches you how to use this information source. Use the CINAHL entry below to test your understanding of CINAHL citing. Answer the questions found underneath the entry.

▽▽▽
Nursing Organizations

Nursing organizations frequently organize speakers, seminars, and workshops on up-to-the-minute nursing topics and related health care topics. These programs are frequently made available to students. Specific nursing organizations are discussed in Chapter 17.

▽▽▽
Community Resources

The city library and museums sometimes sponsor programs and exhibits on topics of interest and use to practical nursing students. Health care facilities such as hospitals and clinics offer lecture series.

▽▽▽
Guest Speakers

Nurses and other health professionals are frequently invited to visit nursing classes as guest speakers. These

---

Using CINAHL

Hypertension: keeping dangerous blood pressure down (Cuddy RP) (CEU, exam questions, tables/charts)
NURSING 1995 Aug; 25(8): 34-43 (4 ref)

Author _____

Title of article _____

Volume and number of periodical _____

Name of periodical _____

Date of article _____

Pages _____

Additional information found in article _____

Are there references in the article? _____

If so, how many? ____ _____

speakers donate their time to present current information on their areas of expertise and updates on specific nursing topics. Often they are released by their employers to visit nursing classes. Students should treat these speakers with respect.

▼▼▼ *S U M M A R Y*

► The hints for using learning strategies and resources found in this chapter will help you obtain the information you need to get better grades on tests and achieve your goal of becoming a practical nurse. The PQRST method of reading a textbook is an effective technique for storing information in your long-term memory so that it is available for recall for tests and can be applied in the clinical area. Specific classroom learning strategies that most probably will be used by the practical nursing student, in addition to textbooks, include mini-lectures, lecture–discussions, and cooperative learning. Additional learning resources include articles from periodicals, the syllabus, course outlines, audiovisual materials, computer-aided instruction, computer simulations, and the learning resource center. Staying current in practical nursing is made possible by using periodical indexes, CD-ROM databases and programs, skills lab, nursing organizations, community resources, and guest speakers. After learning the information you need to be a practical nurse, you must demonstrate that learning has taken place by your performance in the clinical area and on tests.

▼▼▼ *R E F E R E N C E S*

Jerit L, Taylor B. *Towards a Definition of Critical Literacy* (Unpublished paper for Critical Literacy Project of Oakton Community College, Des Plaines, IL), 1991.
Staton T. *How to Study,* 5th ed. Circle Pines, MN: Publisher's Building, American Guidance Service, 1959.

▼▼▼ *B I B L I O G R A P H Y*

Berkman R. *Find It Fast: How to Uncover Expert Information on Any Subject.* New York: Harper Collins, 1994.
Chenevert M. *Mosby's Tour Guide to Nursing School.* St. Louis: Mosby–Year Book, 1991.
DeYoung S, Adams E. Study groups among nursing students. J Nurs Educ 1995; 34(4):190–191.
Kent P. *The Complete Idiot's Guide to the Internet.* Indianapolis: QUE, 1994.
Meltzer M, Palau S. *Reading and Study Strategies for Nursing Students.* Philadelphia: W.B. Saunders, 1993.
Pauk W. *How to Study in College,* 5th ed. Boston: Houghton-Mifflin, 1993.
Sternberger C. Moving past memorization. J Practical Nurs 1995; 45(2):12–15.

Knowing Yourself

 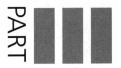
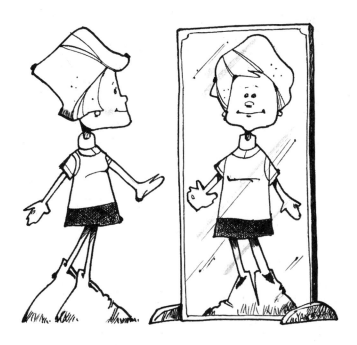

Personal Development

9

▼▼▼ O U T L I N E

Human Needs Theory
Attitude As It Affects Success
   Optimism

How To Change Your Outlook
Motivation
Discipline

Confidence
Getting Along

▼▼▼ K E Y T E R M S

attitude
confidence
discipline

hierarchy
human needs theory
motivation

optimism
physiologic needs

▼▼▼ O B J E C T I V E S

Upon completing this chapter you will be able to:

1. Discuss the human needs theory as it applies to you.

2. Describe how the subconscious records real and imagined images.

3. Discuss how the body acts out what the mind imagines.

4. Discuss four characteristics needed for a positive attitude.

5. Monitor personal self-talk.

6. Explain how positive affirmations and images can be used to develop a positive attitude.

7. Describe "getting along" as a major issue in the workplace.

Personalities develop as people adapt to their physical, emotional, social, and spiritual environments. Personality determines (1) how people cope with feelings and impulses, (2) how they find meaning in relationships, (3) how they respond to their surroundings, and (4) how their value systems develop.

This entire textbook is dedicated to your personal advancement as a current student and as a future nurse. This chapter provides an opportunity for you to look at your own personality development, present and future. On what kind of information are you functioning? How did it get there? Is it real? Can it be changed? How do you feel about yourself? Do you see yourself as being successful? What are your personal goals? Most important, do you have choices, and how can you exercise those choices? These and many other questions will be dealt with. However, before going any further, take the brief test that follows. It will help to personalize the information for you. Once again, answer the questions as honestly as possible, as they relate to you at this point in your life.

> Read the following statements and determine if they are true or false in regard to how you feel right now.
> Write in True or False at the end of each statement.
> 1. I have personal written goals.   _____
> 2. I can usually find alternatives to a problem.   _____
> 3. I say "thank you" to a compliment.   _____
> 4. I work well with groups.   _____
> 5. It is my responsibility to learn.   _____
> 6. I evaluate my own work.   _____
> 7. My parents did the best they could.   _____
> 8. I believe that I can excel.   _____
> 9. I can change how I feel about myself._____
> 10. Self-talk determines my behavior.   _____
> 11. I treat me like a best friend.   _____
> 12. I find something good in everyone.   _____
> 13. I can learn anything I want to.   _____
> 14. I express myself with "I"-centered statements.   _____
> 15. I rarely explain my behavior.   _____
>
> KEY: (count the number of True items)
> 10–15 True = positive attitude
> 0–9 True = need an attitude adjustment

Look closely at the result of the test now, and then look at it again later at the end of the chapter, at which time you are encouraged to write some realistic, time-limited goals for yourself in a special way.

▼▼▼
Human Needs Theory

The human needs theory developed by Maslow (1962) outlines our basic needs in a hierarchy that is useful in understanding ourselves. They are as follows:

> Level 5 Self-actualization needs: self-expression and creativity (highest level)
> Level 4 Self-esteem needs: esteem by others
> Level 3 Love and belongingness needs: group needs
> Level 2 Safety and security needs: protection, one-to-one relationships
> Level 1 Physiologic needs: air, water, food, shelter, sleep, sex (basic level)

Maslow maintained that the most powerful basic needs are those of *physical survival,* such as air, water, food, shelter, sleep, and sex. These needs keep us alive and producing future generations. After these needs are reasonably satisfied you are ready to focus on *safety and security.* This level includes the need for protection. There is a readiness for one-to-one relationships. As these needs are fulfilled the third level of needs for *love and belongingness* emerges. At this level you feel the need to belong to a group. There is a readiness to relate to others beyond a one-to-one relationship. There is a need for acceptance and for being able to give of one's self. You are able to take part in group discussions and activities with limited discomfort. The fourth level focuses on *self-esteem* and addresses the need for feelings of self-reliance, self-respect, confidence, and self-trust. Becoming a part of a vocation or profession that has major responsibilities is possible at this level.

According to Maslow, the first four levels cover basic needs. The remaining level relates to growth needs that center on *self-actualization,* which is the ultimate in needs fulfillment. It is thought that only a few people are fully self-actualized.

It is important to note that progression through these levels is not clear cut. In reality, as most of your needs are met on one level, you are already beginning to check out the next level. When faced with overwhelming difficulties, physical or emotional, some regression takes place. For example,

1. Physiologic needs become a priority if you have lost your job or housing.

2. Safety and security needs become a major issue if you are facing a serious illness or move into an unsafe neighborhood.

Once these issues have been dealt with or resolved, higher needs will emerge once more.

Take a moment to identify where you are functioning now according to Maslow's human needs theory. The result will assist you in understanding some things about your current personality and functioning. Result: More empathy for yourself. This is also a way of looking at your client's current needs. It will help to determine your response to the client. For example, you are not as likely to insist that a psychotic client attend group therapy sessions. After all, even a one-to-one contact with staff is barely tolerable for such a person. See how it works?

▼▼▼
Attitude As It Affects Success

Here is that word again—attitude. But what does it have to do with success? A lot, according to a five-year study supported by the Carnegie Foundation. The research showed that only 15% of a person's ability to get a job, keep a job, and move ahead in that job is due to his or her knowledge; the other 85% is due to attitude. Furthermore, it has been shown that people like to be around positive people and that positive people are more productive on the job because they have more energy and motivation. Knowledge is the key that unlocks a career door; once inside, attitude is the key to success.

There are many people with "good" attitudes, but not all have good goals. Look around you: Some people look like candidates for a good attitude poster contest. They are always grinning. Ask yourself what they *do* with that attitude. Are you picking up another message? Attitude reflects the way you look at the world, your set of beliefs, your values, and the on-going questions you ask yourself. Attitude linked to goals and self-management, including the management of emotions, makes a significant difference for successful nurses. What you think, what you feel, and how you behave need to be congruent (together). Your attitude ultimately reflects how you feel about the work you do in nursing.

The characteristics of optimism, motivation, discipline, and confidence that are a part of a positive attitude will be considered separately. Suggestions for changing a characteristic, if necessary, will be included. All these characteristics are intimately related to getting along with others.

▽▽▽
Optimism

Life is an adventure, and, as pointed out in Isaiah 14:24, "Surely as I think so it shall come to pass." Buddha meant the same when he said, "As the wheel follows the ox behind, we will become what our thoughts have made us." Other great thinkers and philosophers have said the same thing in different words. Immediately, it sounds as though you are responsible for what happens to you. Can this be? Yes, definitely, for you set the tone for each day of your life. For example, think about what you say to yourself when you first awaken. Is it a positive message? Do you anticipate new opportunities for learning and experiences that will prepare you for your career? Do you expect it to be a good day? Do you see the problems that you face as challenges that have solutions? Or do you wake up feeling resentful that you must get up? Do you anticipate problems with class content and tests? Do you just know this will be a bad day because you spilled your juice—"A sign, you know"? Do you immediately personalize the behavior of someone who is cross or ill—"I just can't win"?

Let's take a look at what happens during those first few minutes of your day. All of us are constantly involved in self-talk. That talk and the images it evokes are recorded by the subconscious, the part of our mind below our immediate awareness or conscious mind. Interestingly, it does not matter to our subconscious mind if our perceptions are accurate or inaccurate. It records the messages and images as the truth, and the conscious mind operates on this "truth." In other words, you become what you fear or you become what you expect to be. Life is a self-fulfilling prophecy. With that in mind, go back to what happens when the alarm clock goes off.

> *Scene 1:* "Terrific, it's Monday. I'm going to ace the test. I understand the material."

> *Scene 2:* "Ugh. Monday already? I studied a lot, but I never do well on Monday."

You already know which self-talk is most likely to result in passing the test. Chances are that if the student in Scene 2 does pass the test, it will be dismissed as "just luck."

Optimism has far-reaching effects not only for schoolwork, but for one's overall health and personal relationships as well. Certainly, hereditary and environmental factors are significant. But consider the fact that your conscious mind is trying to follow the messages you provide, to be recording in your subconscious; the body acts out what the mind believes. So, if you provide self-talk messages of "I can't take this much longer," "I'm getting run down," "I usually get a cold when I'm overworked," or "I get a strep infection every year at this time," your body will try to follow directions for what it believes to be the truth. The same is true of personal relationships: Negative self-talk begets negative results. For example, "With my luck, this relationship is bound to fail." "What can you expect? Teenage is a disease to be endured." "That kid cries just to annoy me." "My childhood was so rotten, I don't have a chance." What do you think the outcome will be?

Ideally, you have had a lifetime of self-talk that is optimistic. For those of you who continue to practice negative self-talk leading to pessimism, there is hope.

You can *choose* to become optimistic by changing your self-talk.

The negative self-talk recorded in your subconscious cannot be erased, but you can provide and practice an entirely new script of optimistic self-talk. The subconscious will accept what you give it, and the conscious mind will begin to function based on this new information. You will not experience a difference in feelings right away. Just continue to practice the new self-talk, and your feelings will eventually catch up. After all, your old feelings have been a part of you for quite some time. Maintaining the new scripts with relatively few slip-ups will take a minimum of two to three weeks. More permanent change will take up to a year or more. You will note that as new challenges (formerly called problems) arise, there will be a tendency to return to the old self-talk, that is, "I knew this wouldn't work—not in my life. It's different." Just remind yourself firmly that it will work, and continue practicing the new self-talk. It may feel initially as though you are acting. That's fine. Fake it until you make it. This feeling that you are only acting will go away as your optimism begins to grow and becomes a part of you.

How To Change Your Outlook

Decide on your own positive self-talk. Write it down. For example, "I did a good job today. I will do even better tomorrow." "I will be a terrific nurse." "I can cope with this new challenge." "I'm pleased to have this opportunity to go to school." Overcoming adversity in a positive way helps to build character.

Begin your positive self-talk before going to sleep. For example, "I'm capable and smart." "I'm going to have a great sleep." "I'm lucky to have a teenager who is practicing independence." "We'll make it. There's bound to be a solution." "I grow from every challenge."

Plan what you want to wake up to and take a few minutes to prepare it the night before—a favorite tape, record, radio station, or TV channel, chilled juice, an inspirational saying—whatever is special for you and starts you in a positive way upon awakening.

Greet yourself in the morning with more positive self-talk. For example, "It's going to be a good day for me." "I'm glad to be alive."

Deliberately look for something good in anything that doesn't go just right during the day. It may be necessary, especially at first, to write down daily what you see as problems. Then rewrite these statements of problems as challenges—opportunities to grow and gain inner strength. For example, Problem: Car stalled. Challenge: I proved to myself that I can find a solution to a problem, and I feel stronger because of it.

Treat yourself as you would your best friend. Certainly you would treat him or her with empathy, respect, encouragement, and reassurance that there are alternatives for dealing with the current situation.

Avoid negative people. Those who are involved in criticizing and complaining tend to pull you down, especially when you are attempting to change a pessimistic outlook to an optimistic one. Right now, you need your energy for you. If you do get hooked into complaining, move away from the person or group as soon as you recognize what is happening.

Look for a positive person to be with or to model yourself after, even if being with the person is not possible.

Plan for positive visual and auditory experiences. Play tapes, records, and radio music—inspirational messages that say "I can." When you really listen to many of today's lyrics, they say, "I can't. It won't work, and if it doesn't I'll probably drink, cheat, or kill myself." Meanwhile, your subconscious records it all as you sing along. The same thing happens with television and movies, especially those seen before going to bed. Negative sensory experiences support more negative recording into the subconscious as you sleep.

> **Did you ever have a weird, scary dream after watching a violent TV show and awaken feeling fearful or anxious?**

Look for something good in everyone you meet. This is initially difficult because it is easier to think of people as all good or all bad. Listening carefully to another's viewpoint is a way to begin this process.

> **What is a more realistic way to view every individual that you contact?**

Optimism is closely related to your state of health.

Be aware of the messages to yourself and to others when they ask how you are feeling. Furthermore, you can also influence others' health through your statements to them. Consider the following:

Scene 1

Friend: You're looking good. Looks like you've found positive ways of dealing with your studies.

Student nurse: Thank you. You're right. I'm proud of being able to juggle my life successfully.

Scene 2

Friend: You don't look so good today. Are you getting ill?

Student nurse: Well, I thought I was OK, but maybe you're right. I have been putting in long hours.

Question
What do you think will happen to each of the student nurses in Scenes 1 and 2?

▽▽▽
Motivation

According to Victor Frankl, a well-known psychiatrist and philosopher, what a person really needs in life is struggling for a goal that is worthy of him. Each man knows in his heart what his assignment in life is. Aim at what your conscience wants you to do and success will follow you. That seems to coincide with findings that motivation is one of the major characteristics common to individuals who are outstanding successes in their fields. Interestingly, these individuals have developed personal goals similar to those of major corporations. Far off? Maybe, but it works.

> **Do you have stated goals for your life, or is life just a happening?**

Where does motivation come from? Perhaps you have always looked for someone or something to motivate you from the outside, like a "good" teacher, friend, parent, deadlines, or crisis. It is true that all these people and factors can get you going. But let's face it, that kind of motivation lasts only as long as the teacher is with you, the deadline is met, or the crisis is over—and then it is back to the old habits again.

Motivation means that you are moved from inside, because you have decided that you want to attain certain goals. You will go on to do what needs to be done happily and to the best of your ability because you want to. As Frankl puts it, you will be "struggling for a goal which is worthy of you."

As you consider this characteristic, you may be aware of some internal resistance to change. This resistance to change is named fear, another powerful force in our lives. After all, changing the ending of a story also shakes up your present security. Have you ever noticed how much easier it is to share a story about a crisis with someone when the crisis is a thing of the past and you know the ending, than it is to talk about an ongoing unresolved situation? There is a sense of security in knowing how the crisis in the past ended. So it is with holding on to negative characteristics. You know what the end of the story is. The thought of making a change arouses fear—fear that this new way of behaving will not work out. Your self-talk is a powerful factor in motivation because you do, in fact, do what you think about most.

"Wait a minute," you say, "this is quite a sales pitch. I'm paying my teachers to teach me and to tell me what to learn and whether I'm doing well." Read that statement again. It sounds as if you are creating your own bondage. The instructor is, at best, a facilitator only. He or she sets an example of personal motivation by researching the class content to set up the best course possible. In nursing, this generally means a syllabus or course outline, references, visual aids, clinical guidelines, and student evaluations. The instructor must trust that you will do your part in the instructor–student relationship. It is at this point that internal motivation becomes a significant factor that lets you take control of your learning. A clue: Most courses continue to be based on minimal expectations—that is, the least you can get by on to pass the course. The word minimal tells you that you can learn a great deal more from the course if you are motivated and choose to do so.

> *Economically speaking, how do you get your money's worth from a course? Futuristically speaking, how will you become the nurse best prepared to meet the needs of your clients?*

Consider the following suggestions and apply them as appropriate in ways that will increase personal motivation for you.

1. High achievers have identified their own goals. Write down three things you want in the near future and how you expect to benefit from attaining each one of them. Place the list where you can read it first thing in the morning and the last thing at night.
2. Do the following exercise: Read a single direction and complete it before reading the next direction, and so on.
   a. Take a piece of paper and write "I can't" at the top. Make a list of all the things you think you cannot do.
   b. Cross out "I can't" and replace it with the word "won't." Read your list again. Notice that almost every item on the list, unless related to a severe mental or physical disability, is actually a choice on your part.
   c. Cross out the word "won't" and replace it with "want." Read the list again.
   d. Cross out "want" and replace it with "can." Circle the one item from the list that you desire to accomplish within the next six months.
   e. Write your choice as a positive "I will" statement on an index card that you can carry with you. For example: "I will say no without feeling responsible for other's feelings." "I will speak with a lower, warm, authoritative voice." "I will exercise vigorously for 20 minutes three times per week." "I will weigh 136 pounds." "I will practice rapid relaxation techniques as needed daily."
3. Practice saying the "I will" statement daily, for example, in the shower, in the car, upon arising, before going to sleep, when exercising. What a great idea for a video.

Have you noticed how much of the type of choice discussed in this chapter is yours? You truly do have a choice. The instructor need never know if you have chosen to follow suggestions made to you or if you have chosen to complete the minimum requirements in life. It is indeed, a very personal, private, internal decision.

▽▽▽
Discipline

Think for a moment of how you view discipline. Do you view it as something internal that helps you accomplish your personal goals, or do you view it as something external, imposed by another, which forces you to comply? There is a significant difference between the two. Internal (self) discipline permits you to be in charge of your own life. For example, "I am finally going to have an opportunity to learn about other religions." "I like the idea of learning about home health but would like to visit an agency instead of using the pamphlets as my resource." External discipline, usually referred to as punishment, means that you are dependent on others to make you do what you should or should not do. It also helps to set up a pattern of manipulation between you and the system or other person involved. For example:

> "If she does not ask for a return demonstration, that's one more skill I don't have to worry about."
> "This instructor doesn't care if we come in late or leave early. Good deal."
> "I'll just change the charting. No one will know I did not give the medicine."
> "I'll read the chapters just before the test. She never calls on me in class anyway."
> "I'll just make up my own numbers for the TPR and BP."

Are these far-fetched examples? Not really. There continues to be a tendency, as there was in childhood, to do only what you absolutely have to and to get away with whatever you can until personal discipline becomes an internal reality and therefore, a way of life for you.

Self-discipline means saying: "I have decided that I am going to do whatever is

necessary in order to gain the knowledge, skills, and experience available during school to prepare me for nursing. I am doing it because I choose to do it."

Is discipline related to personal health and interpersonal relationships? Support your answer with an example. The following suggestions are offered to support you as you make an internal decision to excel through personal discipline.

1. Check your vocabulary: What kind of self-talk do you engage in? For example, what do you say to yourself when you are given an assignment or look at a course outline for the first time? Do you say, "Looks like I cannot get out of doing this." Or do you say, "I want to learn about this topic." It does make a difference because the subconscious continues to record, and the message it receives will make a difference in how you act and feel. The power of choice is yours, so pick your self-talk carefully. Avoid phrases like "I cannot get out of this, I should, I should not, I cannot, I have to, they made me, I have no choice." Consciously and deliberately change your self-talk to "I want to, I choose to, I have decided to, I would like to, I am going to, I am doing it for me."

2. Use imagery to support the change you desire to make, whether it relates to study habits, health, or interpersonal relationships. Feelings and thoughts are pulled toward one's mental images. You most often become what you imagine you will become. The nervous system operates on imagery, and your personal images serve as a self-fulfilling prophecy. Images go directly to the nervous system. Images are used for or against yourself. When tired, the negative images seem to make the maximum impression. To counteract this process, create positive images for yourself. Visualize completing the task you have to do successfully. Take time to include enough detail for it to be real to you—smells, sights, sounds. Visualize feeling happy about having completed the task successfully and on time. See yourself being praised for choosing to do the task completely and on time.

3. Take any size note card. Divide it into three columns. In column 1, list the following words: choose,

want, decided. In column 2, list three tasks or projects that have been put off. In column 3, list a completion date specific to each task or project. Look at the sample below.

1	2	3
Choose	Study Chapter 3	Tonight
Want	Nutrition assessment	Monday morning
Decided	Talk to Frank	Sunday afternoon

Read across. You have created three personal guidelines for discipline.

4. Practice, practice, practice. Old habits will want to creep back before the new ones are well established. Don't worry about it. Just reinstate the new behavior immediately where you left off.

▽▽▽
Confidence

Confidence is made up of many factors. Most important among them is how you see yourself and your ability to respect what you see. Ultimately, it is your view of yourself rather than what you are that holds you back. Traditionally, parents and circumstances in childhood have been held responsible for how the individual views himself as an adult. Consider the following opposite views. "I always felt self-conscious because my parents were so poor." And "I grew up in the shadow of successful parents and can't measure up to them." In each example, the individual rationalizes his present internal state by blaming the parents' state of being. It is worth noting that parenting at best is an inexact science, and parents can only give emotionally what they themselves have attained. This in turn is influenced by their interpretation of events. Like you, parents are involved in the adventure of living and continual growth. The positive aspect of all this is that you can be in charge of the rest of your life, usually from age 18 on, and can change (not erase) any of the scripts you do not like. Continuing to go along with current personal scripts that are negative or that you do not like simply provides an excuse for lack of success.

What do you think are the components of developing confidence?

The first component of confidence is knowledge. In this case, *you do not fake it.* Knowledge belongs in the realm of thinking, and it is imperative to have a strong knowledge base on which to make observations and think through decisions based on those observations. Overlearning has already been suggested as a way to learn classroom content. If you are lacking in reading, studying, math, or writing skills, ask the counselor or instructor how to get service in these areas. In many schools, you have already paid for these services through the fees charged at the time you pay tuition. Many schools have learning labs already set up just waiting to serve you. (See Chapter 8 for further information.)

A close second to knowledge skills is clinical practice. Once again, the principles of overlearning apply because it is not always possible to have every experience desired during a clinical assignment. Seek the needed experiences through clinical simulation in the lab and by viewing teaching films and videotapes. It is your responsibility to be actively involved in the learning process. Personal discipline provides the push for developing this aspect of confidence.

Third, deal with negative scripts and feelings that are getting in the way of absorbing the knowledge available to you. Any counseling services you may need are probably already paid for through the fee system. Use them to your advantage. The counselors are prepared to deal with you on issues that face you "here and now" and to look at alternatives that will fit your life style.

Fourth, learn to deal with criticism. In this case, the best defense is a good offense. Decide now to critique your daily work in as objective a manner as possible. It is sometimes said that human objectivity is a myth. This should in no way prevent you from striving for it. To critique yourself objectively, it is necessary to (1) look at what you did well and give yourself credit for it, and

(2) look at areas that need improvement and make an immediate plan to change them. This process should be devoid of emotion. You are simply looking daily at strengths and areas that need improvement. This process is also an excellent prelude to evaluation by the instructor or floor personnel. It is helpful to have the "mind set" that you and the others are critiquing your work to help you be the best possible nurse. If you are accustomed to critiquing yourself, you will be able to be more objective with regard to the comments offered to you by the instructor and others. The following ideas will help you with this process.

1. Remind yourself that this is not an attack on you as a person. Evaluation is meant to look at performance and how to improve it.

2. Consider the information unemotionally, as though it applied to someone else. Evaluate whether it is a valid criticism. If so, ask for suggestions for improvement or offer suggestions of your own. If the error is skill related, ask your instructor for a demonstration. Practice until you do it right. Ask to perform a return demonstration.

3. If the information is based on miscommunication, offer a brief statement of explanation. Be careful not to get on an emotional roller coaster. If the error is yours, avoid over-apologizing. This simply makes it more difficult for all involved to cope. The important issue is the plan of action. Take the blame and go on to other things. Feeling guilty takes energy away from the solution and creates a new problem.

There is an interesting phenomenon that is still a factor in accepting criticism. In our society more males continue to be involved in team sports. They have been conditioned to having their behavior corrected by the team's coach. With this upbringing, many males learn early to separate their personal selves from their actions, which is a preparation for criticism on the job. They listen, make an adjustment, and go on. Some females continue to focus on being liked by others and often receive feedback on their external selves: looks, clothes, and so on. They equate criticism with "You do not like me" (the person) as opposed to "You do not like what I did" (the action).

Fifth is the issue of compliments. Do you accept a compliment by saying "thank you" and allowing yourself to believe it? Do you quickly neutralize the compliment by pointing out your shortcomings? Did it even occur to you that you are insulting the person offering the compliment by not accepting it? You are, as a matter of fact, telling that individual that he is "dumb" in regard to the observation he has made.

Sixth, deal directly with what you fear. The usual outcome is that the issue is not as great as you imagined it to be. Even if the result is not ideal, give yourself ample credit for having dealt with your fear directly. If you have decided to confront someone directly, remember to use "I"-centered statements denoting that you take responsibility for what you are saying. Take responsibility for your side of the conversation only.

Correct: "I feel angry when you criticize me in front of the other students."

Incorrect: "You make me angry when you criticize me in front of the other students" (gives responsibility and power for your personal feelings to the other person). "Maybe you were not aware of doing this" (offers an excuse for the other person's behavior and takes responsibility for both parties involved).

It is also sometimes helpful to imagine the worst possible thing that could happen, in an exaggerated sense, before you take action. For example: "If I tell the instructor I am angry, she might hit me. Then I will have to press charges. She will go to jail, there will be no one to complete the rotation, so I will flunk it, and the other students will be angry with me and picket my house. . . ," etc.

Seventh, learn from someone who is confident and whom you admire. Look at how this person deals with situations. Listen to the tone of voice and observe the body language. Practice techniques that have already been shown to be successful. Approach the individual and ask for tips on how to develop confidence. You have just paid him or her a sincere compliment. Most individuals will be willing to offer information to you. Pick and choose what will work for you.

Table 9–1
How To Build Confidence

1. Study to gain a strong knowledge base
2. Seek clinical experiences
3. Deal with negative feelings that hold you back
4. Learn to deal with criticism
5. Accept compliments graciously
6. Deal with your fears directly
7. Learn by watching confident people
8. Keep your self-talk constructive

Finally, monitor your self-talk. Imagine succeeding in advance. Learn from errors, but do not dwell on them—save your energy for solutions.

▼▼▼
Getting Along

Management continues to spend approximately a full month per year on the problems of employees who do not get along with each other. Consider the losses that occur in productivity, money, and, of course, personal satisfaction and happiness in the workplace.

The four characteristics that influence personal attitude are also the essential ingredients for getting along with others. *Optimism* permits you to see the positive side of yourself and others. Optimistic individuals know that there are alternatives for dealing with current challenges. They use their energy to solve problems. These individuals spend little or no time and energy at the complaint counter.

Motivation provides the impetus for commitment to worthwhile goals. Motivated persons put out their best effort daily. They do their own work and work with others at common worthwhile goals. The bottom line in nursing is the achievement of excellence in client care. They are willing to learn new tasks and are not imprisoned by their own fears.

Discipline provides the internal control to do whatever is necessary to function effectively and to stay current within the field. It also provides the push to deal with issues that arise in the work setting. Unresolved personal issues with peers limit effectiveness and cooperation with others. Discipline also provides the strength to change personal negative self-talk into positive affirmations. How you feel about yourself is reflected in the way you treat others.

Confidence reduces anxiety in those around you, at a peer level and as the one in charge. Confidence says, "I am in charge of me. I do my best at all times. I learn from my errors and go on even stronger on the inside than before." Confident persons are not defensive. They are capable of listening to those they work with and accept critiquing from others. They feel the responsibility to provide feedback to others regarding their client care. Client care becomes, collectively, "our business." Confident individuals are willing to compromise on issues that do not affect the quality of care. They treat others in the same manner they wish to be treated. It is well to remember that confidence is earned, not learned. No one can decree, "Go out and be confident."

Getting Along

Characteristics	How Do I Rate?
1. Optimism	
2. Motivation	
3. Discipline	
4. Confidence	

▼▼▼
Summary

Maslow's human needs theory provides a way to look at our personal needs and how they influence our personality. You are the most powerful force in the continuing development of your personality. Self-talk must be constantly monitored. You become what you imagine you are. Old images cannot be erased, but they can be replaced by new images through positive affirmations.

Knowledge is the key that unlocks a career door. Attitude is the key to success. Characteristics that result in a positive attitude are optimism, motivation, discipline, and confidence. These in turn provide the total package for getting along with others, which is considered a major problem in the workplace.

Walk the walk (i.e., do what you say you will do).

Live up to your promises. Remember to do the little things well. Permit your positive attitude to be translated into action. This is how your personality adds to the total personality of your workplace.

▼▼▼ *R E F E R E N C E S*

Maslow A. A theory of human motivation. Psychol Rev 1943; 50:370.

Frankl V. *An Evening with Victor Frankl.* Milwaukee, WI: Mount Mary College, March 1984.

▼▼▼ *B I B L I O G R A P H Y*

Chopra D. *Quantum Healing.* New York: Bantam Books, 1990.

Chopra D. *Unconditional Life.* New York: Bantam Books, 1992.

Personal Selling Power. 1995; 15(3):14-21, 73–75.

Wellness and Self-Care

CHAPTER 10

▼▼▼ *O U T L I N E*

The Image You Project

Wellness as a Choice and a Responsibility

   Preventing Muscle Injury: Planned Moving

Good Nutrition: Fuel for Your Machine

How to Stay Alive in Nursing: Stress Management

Relaxation Through Meditation

▼▼▼ *K E Y   T E R M S*

accumulative exercise

"colonies"

fat gram budget

personal image

serving sizes

stress management

walk the walk

wellness a choice

willing victim

▼▼▼ *O B J E C T I V E S*

Upon completing this chapter you will be able to:

1. Evaluate your own level of wellness and personal care in regard to:

a. The image you project
b. Present choices regarding wellness
c. Preventing muscle injury
d. Nutrition
e. Stress management

2. Modify present wellness and self-care practices to make the most of what you are and can be.

As a nurse you will model wellness and personal care for your client. The image you project sends a far more powerful message than anything you can attempt to teach verbally. In nursing it is not sufficient to tell the client, "Do not do as I do; do as I say." In nursing, it is important to "walk the walk."

> *What is the relation between the nurse's level of wellness and personal care and the client's willingness to follow postdischarge care directions?*

Consider how you as a client would react to being taken care of by the following nurses:

▶ A nurse who refuses to follow the dress code and looks as if she were put together by a committee
▶ A nurse who smells of last night's gastronomical adventure—garlic bread, and its accompaniments
▶ A nurse with stained hands that smell of tobacco, as does his breath
▶ An overweight nurse who comes in to give directions for a weight-reduction diet
▶ A "high-strung" nurse who cannot cope with the demands of the job and is there to talk to you about stress management
▶ A nurse who helps the client in the next bed but does not wash her hands before she continues with your care

What are some other examples of incongruous nursing behavior?

▼▼▼
The Image You Project

It was the first day of hands-on patient care. Basic nursing lab simulations and demonstrations on each other were over. Professional image had been discussed as part of the personal and vocational issues class.

From a distance it looked as if Martha had followed the guidelines suggested by her instructor; she

▶ was neat and clean
▶ wore a clean, well-fitting uniform
▶ wore long hair pulled back and secured

▶ had nails short and unpolished
▶ wore make-up lightly and tastefully applied
▶ wore small post earrings
▶ and wore a plain band ring and a
▶ watch

As Martha approached, the smell arrived before she did. It was "an exotic oil perfume, a gift from my husband. I always wear a drop or two daily to remind me of him. Why, no one else can even smell it." That was Martha's comment when the instructor asked her not to wear it during her clinical practice with clients.

1. Why is Martha unaware of how overpowering her perfume is?
2. What do you anticipate would be the client's reaction?

▶ Clue A. The client is confined to bed
▶ Clue B. He needs total care this morning
▶ Clue C. His sense of smell is intact
▶ Clue D. He is a nonsmoker
▶ Clue E. He is nonverbal because of a stroke

3. Explain how the clues are connected and how they affect the client's reaction. What did you learn in your Body Structure and Function course about the sense of smell?
4. Would it be possible for a client to have the same reaction to a male nurse's aftershave or to a tobacco smell on a nurse who smokes?

A daily bath and shampoo have a twofold purpose: to minimize transfer of "souvenir illnesses" to yourself and those you live with and to wash away body odors accumulated during the work day. Ideally, bathing takes place shortly after you arrive home, although this is not possible for some of you. At the very least, change shoes and get into "home" clothes. Put the uniform into the wash. Wash your hands thoroughly before tackling home responsibilities.

1. Why are your shoes a source of concern?
2. Why do some work places provide a place for you to leave your shoes and shoe polish?
3. Should you change into a fresh uniform and pair of shoes if you are going from your clinical position to a job at another agency?

Underarm deodorants and antiperspirants are not the same. Deodorants neutralize odors; antiperspirants prevent sweating. The choice should be based on your needs and skin sensitivity. If you have difficulty finding an effective deodorant or antiperspirant, talk directly to a pharmacist and request a special substance made up just for you.

Some of you may experience unpleasant, although normal, all-over body odor, even though you bathe daily. Talk with your physician because there are chlorophyll-based tablets that can be prescribed for this. Most of you do not have to seek these additional solutions. Those who do need to know that alternatives to embarrassment do exist. Sometimes the offending article is a piece of clothing that you are wearing. Material retains body odor even after it has been washed and releases the odor when the article becomes warm and moist when worn. This statement is generally limited to synthetic fabrics that do not have a soil-release component built in. In this case, when special soaps or a vinegar-and-water soak have not solved the problem, you may have to plan a proper burial for the uniform. Before you bury it, try investing in underarm shields. These are hard to find but do exist (e.g., at The Vermont Country Store, P.O. Box 3000, Manchester Ctr., VT 05255-3000). Underarm shields also prevent yellow stains. Try spraying the armpit area of clothes with a prewash solution before laundering it each time. Spray the underarm shields also.

Brushing the teeth after meals solves part of the problem of bad breath. Once a day, teeth must be flossed as taught by a dental hygienist. Bridges and partial bridges must be cleaned. The tongue, roof of the mouth, and insides of the cheeks need to be brushed gently with a clean, soft brush and water. Never mind the gagging when doing the tongue. The white coating that accumulates when you do not brush the tongue becomes a hidden source of halitosis. Unfortunately, mouthwash, mints, and gum are frequently used to mask the odor. This is a temporary solution at best. Daily brushing and flossing will also help to prevent future gum disease.

Dirt under the fingernails and in tiny scratches in the nailpolish are remarkable ways of transporting germs to your sandwich, your mouth, your eyes, your mate, your children, and your dinner salad. Actually, this list should start with the first client, the next client, and so on throughout the day. This is the reason nursing instructors discourage the use of any nail polish, expect you to have short nails, and are such terrors about proper handwashing, which consists of running water, soap, and friction. In some nursing programs, students have the opportunity to culture the material from their nails; they are often surprised at the variety of "colonies" that grow from their "clean nails." Examples of cultured organisms include *Staphylococcus aureus, S. epidermidis, Escherichia coli,* and *Clostridium perfringens.* The organisms involved depend on what the nurse has touched in the course of the day.

> *Where do your "fingers do the walking" during the day? Track the movements of your fingers for one day.*

Some nurses try to make a statement with their hair styles. It is suggested that they wear it up and off the face if it is long. This provides the neat appearance desired by clients and management. There is a hygienic reason for having clean, well-behaved hair. Visualize leaning over a portion of the client's anatomy to change a dressing, insert a catheter, or irrigate a wound. As you lean over, so does your hair. It is like shaking a rug lightly. Whatever is on it falls off. This provides another source of contamination for the client. Furthermore, if you reach up to push your hair back with your hand or do the "whiplash special," you have further increased the chances of contamination.

What about the uniform itself? Some agencies no longer require a white uniform and cap. But they all have a dress code. Adhere to it. A nurse of many years recently noted that she continues to wear her entire uniform, including the cap, and rarely has a client refused any medication, treatment, or direction. "It's a trick, I suppose. So easy. So pleasant. I am greeted with, 'Oh, here comes the nurse,' and a smile." Whatever your dress code, keep in mind, as you dress for the day, that a client—vulnerable, worried, and often in pain—has to look at you and view you as being believable and in charge. The "put-together-by-a-committee" look does not provide that comforting image for the client.

Clingy, skimpy, suggestive garments may provide a topic of conversation and an impetus for inappropriate acting out on the part of the client. This brings to mind the nurse who often wore mini-dresses with fruit prints on them to work and then complained angrily when a confused and disoriented client kept trying to "pick the apples" off her "tree." Think easy care and a professional look. When shopping for items to wear, bend over, stretch, kneel, and crush the fabric in your hand. Go through the motions to which the garment will be subjected. A blend of natural and synthetic fibers is often desirable. For example, a blend of cotton and polyester will provide the comfort of cotton because it breathes and the ease of washing and little or no ironing because of the polyester.

Although undergarments are not meant to be seen, they sometimes are because of the wearer's choice of color and style. Clients and other staff often discover, but will not tell, when they have seen your colorful undergarments when you bend at the knees to pick up an item from the floor. This statement applies to both male and female nurses. Interestingly, beige, not white, is the best choice of color for undergarments beneath a white dress, skirt, or trousers for light-skinned individuals. Many dark-skinned individuals choose black or brown underwear beneath a white dress, skirt, or trousers.

Shoes are the most important investment of all. Invest in a well-fitting pair of leather walking shoes. Your back, legs, feet, and whole body will thank you. If your feet perspire readily, have the shoemaker punch a hole in the instep area. This is an old trick that is good for the shoes and the feet. Perhaps you have already noticed an interesting phenomenon in some nurses of both sexes. They look sharp, and then you notice, from the knees or ankles on down, the rumpled socks, odd-colored hose, or booties with pom-poms in dirty, rundown shoes. The whole effect is destroyed for the client. A nursing student with older, but supple white leather shoes offered information on how to keep the leather from cracking and the color fresh: "I use mink oil periodically to keep the leather soft and polish them at least every other work day. I also bought an extra pair of shoelaces right away. Then I have one to wash and one to wear."

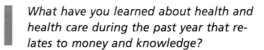

Wellness as a Choice and a Responsibility

A cartoon once showed two people jogging. One asked the other, "How is your health?" The other responded, "I don't know; I'll have to ask my doctor." This not-so-funny cartoon depicts an all-too-common attitude toward wellness. Wellness is something out there; it is out of one's personal control and is the responsibility of someone else. The "someone else" is usually a physician who is looked on as having magical solutions when something goes wrong. Please note that most visits to the doctor are focused on illness, not wellness. The focus is now gradually shifting to include wellness and chronic disease prevention. The shift is driven by two major factors: *money* and *knowledge.*

> *What have you learned about health and health care during the past year that relates to money and knowledge?*

Illness prevention alternatives are being included as a part of total care. This is where personal responsibility and choice come in. You are invited to be a full partner in the process of keeping well.

Research continues to show that life style is responsible for 51% of the deaths due to major chronic diseases (Fig. 10–1).

Life style includes personal behaviors that can be modified such as physical activity, nutrition, stress management, smoking, alcohol consumption, and so on. Can this mean that most of us can no longer hold our genes, environment, and health care solely responsible for our personal health? Hmm. . . .

Consider for a moment how you care for a prized possession. Very carefully! For some of you, this is a car. If you care for it lovingly, you keep up a continual maintenance program to keep it operating at peak performance. This program also helps to avoid costly repair bills. It should be no different with your health. Once you decide that wellness (continual maintenance) is a responsibility and a choice, you can design

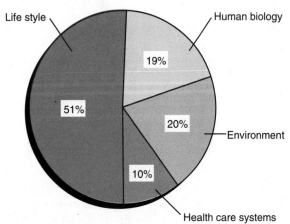

Figure 10–1
Causes of death due to major chronic diseases.
(Based on data from the Centers for Disease
Control and Prevention.)

a life style that will help you maintain your highest
potential for personal health. Wellness does not mean
a lack of imperfection; you can achieve wellness with
a physical handicap or even a chronic condition. What

it does mean is making the most of what you have and
can be.

▽▽▽
Preventing Muscle Injury: Planned Moving

Preventing muscle injury is only one benefit of regular
physical activity. It makes you *feel* better, *look* better, and
work better. Fill in the quiz and test your knowledge
about physical activity.

Plan A

Applaud yourself if aerobic exercise such as jogging,
walking, or swimming is a regular part of your personal
maintenance. Such exercise, which increases the car-
diac and respiratory rate for a period of time, increases
oxygenation and blood circulation to all parts of the
body. If this kind of exercise is already an established
part of your life, stay with it. If you are interested in
beginning regular aerobic exercise and cannot decide

Directions: Check all the statements that are true about physical activity.
1. Feel better

_____ reduces stress   _____ improves sleep

_____ fights anxiety   _____ reduces tension

_____ boosts energy   _____ promotes relaxation

_____ fights depression   _____ improves self-image

_____ reduces the risk of many chronic diseases or conditions such as heart disease, some cancers, diabetes,
stroke, high blood pressure, high blood cholesterol, and obesity
2. Look better

_____ tones muscles

_____ burns more calories: useful for losing or stabilizing weight

_____ helps control appetite

3. Work better

_____ builds strength

_____ increases stamina

_____ helps heart and lungs work better

Answers: All statements are true.

which one to choose, choose walking. If you have a chronic disease or orthopedic condition, call your doctor to see if there are any reasons to be cautious. Chances are that because you passed your preadmission physical exam, you can enjoy the healthful yet inexpensive benefits provided by walking.

Walking is suited for people who consider themselves unathletic and out of shape. It is also effective in improving and maintaining fitness in well-conditioned people. Pain is not considered a gain. Aerobic exercise is based on increasing your heartbeat to its target rate for a sustained period of time. The target heart rate is calculated by using the following formula: $220 - \text{age} \times 70\%$. Periodically check your rate by counting your heart rate for 6 seconds and adding a zero. If you do not have a watch, you know that you are close to the correct target heart rate if you can continue to converse and break into a light sweat. Aim to walk 12 miles a week, and gradually increase your speed until you are walking a mile in 15 to 16 minutes. Walking three miles per day four times a week or walking briskly approximately 45 minutes per day four times a week, excluding warm-up and cool-down, is recommended for cardiovascular benefit. Warm-up includes 5 to 10 minutes of lighter-paced walking to increase your heart rate and body temperature gradually. Cool-down follows your brisk walking. A lighter pace for 5 to 10 minutes decreases your heart rate and prevents blood from pooling in your legs.

The major investment needed for walking is a good pair of walking shoes. Cold muscles are subject to injury. You can begin a bit more slowly and gradually work up to the speed needed to attain the desired pulse rate. Instead, you can do gentle stretching exercises at both the beginning and the end of the walk. Stretching exercises at the end are a must because the muscles, ligaments, and tendons along the back of the legs tighten up during walking.

The key to walking is to be gentle and easy—no bouncing. Plan how to fit walking into your day so that it does not become "just one more thing to do." Some of you will be able to use this exercise as your mode of transportation to work, to run errands, to spend special time with a significant other, to review class information, or to relieve tension after school. Consider your needs.

Plan B

However, if you are among the two out of three of us who are not participating in any aerobic activity—pay attention! The current recommendations for *moderate* physical activity are doable. Researchers looked at what was happening to the heart when we were not able to perform the ideal amount of exercise. They learned that if we do some exercise every day we will be in better health than if we did none (Centers for Disease Control and Prevention, 1994).

 Every adult should accumulate 30 minutes or more of moderate physical activity during most days of the week.

See Table 10–1 for additional information.

A major concern in nursing is the frequency of muscle injuries, especially back injuries. Interestingly, the issue is that of flexibility, not strength. Think of

Table 10–1 Recommendations for Moderate Exercise	
Key Phrase	**What It Means**
Accumulate 30 minutes or more	You get just as much benefit from breaking the 30 minutes up as you do from 30 minutes of continuous exercise
Moderate physical activity	Almost anything as long as you are physically moving. Examples: walking, dancing, playing catch with the kids, gardening, raking, housecleaning. You get the idea!
Over most days	Try to do something every day. If you miss a day or two, don't worry.

From Minnesota Department of Health, 1995. Based on data from the Centers for Disease Control and Prevention, American College of Sports Medicine, in cooperation with the President's Council on Fitness and Sports, 1994.

people whom you consider strong who have been injured because of twisting, bending, or other movements common in nursing. Keeping your muscles flexible is another nursing (and personal) responsibility for you. There is a tendency to skip this responsibility because it is not as obvious initially as your external image. Because it is part of your internal conditioning (and image), there is also a tendency to relate it to such words as willpower or character. This is an issue of keeping your "equipment" ready to use.

A Wisconsin nursing home instituted a stretching program for all care givers at the beginning of each shift. As a result, there were no back injuries for one year. Their insurance company recognized the nursing home for this innovative successful program, which continues today.

Stretching begins at the start of each day and may be necessary periodically throughout the day. It is often the last thing to be done before going to sleep. When you awaken, think "cat." Think about the leisurely stretching process that a cat goes through on awakening. Help those sleepy muscles get ready for the day before you get out of bed. Because nursing involves an additional strain on the back, include some back stretches. Be reasonable in deciding which stretches to do and how often to repeat them. If your initial efforts are too ambitious, chances are you will skip all stretching exercises on the days you feel rushed. Think in terms of a lifelong, manageable routine. And be gentle. Listen to your body. Pain is not gain. Increase repetitions gradually to the number that leaves your muscles feeling alive and ready to face the day.

The bathtub is a wonderful place to relax, especially when there is sufficient warm water and time. Take advantage of the time to stretch the ankles, toes, wrists, and fingers. Make up your own gentle movements. Your feet hold you up all day and obey your commands. Gently massage each foot lovingly and thoroughly. Be aware of any areas that need special care.

What about using the time spent sitting in the classroom? This consumes a major part of some of your days. Here are some ideas for exercises to be done near class time:

▶ Parking lot jaunt—Disappointed not to find a parking place close by? Don't be. In fact, plan to

give yourself five extra minutes and deliberately park farther away. Enjoy a walk to the building
▶ Stairway caper—Unless there is a medical or safety reason not to, choose the stairs over the elevator (or a combination at first, if many flights are involved). Remember to come to class prepared with walking shoes

If there is some television time scheduled during the day, remember that this is a good time to perform stretches of your choice. Young children like to be included, and it models self-care for them.

> **Which stretching exercises are needed and possible as part of your day? Make up a plan that you can begin today.**

▼▼▼ Good Nutrition: Fuel For Your Machine

Here is an interesting dilemma: Nurses receive specific instruction about nutritional needs and yet often have incredibly poor personal eating habits. To which of the following can you relate?

▶ Coffee and a cigarette for breakfast (or for coffee break or lunch)
▶ Over-the-counter diet pills for a quick weight-loss diet
▶ Soda and chips for lunch
▶ Sweet roll and coffee for breakfast
▶ Coffee at the desk and when passing out medications

If you have become a nutritional dropout, get back into good eating patterns by using your head. This (like your daily stretching routine) is important enough to follow through without anyone else's prompting. Continuing a balanced nutritional pattern of eating is more a matter of structure and routine than a test of your character. Pull out a nutrition textbook and look at it from a personal perspective. Recommended food servings have been modified as part of the United States Department of Agriculture (USDA) 1996 Dietary Guidelines. Changes focus on (1) increasing the amounts of fruits, vegetables, grains, and complex carbohydrates, (2) increasing foods higher in fiber, (3) decreasing foods high in fat, especially saturated fats and cholesterol, and (4) limiting (not eliminating) consumption of "goodies" to once in a while.

Research supports the notion that what you eat can reduce your risk of developing chronic diseases including some cancers and cardiovascular diseases. A novel useful slogan: Fight chronic disease with your fork! Figure 10–2 provides a down-to-earth look at current recommendations.

This may sound like a lifetime of boredom with meals, but what it actually suggests is moderation. Put more emphasis on some foods than others. There is no reason to deprive yourself completely of foods that you especially like. Moderation suggests control of the amount you consume and certain "trade-offs," depending on your choices throughout the day. Varying the foods you eat decreases boredom and may open the door to some adventures in eating. In this way, you combine current foods with newer foods that you introduce gradually. Incidentally, do not be fooled by the word "natural" on a label; read the new Food and Drug Association (FDA) product labels to find the actual composition of a product.

By now you may be saying, "Just give me some basics to begin with and forget the hype. I am so busy with school and the rest of my life." No problem.

Breakfast literally means to "break the fast" of your night. It is without doubt the most vital meal of the day. Although breakfast is traditionally thought of as the morning meal, it is really your first meal when you awaken. Depending on what shift you work, someone else's dinnertime may be your breakfast. Plan accordingly. The trendy thing in recent years has been to skip breakfast and settle for a cup of coffee. A vitamin- and mineral-packed substitute in easy-to-manage containers is fresh or canned fruit.

Take along additional fruit to enjoy during break time. During lunch and dinner you will be able to enjoy heavier fare that includes vegetables, starches, and proteins. If you are trying to maintain your weight as opposed to gaining weight, plan to stop eating after 8 PM (or your shift equivalent). This will give your digestive system time to do its assigned task in an uninterrupted fashion. Chances are that you will sleep better. If you still need your coffee, drink it at a nonmeal time.

If you need to lose or stabilize your weight, *diets are out.* Modify your eating habits starting one priority food group at a time. Let modifications become a part of your healthy life style. In turn, it becomes easier to model this behavior for your patients.

1. Plan to lose weight slowly; forget the crash and burn method.

2. Eat more fruits and vegetables including dried peas, beans and lentils, and whole grain products, which are high in nutrients and fiber. The fiber keeps things moving through your digestive system. Some experts recommend at least 20 grams of fiber per day.

3. Track your fat grams. Although calories continue to be important, most people will lose weight by staying within their "fat gram budget" (Table 10–2). The following table is based on averages. Your fat gram budget may vary according to your body weight, activity level, age, and personal health. As always, check with your health provider for additional information.

4. Maintain moderate physical activity. The combination of some food in your stomach and moderate physical activity helps to jump-start your metabolism.

5. Watch those serving sizes. The increase in serving sizes offered at restaurants has provided a false sense of approval. Choose the small muffin or eat half and save the rest for later. Choose the regular hamburger, and so on.

6. Choose snacks with care. Roberts, a registered dietician at Brigham and Women's Hospital, Boston (1992) suggests the following:

▶ Cereal: (except granola) dry or with skim milk any time of the day
▶ Bagels: almost no fat
▶ Fudgesicles: chocolate flavor without the fat. Each contains about 100 calories each, or 35 calories for the diet version
▶ Hershey's chocolate syrup: made from cocoa powder, little fat. Blend with skim milk and ice cubes for a shake or serve over low fat ice-milk for a sundae
▶ Soft pretzels: almost no fat; look in the freezer section

Eat Wisely – Live Well!

 Help yourself to 3-5 servings from the vegetable group and 2-4 servings from the fruit group daily.

Serving size:	VEGETABLE	FRUIT
	1 cup raw leafy	1 med. orange, apple or banana
	½ cup other: cooked, chopped or raw	½ cup chopped, cooked or canned
	¾ cup juice	

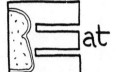 **E**at 6-11 servings from the grain group.

Serving size: 1 slice whole grain bread   1 small muffin, roll or tortilla
½ English muffin or bagel   1 ounce dry cereal
½ cup cooked rice, cereal or pasta

Alcohol beverages supply calories but few or no nutrients. If adults choose to drink, do so in moderation. Moderation is no more than one drink per day for women. No more than two drinks per day for men.

Serving size: 12 ounces of regular beer or 5 ounces of wine or
1.5 ounces 80-proof distilled spirits

Limit your use of fats, oils, sugar and sodium-containing foods--use sparingly.

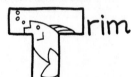 **T**rim fat by eating 2-3 servings from the meat and beans group.

Serving size: 2-3 ounces cooked lean meat, poultry or fish
½ cup cooked dry beans, 1 egg or 2 tablespoons peanut
butter count as 1 ounce of lean meat

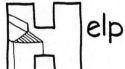 **H**elp yourself to 2-3 servings of low-fat dairy products daily.

Serving size: 1 cup milk or yogurt
1½ ounces natural cheese
2 ounces processed cheese

Children under 2 years should not eat a low-fat diet. Pregnant or breast-feeding women and people with a medical condition should see their health professional for diet information (DHHS and USDA, 1996).

Figure 10–2.

Healthy nutritional choices. (From *Our Nutrition Position.* Two Harbors, MN: Lake County HealthWise Coalition, 1996.)

Table 10–2 Fat Gram Budget			
Women		Men	
Height	Fat Gram Budget	Height	Fat Gram Budget
<5'6"	55 grams or less	<5'10"	70 grams or less
5'6"–6'	65 grams or less	5'10"–6'	75 grams or less
>6'	75 grams or less	>6'	85 grams or less

▶ Pizza: ask for *little* cheese, lots of mushrooms, peppers, and onions. High in calcium and vitamins A, B-complex, and C

1. **List two fruits or vegetables that contain both vitamins A and C.**

   _____   _____

2. **List two vegetables that are a "three star" vegetable (i.e., they contain vitamins A and C and belong to the cabbage family).**

   _____   _____

Clue: Look in your nutrition book.

▼▼▼
How To Stay Alive In Nursing: Stress Management

Client care can be stressful for the nurse. Patients can be demanding and press for answers that you do not have. All clients experience some degree of regression in their behavior during their illness. Some clients are able to express their needs directly. Others express their needs indirectly, through irritability or criticism of your performance. Some clients do not respond to treatment and continue to deteriorate.

Frequently, life and death issues are at stake. Lack of cooperation by the client and his family may cause you to feel angry and frustrated. You may be tempted to blame the client for making you feel helpless and for the client's lack of improvement. Clients may challenge the care they receive and the knowledge base of involved staff members. Family members may call and visit continuously because of concern, lack of understanding, and feelings of helplessness.

Differentiating between feelings of sympathy and empathy in regard to the client is a major consideration in preventing burnout. Empathy is a respectful detached concern. When you empathize, you understand what the client is experiencing but do not experience the emotion with him. Sympathy leaves you vulnerable to identifying with the client and experiencing the emotion as the client experiences it. Consequently, you are no longer in control of the situation and have limited value to the client. A long-term sympathetic response is very stressful. What started out as a caring relationship becomes detrimental to the client and to you because of overinvolvement.

You as a nurse function as a member of an interdisciplinary team. Communication and cooperation are needed to accomplish the very best care for each client. Remember that focus. The focus must be on what is best for the client. If energy is focused primarily on self, there is a limited amount left for the client. If you find yourself saying, "I am shy, I am bashful, I have an inferiority complex," you need to be reminded that this is not synonymous with humility. It is synonymous with conceit. Do something about it.

Mutual trust of a coworker begins with you. This does not mean that you will not be hurt occasionally by those who violate this trust. In a disagreement with a coworker, if you back off in a *passive* way (as opposed to cooling-off time), you may become the willing victim for future attacks. Replying in an *aggressive* way will probably result in a power struggle, and *this* can lead to additional direct or indirect ways of seeking revenge on you. *Manipulation,* or using indirect means to get an individual to behave differently, is encouraged in some cultures. Other cultures encourage dealing directly with the person with regard to the issue at hand. Some basic rules for an *assertive* approach toward a difficult person include: (1) Stand up for yourself; otherwise you will be ignored. (2) Do not worry about being rude. If the other person is interrupting, tell him or her, then keep on talking. (3) Get the individual to sit down. Most people are less aggressive when sitting down. (4) Use I-centered statements. Express how *you* think and feel about the situation. (5) Avoid an all-out fight. Your purpose is to function more effectively. (6) Be ready to be friendly. Once you stand up to a difficult person, the offer is usually genuine.

It is our reaction to a situation rather than the situation itself that causes stress. Everything that happens to you, either pleasant or unpleasant, creates stress. Interpretation of stress as distress or as negative stress depends on one's personal problem-solving skills and the intensity and duration of the situations involved. Ironically, a time of boredom and understimulation is accompanied by high adrenaline levels in the body, as is a time of high stress. In other words, individuals seem to do best with a moderate amount of stress in their lives. What is defined as moderate stress varies from person to person.

Consider, too, that "stress" has become a buzzword for a specific problem. The word seems to explain everything and nothing. Listen and you will hear school children saying "I'm so stressed." Perhaps they and we need to identify more specifically the feeling that is being experienced. Is it anger, fear, sadness, or something else? The next time you think "stress," name the emotion you are experiencing. This may be the first step to finding a solution.

Although work is necessarily commendable and personally satisfying, it is only one part of your life. Recreation is also important and must be a part of your plan for living. Otherwise, it is too easy to brush it aside "because I have too much work to do." The ultimate choice in recreation may not be available to you consistently, but short-term recreational activities are available.

What kinds of recreation do you enjoy? List two that consume a longer time to accomplish and four recreational activities that can be accomplished in a short amount of time or on a continuing basis.

_____

_____

_____

_____

_____

As you look at the answer to the above question, remember that some forms of recreation may be high-stress activities for you. Recreation is not the same as relaxation. Rethink your list and choose one or two short-term recreational activities that you can involve yourself in on an ongoing basis without causing distress in your life. There will be times when you can treat yourself to longer-term recreational activities if you think it through—maybe 9 holes of golf instead of 18. Read your favorite author's work during breaks, while waiting for appointments, at stoplights, on trains, or in the bathtub. Use your imagination.

Relaxation training is one way to manage stress. During a relaxed state, the pulse and respiratory rates decrease, the metabolic rate and blood pressure decline, and muscular tension decreases. Along with the positive physical changes experienced by all except about 3% of the population, there is also a sense of well-being. If you are part of that 3%, there is nothing wrong with you. **It just is.** Think about what activities bring about the physical changes described above for you. For example, one student confided that relaxation exercises made her "ready to climb the walls," whereas rock-and-roll music had a calming effect on her. She insisted on listening to rock-and-roll during the birth of her child.

Many relaxation methods are available and should be tailored to your life style. Decide on a regular practice time. Some of you will want to start your day with a relaxation exercise, and some of you will end your day this way. Because of the stimulant effect of food on the body, relaxation is accomplished most readily before meals or at least two hours after a meal. Caffeine-containing drinks, such as regular coffee and some soft drinks, are best avoided prior to the training session.

Meditation

Ingredients:

> A quiet environment
> A mental device (a word, sound, phrase, or gazing at an object)
> A passive attitude
> A comfortable position

Directions:

Sit quietly in a comfortable position with your eyes closed (or open, if gazing).

Let your muscles relax, beginning at your feet and progressing up to your face.

Breathe through your nose as you breathe out.

Repeat the mental device (or continue to gaze at an object).

For example: Breathe in . . . out . . . (mental device). Eyes may be opened as desired to check the time; simply close your eyes when satisfied, and return to repeating the mental device. Do not worry about being successful. Let distractive thoughts pass through. Simply return to repeating the mental device. In . . . out . . . (mental device). In . . . out . . . (mental device) (based on Benson, 1976, pp. 159–161).

▽▽▽
Relaxation Through Meditation

Meditation is a centuries-old technique that has been repopularized in the United States in the last two decades as an aid to relaxation. Find a quiet spot and follow the directions in the box. A quiet environment helps to eliminate distractions and permits you to concentrate on a mental device of your choosing. A mental device is any sound, word, or phrase that evokes a sense of calm. You repeat the device silently or out loud with your eyes closed. If you prefer to keep your eyes open, you can fix your gaze on an object. Either way, your mind is focusing on one thing. Concentrating on your normal breathing pattern also enhances your repetition of the mental device. A passive attitude is considered most significant for eliciting a successful relaxation response.

Distracting thoughts may occur. Simply let them pass through, and return to the repetition of the mental device. Trying hard usually creates tension. A comfortable position prevents added muscular tension. Sit in a position with good posture, wearing loose-fitting clothes with the shoes off, and the feet on the floor. Lying down is not encouraged because you tend to fall asleep. Benson (1995) suggests that for those who jog, meditation can be part of it. Focus on the cadence of your feet—left, right, left, right—rather than on repetition of a word. Those who use the relaxation response often reach the high point during the first or second mile.

Imagery is another way of relaxing yourself. This kind of imagery is not the guided imagery that is used in psychotherapy and that requires a trained psychotherapist to deal with the symbolic material that may emerge. Some of you are better at imagining than others. Some may see only shadowy figures, whereas others see vivid, technicolor images. Images need not be particularly vivid to be effective. Mental pictures do seem to come more easily when you are relaxed and free of distractions. Begin with a relaxation exercise. If you are very tense, progressive relaxation will be helpful.

Once relaxed, follow with the imagery. Two or three deep breaths are helpful prior to beginning the imagery. In practicing the imagery, it is important to take sufficient time to include enough detail so that you can "get into" the imagery. When ready to conclude the imagery, count from 1 to 10, sit for a while with your eyes closed, open your eyes, and then stretch.

It is worthwhile to remember that if you experience anxiety at any time during the imagery, you need only open your eyes, look around, reorient yourself to your surroundings, and, when satisfied, close your eyes and continue with the imagery. Some of you will be comfortable with your eyes open during the entire process and do not seem to have any problems visualizing. Imagery, like other techniques, takes self-discipline. Daily practice sessions are suggested.

Imagery is an excellent way of learning to relax. Once learned, imagery can be done in less-structured settings, such as during break time. It is also a way of protecting yourself against stressful situations that you may face in the future, by visualizing the situation and how you will move through it successfully. Imagery is also creative and fun. You already do it; you did so before embarking on your present career. What you will learn now is a more controlled way of using imagery.

Imagery: Relieving Anxiety

Design your own favorite place. Whatever is your idea of complete peace, harmony, and joy will do. See yourself, appropriately dressed, in the setting you have created. Take time to look around and visualize your surroundings in great detail. Use all of your senses to experience the sight, sound, smell, touch, and taste available in your special hideaway. See yourself staying there and feeling peaceful and calm. Remember that it is a safe place and that you can return there to rest daily. When you are ready to leave, take one look back, knowing that you can return any time. You will continue to feel relaxed and happy as you return to your daily activities.

Progressive relaxation is a method of tensing and relaxing all of the muscle groups in order, resulting in deep relaxation. The order of relaxation—from head to toes or from toes to head—is a personal choice. Either is effective. If the intent is to fall asleep, then lying down is the position of choice. Otherwise, the general rules for all relaxation techniques can be followed. Sometimes progressive relaxation is enhanced by taped (or natural) sound such as the wind or seashore sounds or by music that is close to body rhythm, such as certain Bach selections, Pachelbel's Canon in D, or Steve Halpern's Zodiac suite. Some experimentation with sound will help you discover if it enhances or distracts.

Brief relaxation techniques are useful throughout the day and can be practiced without special effects. Sometimes just inhaling and exhaling smoothly several times is enough to relax your muscles by creating a wave of calm feeling. Another easy method that can be practiced for two to five minutes several times a day is as follows: Sit down, close your eyes, and imagine your body becoming warm and heavy.

Brief Relaxation

Techniques	Directions	Place
Brief relaxation. This exercise prevents the rush of thought. It can be used to induce on-the-spot relaxation in a public place or to promote sleep.	Part your lips slightly. Place the tip of the tongue behind the lower teeth. Keep it there without pressure for awhile. Continue with normal breathing.	Walking down the hall, in the bathroom, in class, in a meeting. (Not in front of the boss or instructor.) During break, while studying.
Yawning. This is a one-minute tension-release exercise. The lungs expand; the back, jaw, mouth, and tongue relax. More oxygen comes into the system. Nice to do near an open window.	Drop your jaw gently until it feels large enough to take in a whole fruit. As you begin to yawn, it feels as though it will never end. As you yawn, you are taking in a deep breath. When the yawn ends you feel relaxed, clear down into your stomach. Your lungs have expanded, and your back begins to release its tension (Bauer and Hill, 1986, p. 162).	

1. Where can you use these techniques? List at least two places at home, at school, and in the clinical area.

2. What method of relaxation has been successful for you in the past?

3. How can you enhance your current relaxation method?

The preferred way to learn relaxation techniques is with a skilled instructor. Many community education programs include relaxation courses for a modest fee. It is an opportunity to try out and choose a style to fit your needs. T'ai Chi Chih, for example, combines Oriental stretching and breathing movements as well as T'ai Chi movements. This form of relaxation may be especially appealing for those who wish to combine graceful movement and relaxation.

All methods of dealing with personal stress can be sabotaged unless you develop a regular pattern of sleep. Be aware that you can create your own insomnia by taking your worries to bed. Tell yourself firmly that you have done your best for the day and will not think about the issues until you awaken. Any of the techniques can be used to relax before bedtime if needed.

Research on sleep has shown that most people have 90- to 100-minute sleep cycles. To make use of this information, do the following:

1. Go to bed at the same time: Listen to what your body is telling you. Extra early or later than usual is no favor to the body.

2. Most important, when you awaken naturally, get out of bed. Better yet, do your stretching exercises and then get out of bed.

No doubt you have sometimes decided to treat yourself to a few more minutes of sleep and then ended up feeling tired much of the day. Research seems to show that the body is set on a 25-hour clock, and when you get up at a different time, the body tries to "reset" the clock throughout the day. No wonder the "treat" you offered yourself did not work.

1. List three current behaviors in your life style that support lifelong wellness. _____

_____

_____

_____

2. List three behaviors that undermine your wellness. _____

_____

_____

_____

3. List three changes that will improve your wellness and personal care. _____

_____

_____

_____

▼▼▼ S U M M A R Y

▶ It is a nursing responsibility to model wellness and personal care for the client. Therefore, it is imperative for the nurse to make informed decisions about the direction of her personal life early in nursing.

1. The image you project sets the tone for the client's level of confidence, willingness to believe, and cooperation.

2. Health care practices, especially handwashing, decrease the risk of contamination for clients, self, and family members.

3. Wellness is a personal issue that is under your direction and control. Planning needs to be realistic and should be based on your life style. It begins today and is maintained for a lifetime.

▼▼▼ R E F E R E N C E S

Bauer R, Hill S. *Essentials of Mental Health Care: Planning and Interventions.* Philadelphia: W.B. Saunders, 1986.

Benson H. *The Relaxation Response.* New York: Avon, 1976.

Benson H, Stuart E. *The Wellness Book.* New York: Simon & Schuster, 1992, Chapters 4, 5, 8, 9, 10, 16.

Centers for Disease Control and Prevention. *Recommendations for Moderate Exercise.* Atlanta: CDC, 1994.

Our nutrition position. Two Harbors, MN: Lake County Chronic Disease Prevention Project 1995.

Roberts C. The best junk foods now and the worst. Bottom Line 1992; 13(7):10.

Roon K. *Karin Roon's New Way to Relax.* New York: Greystone, 1961.

United States Department of Agriculture. *Dietary Guidelines for America.* Washington, DC: USDA, 1996.

▼▼▼ B I B L I O G R A P H Y

National Dairy Council. *Guide to Good Eating and Daily Food Guide Pyramid.* Rosemont, IL: National Dairy Council, 1994.

Peckenpaugh NJ, Poleman CM. *Nutrition Essentials and Diet Therapy,* 7th ed. Philadelphia: W.B. Saunders, 1995, Chap. 6.

University of California at Berkeley. *The Wellness Encyclopedia,* Parts 2 and 3. Boston: Houghton Mifflin, 1991.

United States Department of Agriculture. Human Nutrition Information Service. Home and Garden Bull. 1993; 253:1–8.

Assertiveness As a Nursing Responsibility

CHAPTER 11

▼▼▼ O U T L I N E

Passive Behavior
Aggressive Behavior
Assertive Behavior

Negative Interactions
Guidelines for Moving Toward
Assertiveness

Problem-Solving Process
Cultural Differences

▼▼▼ K E Y   T E R M S

aggressive
assertive
automatic
choice

compensation
cultural differences
denial
manipulation

passive
problem-solving
projection
rationalization

▼▼▼ O B J E C T I V E S

Upon completing this chapter you
will be able to:

1. Explain why assertiveness is a
   nursing responsibility.
2. Differentiate between assertive,
   aggressive, and passive behavior.

3. Describe three negative interactions in which nurses can get
   involved.
4. Maintain a daily journal that reflects your personal interactions
   and responses.

5. Develop a personal plan for
   change toward assertive
   behavior.
6. Discuss positive manipulation
   as a cultural choice.

Assertiveness is an expectation in nursing—a responsibility for you as a client advocate. Once again you are requested to do a brief exercise before going on with your reading.

> **Directions:** Imagine for the next few minutes that the nurse-client roles are reversed and that you are the client.
>
> **Question.** What are your expectations of the nurse assigned to you? List the rationale for each expectation that you identify.
>
> | Expectation | Rationale |
> | --- | --- |
> | ———————— | ———————— |
> | ———————— | ———————— |
> | ———————— | ———————— |
>
> Completing the above exercise has already begun to give you an insight into the need for assertiveness in the nurse. At the end of this chapter you are encouraged to do this exercise again. Evaluate any changes in expectations.

Three types of communication styles translate into three major behavior patterns. Because communication is both verbal and nonverbal you will both *hear* and *see* the message acted out.

The most effective style is open and honest. It promotes positive relationships and a healthy sense of self. Ineffective communication or behavior is hurtful. It blames, attacks, or denies and is harmful to self as well.

An *assertive* style separates the person from the issue. Most important, *you speak out of choice.* With either an *aggressive* or a *passive* style you are caught by an emotional hook. Both types of responses are *automatic responses.* You no longer respond from choice.

Now let's take a look at the three major behavior styles: passive (nonassertive), aggressive, and assertive. We will also look at negative interactions specific to nursing and at how you can move toward truly assertive behavior.

▼▼▼
Passive Behavior

Passive (nonassertive) behavior is an emotionally dishonest, self-defeating type of behavior. Passive nurses attempt to look the other way, to avoid conflict, and to take what seems to be the easiest way out; they are never fully a participant on the nursing team. *Passive individuals do not express feelings, needs, and ideas when their rights are infringed on, deliberately or accidentally. The overall message is, "I do not count. You count."* This personal pattern of behavior is reflected in their nursing as well. Consequently, they are unable to recognize and meet the client's needs. A number of examples of passive behavior observed in one nurse are given below. With each, the type of behavior is given in parentheses.

▶ Tells another nurse how "stupid" the doctor is for ordering a certain type of treatment (indirect passive behavior)

▶ Limits contact with a client she is uncomfortable with to required care only (indirect passive behavior)

▶ Routinely tells clients who question her about an explanation for the illness, test, medications, or treatment to "ask the doctor" or "ask the RN." Although this answer is advisable some of the time, it certainly is a form of brushoff. Part of the nursing responsibility is to seek answers for the client (takes the easy way out)

▶ Experiences inability to continue with a necessary, uncomfortable treatment ordered for the client (interprets client's expression of discomfort personally ["He will not like me if I make him do this"])

▶ May assume, without checking, that the client wants to skip his daily personal care when a visitor drops in (avoids conflict)

▶ Experiences a feeling of being "devastated" when a client, doctor, nurse, or other staff person criticizes her work (interprets criticism of work as criticism of self)

▶ Responds to client's questions about her personal life and that of other staff (afraid of not being liked)

▶ Client asks her to pick up some personal items on the way home. She frowns but agrees to do so (communicates the real message indirectly)

▶ Becomes angry with the team leader and drops hints to others about her feelings (communicates real message indirectly)

▶ When asked by another nurse to take on the care of her clients, she responds by saying, "Well, uh, I guess I could" although she is already too busy (hesitance, repressing her own wishes)

▶ Needs help with her assignment but says nothing (refrains from expressing her own needs)

▶ After making an error, overexplains and over-apologizes (unaware of the right to make a mistake; should take responsibility for it, learn from the error, and go on)

▶ Plans on finding a new job because she is afraid of approaching the supervisor to tell her side of what has happened (avoids conflict)

▶ When "chewed out" by the doctor in front of the client, the nurse is angry but says nothing (refrains from expressing her opinion)

What are some other examples of passive behavior?

By not taking risks and not being honest, the nonassertive nurse typically feels hurt, misunderstood, anxious, and disappointed and often feels angry and resentful later. Because she does not allow her needs to be known, she is the loser.

▼▼▼
Aggressive Behavior

Outspoken people are often automatically considered assertive when in reality their lack of consideration for others may be a sign of aggressive behavior. Aggressive behavior violates the rights of others. It is an attack on the person rather than on the person's behavior. The purpose of aggressive behavior is to dominate or put the other person down. This behavior, while expressive, is self-defeating because it quickly dis-

tances the aggressor from other staff and clients (Bauer and Hill, 1986, pp. 102–103). The overall message is, "You do not count. I count."

The following examples are some of the ways by which aggressive behavior can be recognized. An explanation is included in parentheses.

▶ You have asked to go to a workshop, and the supervisor tells you, "Why should you go? Everyone else has worked here longer than you have" (attempt to make you feel guilty for making a request)

▶ Another nurse points out your error in front of the other staff and adds, "Where did you say you graduated from?" (attempt to humiliate as a way of controlling)

▶ A peer approaches you with a problem. You don't want to listen and say, "If it isn't one thing, it's another for you. Why don't you get your act together?" (disregard for others' feelings)

▶ A new rule is instituted without requesting input from or informing those whom it will involve. You protest but are told, "That's tough, this is the way it's going to be from now on" (disregard for others' feelings and rights)

▶ The client has had his call light on frequently throughout the morning. You walk in and say, "I have had it. You have had your light on continuously for nothing, all morning. Do not put your light on again unless you are dying or I will take it away" (hostile overreaction out of proportion to the issue at hand)

▶ You attempted to express your feelings to a peer about her behavior toward you. Today she greets you with an icy stare when you say hello (hostile overreaction)

▶ The client tells you, "I thought this was a pretty good hospital, but none of you seem to know what you are doing" (sarcastic, hostile)

▶ You push yourself in front of others in the cafeteria line (rudeness)

▶ Another employee greets you with "I hear you are a real whiz kid. Show us your stuff" (put-down)

What examples of aggressive behavior have you experienced?

Aggressive behavior certainly is a way of saying what you mean at the moment. It often does produce temporary relief from anxiety. However, the feeling does not last. Very often the aggressive person is left with residual angry feelings that simmer until the next stressful situation or person comes along. Interestingly, sometimes an aggressive person was once passive and made a decision that "no one will step on me again." However, instead of practicing assertiveness, such a person practiced and became involved in another form of destructive, self-defeating behavior. The aggressive nurse, like the passive nurse, is unable to function as a true advocate for the client because she is too busy taking care of what she perceives to be her personal needs.

▼▼▼
Assertive Behavior

Assertiveness is a current name for honesty—that is, it is a way to live the truth from your innermost being and to express this truth in thought, word, and deed. The concept seems simple enough, but to practice actually being truthful all the time is difficult. Assertiveness, according to Webster's dictionary, is characterized by taking a positive stand, being confident in your statement, or being positive in a persistent way. You, the nurse, work in a setting that requires speaking frankly and openly to others in such a way that their rights are not violated. Although it is not the nurse's right to hurt others deliberately, it is unrealistic to be inhibited to the point of never hurting anyone. Some people are hurt because they are unreasonably sensitive, and some use their sensitivity to manipulate others.

The nurse has a right to express her own thoughts and feelings. To do otherwise would be insincere. It would also deny clients and other staff the opportunity to learn to deal with their feelings. Assertiveness, then, is a way of expressing oneself without insulting others. It communicates respect for the other person although not necessarily for the other person's behavior (Bauer

and Hill, 1986, p. 103). The overall message is "I count, you count." Being assertive does not guarantee that you will get your way. What it does guarantee is that you will experience a sense of being in control of your emotions and your responses. Win or lose, you gave it your best shot. The real bonus is freedom from residual feelings of anger.

The following examples, with the rationale in parentheses, are expressions of assertive behavior. As an assertive nurse you claim responsibility for your own feelings, thoughts, and actions. Use of "I" in the statements shows acceptance of responsibility for your thinking, feeling, and doing.

► The doctor orders a medication or treatment that seems inappropriate. You request to talk with him privately. Ask about expected outcomes. Present any new information you have that may potentially affect the decision to continue with the order (direct statement of information)

► The client has been giving you a bad time. Pulling up a chair and sitting down, you say, "Mr. Smith, I would be interested in knowing what is going on with you. I have noticed that whatever I do, you are critical of my work." Then listen attentively and with understanding and respond nondefensively (direct statement of feelings, does not interpret client's criticism as a personal attack)

► When the client requests information you are unfamiliar with regarding his illness and treatment, you say, "I do not know but I will find out for you." Follow through by checking with appropriate staff. Determine who is to inform the client (respects the client's right to know)

► The doctor has ordered the client to be walked for 10 minutes out of each hour. She complains that it hurts and asks you not to make her walk. You respond by saying, "I know it is uncomfortable, but I will walk along beside you. We can stop briefly any time you like. I will also teach you how to do a brief relaxation technique that you can use while you are walking." If pain medication is available, you will also make sure that this is given prior to walking and in enough time for the medication to take effect (respects client's feelings but supports the need to carry out doctor's order)

▶ Unexpected visitors arrive when it is time for you to help the client with his personal care. Ask the client directly if he wishes to have his care done now or to postpone it briefly. State the time that you will be available to assist with care (respects the client's right to choose as long as it does not compromise his care)

▶ You have just been criticized for your work. You respond by saying, "Please clarify. I want to be sure I understand." If the error is yours, ask for suggestions to correct it or offer alternatives of your own (separates criticism of performance from criticism of self)

▶ The client asks for personal information about you (or another staff member). You respond by saying, "That information is personal, and I do not choose to discuss it" (stands up for rights without violating rights of others)

▶ Your client asks you to pick up some personal items for him. This would mean doing it on your own time, which is already very full. You respond, "I will not be able to do the errand for you" (direct statement without excuses)

▶ The team leader has been "on your case" constantly, and you think, unfairly. You approach him or her and say, "I want to speak with you privately today before 3 P.M. What time is convenient for you?" (direct statement of wishes)

▶ You are being pressed by other staff members to help with their assignments, but you are too busy to do so. You say, "No, I do not have the time to help today, but try me again on some other day" (direct refusal without feeling guilty. Leaves the door open to help at a future date)

▶ Your day is overwhelming. You approach your team leader and say, "I know you want all of this done today. There is no way I can get it all done. What are your priorities?" (direct statement of information and request for clarification)

▶ The doctor has criticized your work in front of the client. You feel embarrassed and angry. You approach the doctor and tell him you want to speak to him privately. Using I-centered statements, you begin by saying, "I feel both embarrassed and angry because you criticized me in front of the client. Next time, ask to talk to me privately. I will listen to what you have to say" (stands up for your rights without violating the rights of others)

▶ You are ready to leave work when a peer approaches you about a personal problem. You respond by saying, "I have to leave now, but I'll be glad to listen to you during lunch-time tomorrow" (compromise)

▶ Another staff person moves in to the cafeteria line ahead of you with a nod and a smile. You are in a hurry too and feel put-upon. You say firmly, "I do not like it when you get in line ahead of me. Please go back to the end of the line" (stands up for your rights)

> *What examples of assertiveness can you identify in your own behavior or in the behavior of people around you?*

Three rules are helpful overall in being assertive:

1. Own your feelings. Do not blame others for the way you feel.

2. Make your feelings known by being direct. Begin your statements with "I."

3. Be sure that your nonverbal communication matches your verbal message.

▼▼▼
Negative Interactions

With the availability of so many types of preparation for nurses and the lack of differentiation in roles based on preparation, nurses sometimes experience insecurity in their role and the worth of the role as they understand it. This negative interaction involves use of the coping or mental mechanism of *projection*, whereby an individual attributes his own weaknesses to others. The interaction can be characterized as "my education is better than yours" or "I'm more competent than you are" or "You're only a practical nurse," and so on. Unfortunately, this negative, aggressive interaction uses up energy that could be used to provide the client with the care that is being alluded to. Nurses who are confident and assertive enhance each other's knowledge base and legal responsibility. The client benefits.

Another negative interaction is based on a previous unresolved incident between the client and the nurse. The nurse uses the coping or mental mechanism of *rationalization,* in which she offers a logical but untrue reason as an excuse for her behavior. The nurse quickly informs others that this client is a "troublemaker" or a "manipulator" or is "uncooperative." This is a passive, indirect type of behavior on the part of the nurse. Obviously, if other nurses incorporate this information into their transactions with the client, the client will never be seen as his or her true self. Anything that he or she does can be interpreted within the context of the label given by the nurses. A vicious circle can ensue. If the client's needs are not met because of this obstacle, this increases his or her frustration. This in turn is a threat to self, resulting in anxiety. Depending on the client's personal strength at this time, the situation can lead to problem solving, use of coping mental mechanisms, or symptom formation. See Figure 11–1.

An honest, assertive response on the part of the original nurse involved would consist of dealing with the client directly in regard to the previous situation. It would not involve other nurses as allies in "getting this client." An example of an extreme situation resulting from just such a seemingly innocent rationalization occurred at a nursing home. A young man who was paralyzed from the waist down as a result of a car accident was being transferred from one nursing home to another. A transfer form arrived before he did. The information on the form created immediate anxiety for the nurses involved before they had even met the man. The form labeled the man as "manipulative." It explained that "he will be pleasant and polite at first, but watch out because it is a trick. When he has won you over, you will see his 'real colors'." The nurses discussed the prospective admission. They expressed gratitude that they had been warned by their colleagues in the other nursing home. After all, that is what colleagues are for. And now they felt, "forewarned is forearmed."

When the client arrived and attempted to get acquainted, he was dealt with coldly and abruptly and made to wait. The nurses intended to show him that he could not manipulate them. As his frustration and his discomfort increased, he began to demand that his treatments be done on time. He shouted angry comments at the nurses when they finally arrived to assume his care. The nurses called him "demanding" and "hostile." The original title of manipulative was supported when the client asked his roommate to put on the call light to get help to take him to the bathroom. Each day seemed worse than the day before. The showdown finally came when a longtime nurse employee left, saying that she would not come back until the client was transferred to another facility. She would even volunteer to do the transfer note. Other nursing staff threatened to follow suit. Finally the administrator gave in. The client was transferred, and the nurses congratulated each other for having worked together!

1. What factors contributed to the client's behavior?_____

   _____

   _____

2. What factors contributed to the nurses' response to the client?_____

   _____

   _____

3. How could this situation have been handled differently?_____

   _____

   _____

4. Was the behavior of the nurses passive, aggressive, or assertive? Explain your answer.

   _____

   _____

   _____

Another negative transaction involves client rights. This transaction can be known by many titles, depend-

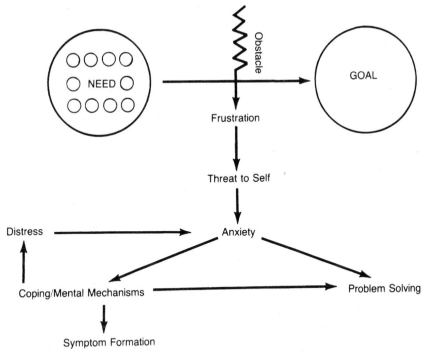

Figure 11–1
Results of interference with goal achievement. (From Bauer B, Hill S. *Essentials of Mental Health Care: Planning and Interventions.* Philadelphia: W.B. Saunders, 1986.)

ing on the issue. It can be called "no guts," "I've got a secret," "it is not my responsibility," "she will be upset," or "she is too weak to know." The responsibility of informing the client about his or her condition or transfer plans is not carried out so that the present staff does not have to deal with the full impact of the client's reaction to the information. The coping or mental mechanism used by the nurses is denial. The nurse refuses to recognize the existence and significance of the client's personal concerns. The nurse further uses denial as a way of excusing her responsibility: "The doctor should tell him" or "It's the team leader's responsibility." Although the decision may not be entirely yours, it is clearly your responsibility to check out what portion of the information is yours to give. You also have the responsibility to check out who is going to present the information and when.

Is the nurse's refusal to take responsibility to seek out the information the client

needs to know a passive, aggressive, or assertive transaction?

Although it has many possible negative interactions, certainly the passive or aggressive game of gossip—i.e., "Did I tell you?" or "I just found out"—is a destructive interaction that has the potential to ruin the reputations of both clients and personnel. The coping or mental mechanism is compensation. The nurse is covering for real or imagined inadequacies in her work by developing what she considers the desirable traits of observation, listening, and reporting. The energy is misguided because reputations are at stake, and time spent socializing while at work is time away from providing quality client care. Listeners can squelch this game by saying assertively, "I will work on a relationship with you and me, but I do not wish to have you talk to me about others." Instead, if the listener, while calling the other nurse a gossip, listens with interest, she supports continuation of this behavior.

1. What other negative interaction between staff or between clients and staff are you familiar with?_____

_____

_____

2. How is the continuation of this type of interaction supported by others?_____

_____

_____

_____

▼▼▼
Guidelines for Moving Toward Assertiveness

The following poem by an anonymous author captures the reason for working toward assertiveness—being able to feel good about yourself as you continue to grow as a person.

Myself
I have to live with myself and so,
I want to be fit for myself to know.
I don't want to stand with the setting sun,
And hate myself for the things I've done.
I want to go out with head erect.
I want to deserve all man's respect,
But here in this struggle for fame and self,
I want to be able to like myself.
I don't want to look at myself and know,
That I'm bluster and bluff and empty show.
I never can fool myself, and so
Whatever happens, I want to grow
More able to be more proud of me,
Self-respecting and conscience free.
—*Author Unknown*

Changing behavior is difficult. After all, the behaviors have been practiced and perfected for years. It is so much easier to tell someone else what they should do to change. The decision to change must come from inside yourself, so that it becomes yours alone.

▽▽▽
Problem-Solving Process

The problem-solving process is a conscious growth-producing method of dealing with this challenge in your life. It is important to note that problem solving is an active process and is more than simply developing an intellectual awareness of the challenge at hand.

Step 1—Define the Problem

Sometimes what is perceived as the problem is not the problem at all. Before making a commitment to change, it is important to look objectively at the gains and losses associated with the present behavior. Your present way of responding to others developed as a response to anxiety-producing situations in life. It usually has its roots in childhood.

Another consideration is that when you change the way you act toward others, you change the way they act toward you. What has been a predictable reaction will no longer be predictable. Initially, the "others" will test you. They will increase their old way of behaving as a way of getting you to give up the new behavior. If you persist with your new way of dealing with and responding to situations, their behavior toward you will also change. This is the only way to influence change in anyone's behavior. No amount of "telling" or "scolding" makes a difference as long as they can count on you to behave in a predictable way.

Defining the problem depends on collecting data for two or three days and writing your problem statement based on this information. Collecting data needs to be done in an objective manner, as though you were observing someone else. Keeping a daily confidential journal helps to pinpoint specific situations. You can track what happened, when it happened, how you felt physically, the emotion you felt, what you would have liked to have done instead, and what kept you from doing it.

Reviewing the data you have collected will give you insight into the pros and cons of your present behavior. The problem statement you develop will have to be personal and specific.

Sample

I am afraid to say what I mean for fear that others will get angry with me.

This behavior is characterized by:

▶ Saying yes to requests to babysit when I need the time for homework.

▶ Not asking for help with household chores even though I am a full-time student plus homemaker.

▶ Saying yes to added requests not related to workload at school that I must complete on my own time.

▶ Feeling tired and resentful much of the time and eventually blowing up over something insignificant.

Step 2—Decide on a Goal

Review the problem statement, and form the question, "So what?" In other words, what do you want to do differently? This can be stated as a single goal. Often it is more useful to break the goal down into a long-term goal and several short-term goals (sometimes called objectives)—the steps needed to attain the desired long-term goal. All goals must be realistic, measurable, and time referenced. At this time, write a goal for yourself.

Sample

Long-Term Goal	Short-Term Goal
Within 6 months I will say what I mean without fear that others will be angry with me (give actual date—this is your best "guesstimate").	Within 2 weeks I will say "no" to babysitting requests when I need the time for homework (give actual date—this is your best "guesstimate").

As you read each of the goals you have written, ask yourself if they are realistic. Are they reasonable to attain? Next, review each goal and ask if it is measurable. Are they so specific that you can use the senses to detect the change? Note that each goal begins with the phrase "I will." This phrase signals a personal commit-

ment to work on the goal. Note that the goals are to be attained within a designated period of time, that is, they are time referenced. This is also the only way to give yourself a personal push to get started.

All the changes are not going to occur exactly by the projected date. You will have to revise the goal dates from time to time. But most important, they provide target dates to strive for. As you accomplish each short-term goal, cross it out and go on to the next one. Do not be alarmed if you find yourself working on more than one goal at a time. This is possible and even desirable when the opportunity presents itself. It is important to continue recording your progress in the confidential journal that was begun initially to obtain data. Its value now lies in keeping a record of the process you are going through and in seeing the changes taking place. Unless you do this, you may not fully appreciate your work and its progress. Many changes will be subtle and will not be accompanied by bells and claps of thunder.

Step 3—Choose Alternatives

Alternatives are the approaches that you will be using to attain each of the established goals. When you make a list of alternatives in your journal, let your imagination run wild. Consider all the possible solutions, from serious to humorous. This may even provide some comic relief to the serious challenge with which you are dealing. Remember to include "Do nothing" in the list of alternatives. Doing nothing is a *choice* and therefore an alternative. Look at each of the goals and think of specific things you can do or say to help support the goal.

Sample

Approach: Practice in front of a mirror. In an even tone of voice say, "No, I will not be able to babysit tonight, but try again another time." If she persists, say "No, I do not have the time tonight." Repeat as needed until heard. Compliment yourself for not giving in.

Do you see how the approach (alternative) corresponds specifically to the short-term goal?

Step 4—Try Out The Alternatives

The initial plan has been made. It is time to put the plan into action. For many of you the paperwork is far easier than taking the first step to make the "paper trip" become a reality. You may also have discovered that it is far easier to offer ideas to peers than to take the first step into action with your own plan.

> *What are you gaining from staying nonassertive? What are you losing from staying nonassertive?*

The answer belongs in your confidential journal. Whether you are writing or tape recording a journal depends on your learning style. Regardless of the journal method used, it should by now have become an important part of the learning process.

It is a good idea to build in an incentive to continue using the new assertive approaches. Promise yourself something that is worthy of you (a worthy goal). As you go along, you will sometimes slip back into old familiar ways of behaving. Do not be dismayed. This is normal. Simply reinstitute the newly planned approaches immediately and continue. The more you practice the new approaches, the more they will become part of you. Ultimately, new assertive behaviors will replace old passive or aggressive behaviors.

Step 5—Evaluate the Effectiveness of Your Approach

The evaluation mechanism is built into the overall plan for change by making the goals time limited. This tells you that each goal, along with the alternatives you have chosen, will be evaluated at the time indicated. Do not change a goal or approach too quickly. Give it at least two to three weeks. There are two reasons for this: (1) The negative behaviors of other individuals toward you will increase initially as they attempt to resist change created by the change in you. (2) It takes a minimum of two to three weeks for the new behavior to catch on. It takes approximately a year for a new behavior to become part of you. As a part of the evaluation process, review your entire confidential journal. This is an excellent source of information for

what happened, how you dealt with it, and whether the present course is effective.

Step 6—Repeat the Process if the Solution Is Not Effective

Step 5 gives you information about whether or not to pursue the established course of action. If changes are needed, go back to step 3. Identify additional alternatives or perhaps choose alternatives that you originally identified but did not use. Then go through the rest of the steps as before.

As you pursue an assertive way of behaving, monitor your nonverbal messages. The nonverbal communication you provide is even more powerful than your words. It is possible to have the words just right but to sabotage them by hesitating, a sarcastic tone of voice, or emphasis on certain words. Practice in front of a mirror. Busy schedule? Try bath time. Listen to the way you sound. A tape is helpful, as is speaking into an empty corner and hearing your words bounce back. Try lowering your tone of voice. Be sure that the last word of a sentence is no higher than the one before. Listen for this in others. It makes a statement sound like a question. Posture plays an important role. Sit up straight, walk with the shoulders back and a confident stride. Make eye contact when speaking. If this is new and difficult for you, look at the area between the eyes of the person you are addressing. This provides an illusion of eye contact. Periodically look away so that it does not look as though you are staring. Avoid annoying characteristics such as nail biting, finger or foot tapping or jiggling, playing with your hair, chewing on a pencil or glasses, and artificial laughter. When someone asks you what you think of an issue or what you would like to do, answer them instead of saying "I really do not know" or "Whatever you like. It does not matter." Life is an adventure. All of it, including your ideas, counts.

▼▼▼
Cultural Differences

With feedback from valued teachers, students, and reviewers, the authors have learned that it is not safe to assume that all cultures are focused on moving toward assertive behavior. In some cultures manipulation is an accepted norm. Although the term manipulation has a negative connotation in our society, manipulation in itself is not a maladaptive behavior. In some cultures it is taught and is accepted as a purposeful way of meeting one's needs. Skillful manipulation is especially applauded.

It is easy to jump to the conclusion that a manipulative person is trying to "trick" you because you do not share the same cultural background. Make time to talk. The differences will be interesting and revealing for both of you.

Manipulation is considered maladaptive if (1) the feelings and needs of others are disregarded or (2) other people are treated as objects to fulfill the needs of the manipulator. The following examples of negative manipulative interactions show a lack of consideration for others' feelings and needs.

The *seducer* initiates a relationship with someone (for example, a nurse with a supervisor). They share what seem to be common goals and insights. Ultimately, the seducer asks for special favors or privileges. If denied, the seducer pushes the guilt button: "I thought you liked me," or, "I thought we understood each other." The other person is left feeling guilty or angry or both.

The *passive-aggressive* manipulator focuses on the other person's weaknesses. He or she uses this knowledge to exploit or to create anxiety for the victim. For example, a physician might point out a nurse's errors or personal or professional problems in front of a client or other staff. The nurse is left feeling guilty, angry, embarrassed, or all of these.

The *divide-and-conquer* manipulator "confides" half-truths, rumors, gossip, and innuendo. A skilled manipulator can sever work relationships by sowing seeds of distrust. As the staff squabbles there is less energy to unite and focus on common client issues. For example, a *divide-and-conquer* manipulator who is an established member of the community might "confide" to another department head that a newer employee cannot be trusted. By the time this information proves to be untrue, valuable time has been lost in client planning and care. Meanwhile, the divide-and-conquer manipulator has continued to tell the same story to other listeners. Because the feelings and needs of others are not considered, they are left with anger and seeds of distrust.

Dealing with a negative manipulator is difficult. An assertive approach is the best recourse. This will, however, be met with resistance and resentment. You may end up backing off if the problem cannot be worked out. Set limits on any inappropriate manipulative behavior toward you. Refuse to play the game any more.

▼▼▼ *S U M M A R Y*

- ▶ Communication translates into behavior. Assertiveness is honest and open behavior. It considers others' feelings and needs. It is based on *choice*. Both passive and aggressive behaviors are based on *emotional hooks*. These styles are ultimately damaging to both parties involved. The end result is usually resentment and anger.
- ▶ In some cultures, skillful positive manipulation is practiced successfully. Positive manipulation involves consideration of others' needs and feelings. Furthermore, other individuals are treated with respect rather than as objects to be used for personal gain.
- ▶ Undesirable behaviors and interactions can be changed through using the steps of the problem-solving process. Both verbal and nonverbal interactions must be dealt with during this change.

▼▼▼ *R E F E R E N C E S*

Bauer B, Hill S. *Essentials of Mental Health Care: Planning and Interventions.* Philadelphia: W.B. Saunders, 1986.

▼▼▼ *B I B L I O G R A P H Y*

Alberti RE. *Your Perfect Right: A Guide to Assertive Behavior,* 6th ed. Broomfield, CO: Impact Publishers, 1990.

Benson H, Stuart E. *The Wellness Book.* New York: Simon & Schuster, 1992, Chapter 4.

Branden N. *The Six Pillars of Self-Esteem.* New York: Bantam Books, 1995.

Hopkins E. How to train friends and influence people. Mademoiselle 1991; May: 200–243.

Varcarolis E. *Foundations of Psychiatric Mental Health Nursing,* 2nd ed. Philadelphia: W.B. Saunders, 1994.

Pitfalls to Success in Practical Nursing

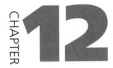

▼▼▼ KEY TERMS

apple-shaped
burnout
caring
codependency
creative communication
crime alert

empathetic approach
hepatitis B
HIV/AIDS
humor
impaired nurse

pear-shaped
smoking prevalence rate of 32%
sympathetic reaction
understanding
universal precautions

▼▼▼   O B J E C T I V E S

Upon completing this chapter you will be able to:

1. *Discuss two ways to prevent burnout in nurses.*

2. *Describe abuse of alcohol or other drugs as a path to the label of Impaired Nurse.*

3. *Explain the effect of smoking tobacco by the nurse on the nurse and the client.*

4. *Identify the need for personal weight management as a health issue for the nurse.*

5. *Describe fears of occupational risk such as AIDS, tuberculosis, and hepatitis.*
   a. *myths and facts about AIDS*
   b. *the connection between tuberculosis and AIDS*
   c. *hepatitis: what are the risks?*
   d. *universal precautions as a way of life in nursing*

6. *Discuss codependent behavior as an obstacle to success.*

7. *Discuss violence in the workplace.*

8. *Identify specific pitfalls, if any, that may prevent your success in practical nursing.*

As a nurse you must learn to take care of yourself. In turn, you can be more effective in meeting your client's nursing needs. In taking care of yourself positively, you serve as a positive role model for both your coworkers and your clients. Stress is involved in caring for clients. However, it is not the event itself; it is how you view the event that determines the amount and kind of stress you experience. The difference between success and failure in nursing comes down to being able to manage your emotions. Remember the word congruent? All that you think, feel, value, and believe in come together as you move toward your goals in nursing.

> 1. **What current situation in your life is creating negative stress?**
> 2. **In what way can you view the event in a more positive way?**

▼▼▼
Burnout

Burnout is like looking at your career world through black glasses. The positive attitude you held about nursing, working with clients, and self-care begins to change. Attitude and behavioral changes may include:

1. Lack of respect for clients.
2. Blaming patients for their illness.
3. Taking a cynical view of clients, your place of employment, and management.

4. Personal feeling of emotional exhaustion.
5. Lack of self-care that may include an increase in the use of alcohol and other drugs.
6. A negative self-view.
7. More conflicts at home.

Differentiating between feelings of empathy and sympathy in regard to your client is a major consideration in preventing burnout. Empathy is a respectful, detached concern. As a nurse, you understand what your client is experiencing but do not experience the emotion with him. Clients entering a medical facility are out of their own element. The stress they experience can be picked up by you as a sympathetic response.

The client may be demanding a magical, dramatic change in his or her condition. Regression almost always is present in the client. Needs are often expressed indirectly, perhaps through irritable comments or requests. The client's emotional responses may elicit negative emotional responses in the sympathetic nurse.

Some clients do not respond to treatment no matter how hard they and you try. They may continue to go downhill to the point of death. Meanwhile, other clients may not cooperate, and your sympathetic response of anger and frustration will get in the way of a therapeutic relationship with them. Some clients are negative in their responses to staff or constantly ask questions in a challenging way. The families must be dealt with also, and at times they are equally or more challenging than the clients. Maybe you are beginning to think in terms of who does and does not deserve care.

A sympathetic reaction leaves you vulnerable to identifying with and experiencing the emotion along with the client. This means that you are no longer in control of the situation, and your therapeutic value as a nurse will be limited. A long-term sympathetic response is very stressful. What starts out as a caring relationship can become detrimental to you and your client because of your overinvolvement.

Another significant step in preventing burnout is to develop a detached way of evaluating your daily personal performance. Waiting for a client, doctor, or nurse manager to notice your performance is rarely helpful or rewarding. Perhaps they notice only what is missing. However, a detached, daily evaluation of your performance leaves you free to credit yourself for what you have done well. Furthermore, it alerts you to areas in which you need more study, assistance, or practice. *You are your most effective boss!*

Time management is another important factor in dealing with both the personal and the professional areas of your life. Because of its significance, Chapter 5 is devoted to this topic.

> *What changes have you made using information from the chapter on time management? If you said none, read the chapter again. Repetition reinforces learning.*

Humor—do not forget humor. No matter how seriously you take yourself, you are never going to get out of this life alive. So lighten up. There are many things that happen in a nursing situation that can be lightened up through humor. Case in point: The nursing instructor walked into the room to see how the student nurse was doing with her client. As she approached the client, she extended her hand and greeted the client by name. As he opened his mouth to speak, he simultaneously expelled flatus—a thunderous clap! The client's eyes opened wide, there was a momentary silence, the student looked shocked, and then the instructor chuckled! "It happens," she said with a shrug. Soon all three were laughing; the embarrassment was gone. The real issue of the client's condition and nursing care was again the priority.

Maintaining nursing skills is essential. Even if you are in a situation that requires less hands-on care, make time to perform nursing procedures. Learn how to perform new procedures as they are introduced to your facility. This helps to feed your self-esteem and makes you a more valuable employee, an issue that is closely related to preventing burnout. Otherwise, you may develop a secret fear of being put on the spot and perhaps will lie your way out of requests to demonstrate or assist.

Some final tips for staying alive and well in nursing:

1. Set clear goals with realistic expectations.
2. Know your limits.
3. Work within your team structure.
4. Keep in mind that you cannot be all things to all people.
5. Maintain a clear understanding of what constitutes a professional relationship. Demonstrate professional—detached and somewhat limited—caring. A different kind will end in burnout because it becomes too burdensome.
6. Do not personalize the client's response to you. Keep the client in the client role. Maintain a professional outlook. See that the client responds out of the client's own needs. If you do this you will experience less guilt or anger.
7. Maintain a positive attitude, i.e., warm, caring, and hopeful, even if the client is dying. The client and the family will feel less hopeless.
8. Understand your own needs, both professionally and personally. You need to maintain a balance and a clear distinction between your work and your personal role.
9. Be alert to signs of burnout. Lack of caring is a real danger signal.
10. Maintain perspective about your work. Sometimes the whole world looks ill and grim! Remind yourself that you have a choice: Nursing can be a limited part of your life or the dominant goal in your life. You choose.

> 1. *Do you find yourself frequently focusing on home issues when at work?*
> 2. *Are you talking often about work when you are with your friends and family?*
> 3. *Name one change that you will begin to work on starting now.*

▼▼▼
Impaired Nurse

Impaired and nurse sound like contradictory terms. Some nurses, however, become chemically dependent on alcohol or other drugs. You may be one of them.

Alcohol is a drug that acts like a depressant. Because of the loss of inhibition, the person who drinks may initially experience a sense of "loosening up." Unlike food, alcohol does not have to be digested. It is absorbed directly into the bloodstream from the stomach and small intestine. It reaches every tissue and organ of the body and slows the activity of the cells.

Alcohol is processed by the body at the rate of ¼ to ½ ounce per hour. This is the amount of alcohol in one 12-ounce can of beer or one 5-ounce glass of wine. The liver processes most of the alcohol: A small amount is processed in the testis and eyes. The remainder is excreted by the kidneys, sweat glands, and lungs.

What is the difference between alcohol abuse and alcoholism? Abuse is drinking so much that you get drunk. Alcoholism is an addiction. The body craves alcohol, and physical effects result from its withdrawal. For you as a nurse, either way impairs your judgment and places your client in danger. Early intervention is essential. Not only are your health and life at stake, but so are the lives and health of your clients.

The most telling sign of any chemical dependency is a gradual decline in performance, which usually becomes noticeable in three to six months. Behaviors that need to be checked out include:

1. Complaints by staff and clients.

2. Accidents, errors in documentation, a greater number of injuries caused while moving clients or equipment, errors in practice.

3. Increased visits to the employee health department or emergency room.

4. Increased volunteering to take call for others.

5. Arriving early or staying late to assist in the narcotic count.

6. Frequent absenteeism after days off and for personal emergencies, especially on a Monday.

7. Irritability and mood swings.

8. Performing only the minimum amount of work required.

9. Inability to perform psychomotor skills owing to intoxication or tremors (Abbott, 1987, p. 1108).

Two emotional characteristics of chemical dependency make it difficult to begin treatment. The denial system is very strong, and the person who drinks is usually a skilled manipulator. A recovering alcoholic who is a commercial photographer explained, "I was always drinking with the finest professionals. My companions included a judge, a lawyer, the town's top surgeon and the police chief. Obviously *they* weren't alcoholics. Anyway there was always someone in a more advanced stage than I was. As my alcoholism continued to progress I would point to someone in a more advanced stage and say, 'look at them. I'm not doing that. I'm not an alcoholic.' And then one day I almost died after I fell down a flight of stairs. I finally heard when the doctor said, 'Either you quit drinking or you will die.'" Unlike Michael L., it is not necessary to hit bottom to intervene.

1. Do I turn to alcohol and/or other chemicals for relief from pain or stress on a regular basis? _____

2. If the answer to question one is yes, to whom will you go to seek intervention? _____

_____

3. List the names of some facilities and persons in your area who assist with chemical dependency issues.

_____

_____

_____

4. If you realize that a coworker is drinking and is impaired while on duty, what is your responsibility to the client in this matter?

_____

_____

_____

You can seek help from counselors, treatment centers, Alcoholics Anonymous, Narcotics Anonymous, and other local resources. The yellow pages in your phone book list resource numbers under Alcohol Abuse Information and Treatment and Drug Abuse Information and Treatment. You can also look in the white pages under Business and Professional Listings for alcohol or drug abuse services and helpline and hotline numbers. It is worth the risk making a phone call to obtain information on your own or a friend's behalf.

▼▼▼
Smoking

Nurses and smoking are another set of contradictory terms. "None of the habits that can damage the health of human beings has been as clearly documented or as widely publicized as smoking. There is simply no room for debate: Smoking promotes heart disease and cancer and is the major cause of premature, preventable deaths in the United States. Smoking can make you sick if you're healthy, and make it harder to recover if you do get sick" (University of California, Berkeley, 1991, p. 53).

As a nurse you will be asked to encourage your clients to decrease or discontinue their use of tobacco.

Visualize the contradiction that will occur if you, too, are a smoker. Your breath, hair, skin, clothes, and hands will quickly make your words unconvincing. A 1994 report on smoking prevalence by occupation in the United States identified physicians as the occupation having the lowest rate (approximately 5.5%). Licensed practical nurses had a prevalence rate of approximately 32%, and registered nurses had a rate of approximately 22% (Nelson et al, 1994, pp. 516–525). All nurses still have some way to go to internalize and practice what they now know about smoking.

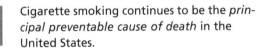

Cigarette smoking continues to be the *principal preventable cause of death* in the United States.

It is interesting to note that the rate of smoking in men has continued to decrease, but the rate of smoking in women has increased. Approximately half of American smokers who have ever smoked have quit. Most heavy smokers continue to smoke even after a life-threatening illness occurs. It is thought that many of these smokers are physically addicted to the nicotine in tobacco. Meanwhile, approximately 3000 young people begin to smoke each day. If you are a smoker, take the following test.

Why Do You Smoke?

I smoke (true or false):

_____ 1. because I light up automatically and don't know I'm doing it.

_____ 2. because it's relaxing.

_____ 3. because I like handling cigarettes, matches, and lighters.

_____ 4. to help deal with anger.

_____ 5. to keep from slowing down.

_____ 6. because it's unbearable not to.

_____ 7. because I enjoy watching the smoke as I exhale it.

_____ 8. to take my mind off my troubles.

_____ 9. because I really enjoy it.

_____ 10. because I feel uncomfortable without a cigarette in my hand.

_____ 11. to give myself a lift.

_____ 12. without planning to—it's just part of my routine.

Results: True answers to questions 5 and 11 indicate that you smoke for stimulation; to 3 and 7, that the pleasure of handling cigarettes is important; to 2 and 9, that you seek relaxation; to 4 and 8, that you need a tension-reducing crutch; to 6 and 10, that you have a physiologic addiction; to 1 and 12, that you smoke from habit. No doubt you smoke for a combination of these reasons.

From U.S. Department of Health and Human Services.

Nicotine, a drug, occurs naturally in tobacco leaves. When smoke is inhaled, it is absorbed into the blood through the lung lining. Arteries transport the nicotine-containing blood directly to the brain. Nicotine is a seductive drug that can either calm you down or pick you up. Addiction to nicotine occurs in about six weeks. Consider that many who smoke started at the age of 12 to 13 years.

There is also a psychological addiction to smoking. Nicotine becomes the friend who is always there at any time of the day or night. Finally, there is the habit. Perhaps it goes with coffee or a soft drink, a phone call to a friend, or on the way to work.

What do you do with your hands when the cigarette is no longer there?

Any one of the three aspects of addiction is difficult to contend with: physical addiction to nicotine, the loss of a friend, or the loss of a habit. For some individuals, the use of nicotine patches in graduated doses plus classes in smoking cessation have been helpful. The patch provides a sustained level of nicotine in the blood and takes care of physical withdrawal. Classes provide information and support on how to deal with the loss of a "friend" and a "habit." Patches are available now but are not for everyone.

Because there is no safe way to smoke, it is important that you quit, for your sake and for your clients' sakes. "Nothing you do for your health—not even dieting and exercise—pays as many dividends so quickly as giving up smoking" (University of California, Berkeley, 1991, p. 55). Benefits to the heart show up so quickly that in 2 years much of your risk of heart disease has disappeared. In 5 to 10 years the risk will be the same as if you had never smoked. The risk of lung cancer and other malignancies begins to decrease steadily when you quit smoking. After 10 years your risk is almost as low as that of a nonsmoker. If you have bronchitis or emphysema you can expect to see an improvement in breathing almost at once. Plus, nonsmokers have stronger bones and less chance of getting osteoporosis (University of California, Berkeley, 1991, p. 55).

Even nonsmokers are at risk. People who have never smoked before can suffer illnesses by breathing other people's "secondhand" smoke.

Whether you are helping your client quit smoking or doing it yourself, the method used must meet the needs of the individual. Talk to your physician to help you identify resources. Contact the American Cancer Society or the American Lung Association for information about classes on how to stop smoking.

▼▼▼
Weight Management

Too little weight or too much weight? Either has possible implications for energy, strength, and personal health.

1. At what weight do you feel most healthy? _____

2. At what weight do you experience the greatest amount of strength and energy? _____

3. Do you have any illnesses or injuries that may be related to overweight or underweight? _____

   _____

4. Are you able to do the nursing work assigned to you without excessive tiredness or soreness? Too much weight is a health risk. The 1996 USDA Guidelines recommend maintaining your weight within a healthy range, i.e., less than a 10-pound gain since you reached adult height and are otherwise healthy.

Studies show that relationships exist between obesity and hypertension, high blood cholesterol levels, heart disease, heart attacks, and possibly diabetes. Also connected are certain cancers—colon and prostate cancer for men and uterus and breast cancer for women. There is also a direct relationship between too much and too little weight and back and joint injuries.

You may have heard references to pear-shaped and apple-shaped bodies. *Pear-shaped* refers to fat located primarily in the hips, buttocks, and thighs. This fat is stored primarily under the skin. *Apple-shaped* refers to fat located primarily in the abdominal area. The apple shape, abdominal fat, is stored deeper inside the body. It is theorized that more fatty acids are released into the system of the apple-shaped person, who becomes more susceptible to the aforementioned illnesses.

In Chapter 10 you learned about a common-sense approach to combining good nutrition with exercise. Good nutrition fuels the body. Exercise strengthens the body and aids with flexibility. As a nurse, you promote or do not promote health, just by being. So take time to review how you manage your weight and if necessary, set some reasonable, reachable goals. No personal badgering is allowed. See Table 12–1.

▼▼▼
Occupational Risks

You come into nursing knowing that you will be expected to provide nursing care for clients with infectious or contagious disorders. In fact, there are times when a client is admitted, and the diagnosis is unknown until a series of tests have been completed. To protect

Table 12–1
Healthy Weight Ranges for Men and Women

Height	Weight (in Pounds)
4'10"	91–119
4'11"	94–124
5'0"	97–128
5'1"	101–132
5'2"	104–137
5'3"	107–141
5'4"	111–146
5'5"	114–150
5'6"	118–155
5'7"	121–160
5'8"	125–164
5'9"	129–169
5'10"	132–174
5'11"	136–179
6'0"	140–184
6'1"	144–189
6'2"	148–195
6'3"	152–200
6'4"	156–205
6'5"	160–211
6'6"	164–216

Weights above this range are less healthy for most people. The further you are above the healthy weight range for your height, the higher your weight-related risk. Weights slightly below the range may be healthy for some people but are sometimes the result of health problems, especially when weight loss is unintentional.

From U.S. Department of Agriculture. *Dietary Guidelines for Americans*. Washington, DC: U.S. Dept. of Agriculture, 1996.

yourself and your clients, you need to perfect your technique for following universal precautions or sterile technique when needed. Basic nursing instructors traditionally will not pass you on either of these skills unless you demonstrate perfection. Once out of the classroom, it is up to you to maintain technique.

Although the human immunodeficiency virus (HIV) is a fragile virus, a great deal of misinformation about it continues to instill fear in nurses. It seems prudent to review the facts as we know them today. Casual contact is not a risk. You will not be infected by touching or being near a client or coworker who is infected with HIV. There is no evidence that HIV is spread by sharing facilities or equipment. This includes phones, computers, pencils, cups, and bathrooms. Nor is the virus passed through the air by coughing and sneezing. Furthermore, you will not pick up HIV infection through casual social contact. Nor will you get it from a food handler or a waitress. You will not get it from eating utensils, drinking fountains, or swimming pools. Sitting next to an infected person in a bus, car, or plane does not put you at risk. There is no evidence that a child will be infected by sitting near or playing with a child infected with HIV or the acquired immunodeficiency syndrome (AIDS).

To understand the nurse's role in preventing transmission of AIDS, it is helpful to review what is currently known about this illness. HIV is transmitted from one person to another through blood and body fluids. The most common methods of transmission are sexual intercourse and sharing needles during intravenous drug use. During sexual intercourse, HIV in the semen, vaginal fluid, or blood of the infected person infects the bloodstream of the other person through the tissue lining the rectum, vagina, penis, or mouth. In intravenous drug users, HIV enters the bloodstream through a puncture made by a needle contaminated with infected blood. Less common means of transmission include passage of the virus from an infected woman to her child during pregnancy or birth, breastfeeding by an infected woman (rare), and blood transfusions. The current risk of transmission through blood transfusion is small because donated blood is tested. You cannot be infected with HIV by donating blood. All equipment is sterile and is used only once.

AIDS is not a single disease. The body reacts in a variety of ways to the virus, ranging from no symptoms at all to death. An attempt has been made to assign stages to the infection, such as HIV infection, HIV disease, and end-stage AIDS. Some people progress rapidly to death, whereas others do not. These latter individuals are termed long-term survivors or nonprogressors. Some scientists now believe that HIV is not dormant at all, even when symptoms take years to appear. They believe that the body's immune defenses start fighting the virus at the beginning of the infection. In some people, the immune system can keep the virus in check for years. In some long-term survivors, the immune system finally exhausts itself. The mystery about what keeps nonprogressors so healthy continues. Currently, a person is considered to have AIDS when the T-lymphocyte (T-cell) count is less than $200/mm^3$.

What is the role of the T cells in the immune system?

Persistent symptoms may develop in the infected person. These may include severe fatigue, swollen lymph glands, night sweats, fever, cough, diarrhea, or weight loss. The symptoms are often mild at first but become progressively worse. Thrush, composed of white curdlike patches, may coat the mouth and esophagus. Esophageal thrush is considered specific to AIDS. Hairy leukoplakia, grayish white patchy discolorations, may erupt on each side of the tongue.

Pneumocystis carinii pneumonia, an unusual form of pneumonia, is another defining characteristic of AIDS. It is the most frequent life-threatening infection in patients with AIDS. Kaposi's sarcoma, a rare form of cancer, may present with spots ranging in size from an insect bite to large nodules or plaques. The infected person may also have a variety of nervous system disorders, ranging from depression to dementia.

AIDS is a preventable disease that continues to be spread primarily through risky and careless behaviors. Confidential testing is available. Testing for HIV is a difficult procedure. The primary test methods are HIV antibody tests and viral cultures. It takes approximately six weeks to six months after infection for HIV antibodies to appear in the blood. Antibody testing continues to be the method of choice for rapid confirmation of HIV. It is important to remember that antibody testing alone is not diagnostic of AIDS. Viral cultures continue to be expensive and time consuming.

The HIV virus is fragile. It can be destroyed readily by following recommended cleaning and sterilization procedures. Special client isolation procedures are used only in those with conditions such as infectious diarrhea, tuberculosis, or other communicable diseases.

Nurses should continue to follow universal precautions and treat all clients as if they were HIV positive. Review the universal precautions recommended by the Centers for Disease Control and Prevention (CDC) in the box following. Check your basic nursing notes.

A. Use barrier precautions to prevent skin or mucous membrane exposure to blood or body fluids.

   1. When do you use gloves? _____

   2. When do you use masks or face shields? _____

   _____

   3. Why are gloves not washed and reused even with the same patient? _____

   _____

B. Handwashing

   When, why, and how? _____

   _____

C. Sharps and needle stick protection

   What is the established protocol? _____

   _____

   _____

D. Saliva

   1. Is saliva implicated as a source of transmission of HIV? _____

   2. Are you required to exercise universal precautions in regard to saliva? _____

E. Weeping dermatitis or exudative lesions

   What are the recommendations for the nurse with weeping dermatitis or exudative lesions? _____

   _____

   _____

F. Pregnant care givers

   Are pregnant care givers more at risk for contacting HIV during contact with clients? _____

   _____

G. List additional protective precautions that you follow as a result of what you learned during basic nursing

   courses. _____

   _____

   _____

Are there risks for you as a nurse? Perhaps. But not in the way you think. Rarely is the client with HIV infection or AIDS a source of transmission unless there has been a serious break in technique. Do not try to second guess whether a person has an infectious disease by how they look or who they are. Resolve to follow universal precautions and blood-borne pathogen standards with every contact with clients.

Some clues as to who may be at risk may be found by thinking back to the 1970s. This is when HIV first started spreading in the United States. Those at risk include persons who have been sexually active, who have not been in a mutually monogamous relationship since then, who have shared intravenous drugs (or their partners have shared them), or who have received a blood transfusion or blood product prior to 1978. Encourage these at-risk persons to be tested.

▽▽▽
The Connection Between Tuberculosis and Human Immunodeficiency Virus

Tuberculosis (TB) is occurring more often in persons infected with HIV and other diseases that compromise the immune system. When the disease is not recognized or treated, it provides a potential hazard to nurses and other health care workers.

Tuberculosis is spread from person to person through tiny airborne droplets that contain the tubercle bacilli. The person with active pulmonary TB coughs up these particles. A susceptible individual who shares the same airspace for a prolonged time inhales the bacilli. The organisms travel to the lungs. If they reach the air sacs and multiply, TB begins.

Most individuals who become infected with TB do not develop active TB. A healthy immune system can often keep it in check. However, even a healthy immune system cannot kill all of the TB organisms. Therefore, infected individuals remain at risk of developing active TB when the body's immune system is weakened. Because HIV weakens the body's immune system, it is far more likely that active TB will develop in an individual with latent TB infection. This can be thought of as an **internal** source, because

the infection arises from within the body. Individuals can also pick up TB from an external source. For example, an LPN who had not been previously infected (she had a negative Mantoux test and a negative x-ray) picked up a primary TB infection at work. The LPN worked evenings in a nursing home. An elderly client had been admitted from a local hospital. She had a fever of 102°F and a productive cough. The LPN tucked her in and gave her a good night kiss on the cheek every night. Active TB was finally diagnosed in this client. The LPN became ill, and active TB was diagnosed in her also.

Incomplete treatment of persons with TB has resulted in drug-resistant TB—a new concern for nurses. Homelessness is thought to be a contributing factor to noncompliance with treatment regimens and also for an inability to track persons with TB to ensure complete treatment. The medications developed in the 1950s and 1960s are ineffective in treating drug-resistant TB.

The most common site for TB is the lungs, that is, pulmonary TB. However, it can occur in any site in the body. Tuberculosis of the lymph nodes and miliary (disseminated) TB are also commonly seen in patients with HIV. Characteristic symptoms of active pulmonary TB include cough, fever, night sweats, weight loss, and fatigue. Symptoms of extrapulmonary TB (other body sites) depend on the site that is affected.

In 1989, the Centers for Disease Control and Prevention (CDC) in Atlanta, Georgia recommended that all persons who are HIV seropositive should be given a Mantoux tuberculin skin test. Similarly, persons with high-risk behaviors, such as intravenous drug users, should also be tested for TB.

Some persons with both HIV and TB may show falsely positive skin tests. Chest x-ray and other studies may be needed to confirm a diagnosis of TB. Meanwhile, it is important for the nurse to practice infection-control techniques for preventing the spread of airborne infections. The basic nursing course is a dress rehearsal for real life on the clinical unit. Teach your client to cover the mouth and nose when coughing, sneezing, or expectorating. Dispose of tissues properly, just the way you learned in basic nursing. Adequate ventilation helps to keep the TB organism count down.

▼▼▼ Hepatitis

The greatest bloodborne risk faced by health care workers is hepatitis B virus (HBV). According to Assistant Labor Secretary Gerald Scannell, occupational exposures alone accounts for 5900 to 7400 cases of hepatitis B infection a year (Scannell, 1992, p. 82).

During 1985, the CDC first recommended universal precautions. However, their guidelines were not legally binding. Consequently, during December 1991, the Occupational Safety and Health Administration (OSHA) developed a standard for bloodborne pathogens (HIV, HBV, and others). The standard makes universal precautions mandatory in all health care settings. The new rules also order employers to offer hepatitis B vaccine free of charge to every employee who can be "reasonably anticipated" to have "skin, eye, mucous membrane or parenteral contact" with blood or other potentially infectious materials. Besides being free, the vaccine must be offered "at a reasonable time and place" and "within 10 working days of initial assignment." OSHA is able to back up their standards with fines of up to $10,000 for "serious or willful" violations (Scannell, 1992).

The term hepatitis means inflammation of the liver. Its numerous causes include bacteria, drugs, alcohol, and other toxins. Of serious concern is hepatitis caused by hepatitis viruses that infect the liver. There are at least five types of hepatitis caused by different hepatitis viruses. They are currently known as hepatitis A through E. Study Table 12–2. Focus especially on hepatitis viruses B, C, and D.

▼▼▼ Codependency

Before you read any further, answer the following questions:

1. What is your reason for making nursing your career choice?

2. Who supplies the most important critique of your day's work?

3. How do you feel if the client does not tell you that you did a good job?

> *"A codependent person is one who has let another person's behavior affect him or her, and who is obsessed with controlling that person's behavior" (Beattie, 1992, p. 36).*

Some writers have speculated that a significant number of nurses may be codependent (Cavello, 1991, p. 132). Cavello explains codependency as follows: "The codependent nurse has a pathological need to be needed." Codependent nurses relate to their clients and their coworkers in unhealthy ways. For some, a painful childhood that included sexual abuse, violence, or chemical abuse may have paved the way to codependency.

Whenever a definition of a behavior provides a tinge of truth, it is followed by denial or harsh self-criticism. However, the intent is to inform—to allow you to evaluate yourself and modify codependent behaviors *if* they exist. Some characteristics of the codependent nurse follow.

Codependent people "fix" things and right wrongs. They react too quickly to feelings with a sense of intensity and urgency. Clients are viewed disrespectfully, i.e., they are thought to be incapable of participating in their own care. This viewpoint takes away clients' sense of personal control and may give them the message that they are more ill than initially perceived.

The following true incident illustrates codependency in a nurse. A man and his fiancée, both in their twenties, were involved in a car accident. The woman experienced serious injuries and was placed in traction. The man was admitted for observation. He was not placed on bed rest. The following morning a nursing student working as an aide during her summer break was assigned to him. Later in the day, other aides were overheard talking about the male client's description of his morning care. "He told me that it was the best care he had ever received. She (the aide) insisted that he have a bedbath. She scrubbed him from top to bottom—and I do mean bottom! She even powdered his penis!" This aide interfered with the client's autonomy.

Using denial and manipulation to gain satisfaction

Table 12–2
Hepatitis

	Hepatitis A (HAV)	Hepatitis B (HBV)	Hepatitis C (HCV)	Hepatitis D (HDV)	Hepatitis E (HEV)
Former name	Infectious hepatitis	Serum hepatitis	Non-A, non-B hepatitis	Delta hepatitis	Epidemic or water-borne non-A, non-B hepatitis
Mode of transmission	Excreted in feces; passed on unwashed hands to food and other items that go into mouth; may contaminate drinking water or food, including raw or steamed clams, oysters, and mussels	Found in all body fluids in infected people, including blood, semen, saliva, and urine. Spread by (1) intimate contact with infected people and exposure to body fluids; (2) piercing of skin by contaminated instruments: tattooing, ear piercing, acupuncture, dental, or medical procedures; (3) intravenous drug use; (4) sexual intercourse; (5) spread to babies at birth by infected mothers	Spread by transfused blood, intimate contact, IV drug use, other percutaneous exposures. Maternal transmission low; heterosexual transmission less common than with HBV. Does not appear to be associated with homosexual activity	Must have hepatitis B before being infected. Combination of two diseases is more severe than hepatitis B alone. Transmission same as HBV; in U.S. occurs primarily in those receiving blood products (i.e., through dialysis, by hemophiliacs, through IV intravenous drug use)	Ingestion of contaminated water or food; most outbreaks associated with water contamination
At risk	Persons exposed to unsanitary conditions, i.e., those who consume virus-	Health care workers; patients and staff on units where blood is handled; staff of institu-	Anyone who receives transfused blood or blood products (6%). Employment-related	Anyone who already has hepatitis B	Same as hepatitis A; to date all cases in U.S. have been imported by immigrants or visitors

contaminated food or water. Common in day care centers or nurseries; infected children and/or contaminated care givers transmit disease quickly to others	tions for mentally handicapped. Certain military personnel Those who have personal contact with infected persons · Morticians and embalmers Blood bank workers Anyone with risk-taking sexual behaviors Intravenous drug users People of Asian, African, Eastern European, Caribbean, Pacific Island, American Indian, Native Alaskan, or South American descent	exposure Exposure related to tattoos, acupuncture treatments, non-medication treatments such vitamins and minerals 40% of cases related to two ambiguous categories: (1) low socioeconomic status, and (2) no identifiable risk factors		from epidemic areas, including Mexico, and a large number of developing nations; no outbreaks have been reported in U.S., Canada, or any developed nation of Europe or Asia
Prevention	If exposed and not vaccinated: gamma globulin HAV vaccine (HAVRN) Vaccine recommended if: (1) travel outside of U.S. except Australia, Canada, Japan, New Zealand,	HBV vaccine If exposed and not vaccinated: HBIG (hepatitis B immune globulin)	Little progress toward developing a vaccine	HBV vaccine CDC recommends universal HBV vaccination of newborns	No vaccine

Table continued on following page

Table 12–2
Hepatitis (Continued)

	Hepatitis A (HAV)	Hepatitis B (HBV)	Hepatitis C (HCV)	Hepatitis D (HDV)	Hepatitis E (HEV)
	and western Europe; (2) have chronic liver disease; (3) community experiencing outbreak of HAV; (4) contact with someone with the disease; (5) infected medicines used; (6) male with a male sex partner				
Diagnoses	Blood test	Blood test	Blood test	Blood test	—
Outcome	Usually resolves without long-term effects	Complete recovery Death (less than 1%) Chronic liver disease that may progress to liver cancer in 5% to 10%	50 to 60% chance of lifelong liver disease Long term: Mortality low but 20% of patients with chronic infection may develop cirrhosis; up to 70% develop chronic hepatitis; liver cancer a possibility Significant public health problem that may match or exceed HBV	Generally progresses to chronic active disease or death due to severe hepatitis	In developing countries, leading cause of acute viral hepatitis Mortality rate in infected pregnant women nearly 20%

Codependent Nurse	Possible Behavior
1. Says "yes"—really means "no."	Agrees to help another staff member and then complains to someone else about being taken advantage of.
2. Feels the fate of nursing care rests on her shoulders.	Takes on nonnursing duties that belong to other departments.
3. Feels responsible to solve other's problems.	Sympathetic, rather than empathetic response to patients and other staff.
4. Competes for attention rather than supporting coworkers.	Engages in one-upmanship and intershift rivalries over patient care.
5. Often feels angry, unappreciated, and used.	Comes in early and works late. Works extra shifts to "help" coworkers.
6. Does not support patient's need for autonomy and return to self-sufficiency.	Does for the patient what he needs to do in order to regain optimal health and self-confidence.
7. Makes excuses and conceals negative practices rather than working for change.	Feels powerless. Takes on extra duties because of chronic understaffing.
8. Shows feelings of anger indirectly.	Pouts, procrastinates, forgets, gets sick, or is late.
9. Perfectionistic: gossips and judges.	Unrealistic expectations of others.
10. Avoids conflict.	Too nice, loving, and forgiving. Smiles when having negative feelings.

in unhealthy ways has usually been practiced for many years. It takes special courage to really look at oneself to see if any of these behaviors are present. Both self-help groups and books are available. How about codependency as a topic of discussion during class in relation to personal life or one's relationships with classmates? Replace the words "client," "coworkers," and "staff member" with "others" in the preceding characterization. Determine your codependency traits outside of nursing.

Beattie (1992, p. 83) compares codependent behavior to the sides of Karpman's drama triangle. Since codependents are caretakers or rescuers, they rescue, then persecute, and ultimately end up feeling victimized.

1. *Do your behaviors in regard to clients fit this pattern?*
2. *Are you looking for happiness through your relationship with the client?*
3. *Do you maintain focus on clients' needs, i.e., medical or nursing orders?*

▼▼▼
Crime Alert: Violence in the Workplace

Workplace violence has always been here. It is the increase in violence that is making nurses take notice. Homicide is the third work-related cause of death in the United States. The U.S. Bureau of Labor statistics reports homicide as the leading cause of death for women at work.

Violence is typed according to four categories:

1. Employee: Violence is directed toward supervisors or management.
2. Domestic: The issue is personal, but the violent act takes place in the workplace.
3. Property: Violence is directed against the employee's or employer's property.
4. Commercial: The employee engages in activities such as stealing from employers. Violence may ensue as a result of the activity.

Be alert to signs of violence. Early signs might include:

▶ Unusual behavioral change
▶ Lack of cooperation with nursing supervisors
▶ Cursing and other hostile forms of communications
▶ Short fuse and frequent arguments
▶ Spreading gossip or rumors to harm others deliberately
▶ Uninvited sexual remarks
▶ Hostile responses to other nurses, clients, or family members
▶ Sleep disturbances mentioned at work
▶ Increase in irritability and anxiety

The next stage might include:

▶ Conversation focused on "poor me, the victim"
▶ Notes with threats or violent or sexual content
▶ Verbalization that includes plans or a desire to harm someone
▶ Ignoring workplace policies
▶ Stealing workplace property
▶ Less interest in work and follow-through on assignments
▶ Increase in arguments
▶ Increase in physical accidents or injuries

As the anger intensifies and if conflicts remain unresolved, the result can be violence against self or others.

▶ Behaviors directed toward self might include depression or suicidal threats
▶ Behaviors directed toward others might include physical fighting, property destruction, or use of a weapon to harm others.

Prevention begins when each nurse makes a personal commitment to practice prevention guidelines. There are policies in every workplace that cover harassment and other forms of violence. Check them out. Be alert to warning signs. Think through what you can do. Take all threats seriously. Report them to management. Some general safeguards include:

1. Doing your part to promote a supportive, congenial, yet professional work environment.

2. Whenever possible, resolve conflicts as they arise. Know that there are times when you have to back off. *However,* most of the time people want to have their point of view understood, to be listened to. A technique called *creative communication* encourages you to:
   a. Listen carefully to the other person's point of view.
   b. Ask questions to clarify what you do not understand. (Remember that this step is not a sneaky way to argue or to interject your own opinion!)
   c. Tell the person what you think they said and what you think they are feeling. If your version is inaccurate, have them repeat the explanation. When you can repeat back accurately what they *think* and *feel,* it is your turn to present your view. Steps a, b, and c work for you as well.

3. Deal directly with harassment including uninvited sexual advances. Review your own behavior to determine if:
   a. A clarification of the person's signals is in order, or
   b. Limits must be stated clearly and firmly on what you consider unacceptable behavior, or
   c. Supervisor or management intervention is needed.

4. Get to know your fellow workers and look out for each other.

5. Promote workplace integrity. Treat each other, your clients, and their families with respect, courtesy, and professionalism. Negative comments by clients and relatives usually are a response to their fear of the unknown. Rarely are the comments meant to be personal. Check out the fear. What are the questions? What can you do to help find answers?

6. Be alert to changes in behavior that may signal violence.

7. Avoid putting yourself in obvious danger. Make use of security guards for escort to parking lots and out-of-the way areas. *Listen to your intuition.*

▌ *What are additional ways that you know of to diffuse or prevent violence?* **▌**

▼▼▼ *S U M M A R Y*

▶ Major pitfalls to success in practical nursing are most often personal rather than work-related. As a nurse it is essential to take care of yourself. By doing so, you give permission for others to take care of themselves. "Should" and "ought" type of messages need to be replaced with messages conveying "I choose to" or "I choose not to." Maintaining and practicing nursing skills such as universal precautions are an expected part of nursing.

▶ How you see your client gives you important clues about your needs. If you are able to separate your personal and professional lives, develop an empathetic approach to client care, and be your own best friend and boss, chances are nursing will continue to excite you.

▶ Behaviors that impair nurses are harmful not only to the nurse but are potentially dangerous to the client as well. Codependent behaviors encourage patients to become dependent rather than to regain control of their own lives. Neither you nor your client is satisfied. Nursing is a wonderful vocation. Take time to evaluate your behaviors at this time. If changes need to be made, reach out. You will find that there is someone out there ready to reach out to you.

▶ Violence in the workplace has always been there, but it is on the increase in some areas. Most agencies have established policies and security measures for your benefit. Know what they are and follow them.

▼▼▼ *R E F E R E N C E S*

Abbott C. The impaired nurse. AORN J 1987; 46:1104–1108.

Beattie M. *Codependent No More,* 2nd ed. Center City, MN: Hazelton, 1992.

Cavello B. Codependency paints nursing's goals. RN 1991; 54:132.

Nelson D, et al. Cigarette smoking prevalence by occupation in the United States: A comparison between 1978 to 1980 and 1987 to 1990. JOM 1994; 36(5): 516–525.

University of California, Berkeley. *The Wellness Encyclopedia.* Boston: Houghton-Mifflin Company, 1991, pp. 53–59.

United States Department of Agriculture. Healthy weight ranges for men and women. *Dietary Guidelines for America.* Washington DC: U.S. Superintendant of Documents, 1996.

▼▼▼ *B I B L I O G R A P H Y*

Barker T. How to prevent violence in the workplace, Safety and Health 1994; July, pp. 32–38.

Bonneville G. Diagnosis violence. University of Minnesota Health Sciences 1995; spring, pp. 2–7.

Centers for Disease Control and Prevention. *Guidelines for Preventing the Transmission of Mycobacterium tuberculosis in Health Care Facilities.* Atlanta. CDC, 1994, pp. 516–525.

Coming to Terms With Obesity. Harvard Womens Health Watch, 1994; 2(3): 4–5.

Czarnecki G. Presented at The Hurt and the Healing, a workshop on codependency, at the University of Wisconsin, Green Bay, Green Bay, WI, October, 1991.

Does alcohol really prevent heart disease? University of California at Berkeley Wellness Letter, 1991; November: p. 1.

Flaskerud J, Ungvarski P. *HIV/AIDS: A Guide to Nursing Care,* 2nd ed. Philadelphia: W.B. Saunders, 1992.

Franklin F. Hooked. Health 1990; November/December: pp. 39–52.

Grainger R. The genie in the bottle. Am J Nurs 1993; March: p. 18.

Hughes T, Smith L. Is your colleague chemically dependent? Am J Nurs 1994; 94: 31–35.

Long P. Great weight debate. Health 1992; February/March: pp. 42–47.

Mallory G, Berkery A. Codependency: A feminist perspective. J Psychosoc Nurs 1993; 31(4):15–18.

Morrow L. A nation of finger pointers. Time 1991; August 12:14–23.

Regs put new legal force behind universal precautions. Am J Nurs 1992; 92:82–84.

Scannell G. OSHA stiffens bloodborne rules, decrees free hepatitis B vaccine. Am J Nurs 1992; 92:82.

Yates J, McDaniel J. Are you losing yourself in codependency? Am J Nurs 1993; 93:32–36.

Knowing Others

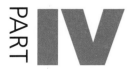
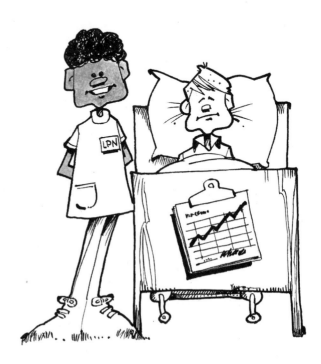

Communicating for Success

Judith A. Mix

CHAPTER **13**

▼▼▼ *OUTLINE*

▼▼▼ *KEY TERMS*

caring

empathy

rapport

therapeutic

trust

nonverbal messages

body language

barriers

sensory-deprivation

culture

"talking stick"

listening

personal space

β-endorphins

networking

collaboration

Alzheimer's disease

computer literate

▼▼▼ O B J E C T I V E S

Upon completing this chapter you will be able to:

1. Explain the significance of effective communication skills (verbal and nonverbal) in health care.

2. Describe the communication process and its components.

3. Describe the purposes of communication in nursing.

4. Contrast verbal and nonverbal communication.

5. List seven examples of nonverbal communication.

6. Develop verbal communication skills: speaking, reading, and writing.

7. Discuss factors that influence the communication process.

8. Develop or enhance beginning listening skills.

9. Describe the significance of the use of humor in client interactions.

10. Utilize and explain the rationale for therapeutic communication techniques.

11. Identify and explain the effect of blocks to therapeutic communication.

12. Describe the significance of effective communication with colleagues and the benefit of transactional analysis in this interaction.

13. Describe techniques that may be useful when communicating with children and the elderly.

14. Explain why it is essential for nurses to be computer literate and have computer skills.

15. Evaluate the effectiveness of your communication skills.

16. Improve your therapeutic communication skills.

▼▼▼
Significance of Communication

Imagine that suddenly you find yourself in an environment where all human communication has ceased. There is no verbal or written language. Humans in this environment do not use gestures or facial expressions to communicate. There are no newspapers, books, radios, television sets, computers, or videocassette recorders. Fortunately, it is highly unlikely that an environment totally lacking in communication exists anywhere because communication is necessary for physical as well as emotional, social, spiritual, and cultural survival.

Your waking day is almost totally consumed in some form of communication. Communication activities link you to the environment and to people in our environment. These activities include reading, speaking, writing, listening, watching television and other forms of audiovisual media, satellite communications, computer use, word processing, E-mail, and nonverbal methods such as body movements and facial gestures (body language). Expressions of love and acceptance, or dislike and nonacceptance, are communicated mainly by nonverbal means. Touch is

a powerful communicator of how you feel about another human.

Communication (verbal and nonverbal) is essential to formal and informal learning. We learned how to function as humans by utilizing all of the communication activities available to us as well as by listening to others, observing their behaviors, and processing information. Communication enables you and others to work and play together and to establish harmonious and productive relationships. Poor communication leads to problems in human relationships and consequently to social problems. Effective communication skills are essential tools for the nurse. You are encouraged to assess your understanding of the ideas presented, noting your strengths and weaknesses, and to work on improving your communication skills. Keep in mind the objectives at the beginning of this chapter and evaluate your abilities in relation to these objectives.

The forerunner of effective communication is establishing rapport. Clients will confide in you only after a trusting relationship has been developed. How do you establish a rapport or a trusting relationship with another person? You can enhance your communication skills by actively studying the concepts and the techniques in this chapter. Effective relationships with coworkers are essential to teamwork and the attainment of the team's or the institution's goals. Effective communication skills assist us in our interactions with others by helping us to present ideas clearly and by helping us to understand another person's message.

This chapter includes a discussion of what communication is and is not, the elements of communication, types of communication (verbal and nonverbal), barriers to communication, techniques of therapeutic communication, blocks to effective communication, listening techniques, transactional analysis, and computer communication in health care.

▼▼▼ Communication Defined

Language is the basis for communication. It enables us to formulate thoughts, ideas, and feelings and to relate these thoughts, ideas, and feelings to others.

Communication is a dynamic, changing, and never-ending process. You communicate through the senses of sight, sound, taste, smell, and touch. How well you communicate with other human beings depends on mutual understanding of verbal and nonverbal signs and symbols. If I say, "It looks reddened, feels soft, sounds like a doorbell, tastes sweet, smells like a rose," you need to have the same image that I do for effective communication to occur. We express what we have sensed in a verbal or nonverbal manner. When you feel something hot, such as the vinyl seat covers in your car on a hot summer day, you respond by sitting down slowly or by jumping off the seat. A small child communicates fear and pain by crying in a particular way. We recognize and understand the signal. When the signal is not understood, communication has not occurred.

Communication is the conveyance of a thought or an idea from a sender to a receiver. It means making something known to another person or asking for information from another person. It can be done verbally (by speaking or writing) or nonverbally (through the expression of feelings, attitudes, or thoughts). Communication requires two people or more who interact for some reason. People who communicate also interact, and by doing so, they respond to messages they receive. Communication is usually purposeful.

▼▼▼ Elements of Communication: A Model

The essential elements of communication are the sender (the person conveying an idea or asking a question), the message (the idea or question), and the receiver (the person or group for whom the message is intended). Communication is an active process and requires a vehicle or channel to transmit the idea or question. The sender uses the senses to convey messages verbally (spoken or written) or nonverbally through body language. The receiver receives and interprets the message. The receiver frequently gives the sender feedback about his or her understanding of the message. As the sender, you can ask for feedback of the message from the receiver if the receiver does not respond or if you are uncertain whether your message has been understood. When you are the receiver you can ensure that your understanding of the message is correct by saying to the sender, "Is this what you are asking?" Figure 13–1 illustrates the communication process.

Exchanging messages requires knowledge. The sender must have knowledge about the topic to send the message, and the receiver must have basically the same knowledge to understand the message. The sender must use language and terminology that the receiver will understand and should check for understanding. The past experiences of the sender and the receiver influence messages sent and received. If you have not experienced an event such as a loss, childbirth, or hospitalization, it is difficult to understand those experiences. Unless the sender and the receiver have similar past experiences and knowledge, communication can be difficult.

Communication is influenced by feelings and values. That is, if you think a topic is important or not

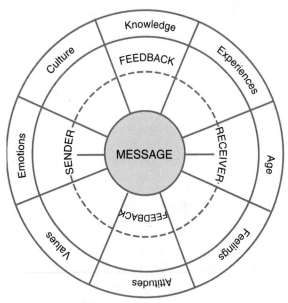

Figure 13–1
Mix communication model.

important you will communicate that feeling or value to the receiver. For example, it would be extremely difficult to encourage another person to stop smoking if you yourself are a smoker. Cultural biases and opinions are communicated readily, sometimes unknowingly.

▼▼▼
Purposes of Communication

Reasons for communicating are usually one of the following: social or therapeutic, relationship development, receiving information, giving information, clarifying and validating information, and conveying feelings. If you are going to be therapeutic, you need first to determine what the purpose of communication is before you can communicate with clients. Nonpurposeful conversation can actually be nontherapeutic and even destructive. The nurse uses the communication process for multiple purposes, including social reasons. You may be the only family that an elderly person in a nursing home has. In that situation you are being therapeutic by spending some time talking to the individual. Close relationships are frequently devel-

oped when clients and nurses interact for an extended period.

▼▼▼
Communication and the Nursing Process

Nurses use communication skills during each step of the nursing process. Communication between the client, the client's family, and the health care team is essential to the effectiveness of each step of the nursing process. Assessment involves the collection of data, which requires completeness and accuracy. Communication skills greatly affect the ability of the nurse to collect reliable, accurate, and adequate data.

The licensed practical nurse's role is to collect data that the registered nurse combines with other collected data to assess a client's status, to develop nursing diagnoses, and to evaluate the care provided. If the data collected are not accurate or are incomplete, the nursing care plan could be inappropriate for the client and consequently may lead to inappropriate, ineffective, or unsafe care. The implementation of care requires cooperation from the client. The nurse must use communication skills to explain what needs to be done and to solicit the client's consent and cooperation. The evaluation part of the nursing process requires that the nurse validate the effectiveness of care through communication (verbal and nonverbal) with and observation of the client.

▼▼▼
Nonverbal Communication

What is nonverbal communication? What is its significance in the communication process? Without words people can show feelings: love, pain, joy, contentment, peacefulness. Have you ever noticed that sometimes what a person says does not match what is being communicated nonverbally? For example, you ask a person how things are going. The reply is "Great, things are great." However, you get the idea that things are not so great when the person starts to cry or clenches his teeth.

Nonverbal behavior does not always have the same meaning for all people. Cultural differences, age, sex, past experiences, and individual responses to situations can vary the meaning. For example, men in many societies have been conditioned to believe that they should always be strong, both physically and emotionally. Some men as well as some women will have difficulty in admitting that they are in pain or have other physical or emotional problems. Consequently, they may not seek assistance when needed and may mask nonverbal expressions of pain as much as possible. In this situation, you need to be attentive to subtle nonverbal communications. What, specifically, should you observe to assess nonverbal communication? What precautions can you take to avoid miscommunication of nonverbal cues, and what can you do to avoid sending undesirable or nontherapeutic nonverbal messages? Body language is another term for nonverbal communication. The following topics represent body language.

▽▽▽
Eye Contact

Eye contact suggests a willingness to communicate. Eye contact is an important step in the development of a relationship. It tells another person you are giving them your attention and are ready to listen. Lack of eye contact may suggest that a person is shy, embarrassed, nervous, about to tell you something that is emotionally difficult to say, anxious, or defenseless, or has low self-esteem or does not wish to communicate. The eyes carry other messages, such as sorrow when crying, anger by means of a fixed stare, and disgust when a narrowing of the eyes is noted. In some cultures, eye contact may be a sign of respect, and in other cultures it is a sign of disrespect or implies sexual consent. Therefore, the actual meaning should be checked out verbally.

▽▽▽
Facial Expressions

The face tells others much of what we are feeling. The complex and unique musculature of the face enables us to smile, frown, and express joy, sorrow, surprise, anger, frustration, disbelief, preoccupation, anxiety, fear, sus-picion, pain, and contempt. The facial expressions used to communicate these different feelings and emotions are unique, so that many times you can recognize what the other person is feeling without asking him or her to verbalize. To be certain, you need to check out nonverbal communication in a verbal manner to ensure clarity. Nonverbal cues are indicators to the nurse but do not always clearly indicate exact meaning.

▽▽▽
Posture, Gestures, and Gait

A person's posture reveals a great deal about attitude, feelings, and how the person is getting along both physically and emotionally. A person with high self-esteem who is in good physical and emotional health holds his or her body erect and in good alignment. A slouched body position may indicate physical pain, a disability, depression, or boredom. Holding the body tensely suggests that the person is in pain, extremely shy, or closed to communication.

Feelings of authority and domination are expressed through body position, such as standing above another person or leaning back in a chair with hands behind the head (Fig. 13–2). To avoid giving this impression, seek the other person's level when talking. In the clinical situation, you could sit on a chair. To minimize the feeling of subservience that occurs when someone else is nonverbally communicating authority and dominance and the desired relationship is that of colleague or peer, stand up if the other person is standing so that you are at or close to eye level. Many times, short people have problems in achieving eye level and need to use other means to achieve equality. Refer to Chapter 11 on assertiveness for suggestions.

Provide space to avoid intimidating the person with whom you are communicating. Give consideration to the idea that because of cultural and personal differences, some people prefer closeness and others need more space.

Body gestures carry messages. One example is tapping the fingers on a table. This gesture indicates boredom, impatience, discomfort (physical or emotional), anxiety, or anger. Wringing of the hands may communicate pain, fear, or anxiety. A clenched fist communicates anger or pain. You need to check out your obser-

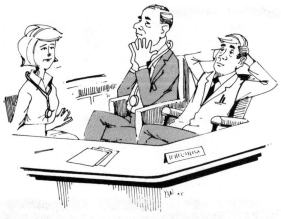

Figure 13–2
Body position.

vation verbally with the other person because one gesture may communicate two or more conflicting messages. The steepled hands of the man (high position) in Figure 13–2 communicate authority, domination, and superiority. The steepled hands of the nurse (low position) indicate feelings of low self-esteem. A slouched posture also indicates feelings of low self-esteem. What can you do about your posture and body gestures to project an impression of high self-esteem even when you do not really feel that way?

The manner in which a person moves about (gait) carries a message of wellness or illness and high or low self-esteem. A deliberate, brisk gait communicates a different message from a slow, aimless one. The former indicates wellness and high self-esteem, while the latter indicates illness or low self-esteem.

▽▽▽
Personal Appearance

A person's (the client's or the nurse's) physical appearance, personal hygiene, and grooming convey significant nonverbal messages. Healthy persons with good self-esteem tend to be concerned about their general appearance and consequently attend to details of nutrition, hygiene, dress, and grooming. Persons with low self-esteem frequently convey their feelings about themselves through inattention to general appearance. Sometimes very ill persons do not have the energy to

attend to these needs and depend on the nurse for assistance. Attention to or concern about personal appearance is one indicator of improving wellness. An emotionally ill person's progress can be measured by the degree to which the person attends to the aspects of general appearance.

Frequently, illnesses and therapies cause general changes such as skin changes (dryness, rashes), loss of muscle tone, and changes in awareness and alertness. These changes must be detected and evaluated to determine the progress of the client and the effectiveness of the therapies. The person's body response communicates significant messages to you, the nurse.

▽▽▽
Vocal Nonverbal Communication

Sounds such as crying, sobbing, sniffling, and sighing are considered nonverbal communication. Their meanings are not specific. Tears may be due to sadness, joy, or fear. A sigh may indicate relief or reluctance. However, these sounds are significant and should be attended to by the nurse. The client is communicating. The loudness and the pitch of the voice (inflection) carry messages of joy, fear, discomfort, and excitement.

▽▽▽
Touch

Touch communicates feelings of acceptance or nonacceptance. Failure to touch in appropriate situations, such as in care giving, can communicate rejection by the nurse.

Healing through touch is an ancient belief—"the laying on of hands." Western culture socializes us not to touch others, particularly strangers. Therefore, touching in care giving can be viewed as an invasion of privacy or a sexual advance by the client or the nurse. People who are anxious, dependent, or lonely generally need to have verbal support before nonverbal support is welcomed. All people need personal space and being touched at times can be threatening and not appreciated. You need to establish a rapport with a person before using touch.

Touch is therapeutic. The skin is our outer boundary; it receives messages from and is in constant communication with the environment. To touch and be touched are human needs. Holding and touching an infant are important actions because they can communicate love and caring. Infants who are not touched and held in a loving, caring manner fail to thrive. This may cause retardation in their growth and development. The elderly have a great need for human touch and the communication of acceptance. In some cases, touch may be the only sensation a client is aware of, and it will arouse and stimulate the other senses. The skin also communicates outwardly in the form of rashes, goose bumps, warmth and coldness, and moistness and dryness. Therapists have found that touch is sometimes an effective therapy for clients who are mentally ill or retarded.

Touch can communicate affection and closeness by hugging, kissing, handshakes, and touching the arm. Again, the form of touch used should be appropriate for the situation. Some people are comfortable with touch and others are uncomfortable. Some family members or entire families do not feel comfortable hugging and kissing, whereas others always kiss and hug when they see one another. Touch can also convey dislike, anger, and physical aggression, depending on how it is done. This form of touch is never appropriate and is certainly never therapeutic.

Studies indicate that people who have been or are deprived of touch and physical affection have more physical and emotional illnesses. Hospitals and long-term care facilities are sensory-deprivation situations because clients are being cared for by strangers, and their loved ones sometimes tend to touch them less. Clients who tend to be touched less by nurses are the seriously ill, those with communicable illnesses, those over 65 years of age, and adolescents. Lack of touching generally makes them feel less worthwhile. In seriously ill or semicomatose patients, touch is the person's only contact with the outside world. If you deprive them of touch, they may not progress as rapidly as they would with the stimulation of touching.

▽▽▽
Smell

How does the sense of smell affect our personal relationships with others and our therapeutic relationships with clients? Americans, unlike people of many other cultures, are embarrassed and offended by various body odors. We use many hygiene products and colognes to ward off offensive odors. Advertisers tell us we can improve our relationships with others if we use their products.

Have you ever moved away from or avoided someone with body odor or bad breath? The client frequently cannot move away from or avoid the care giver. Therefore, it is obvious that you, the nurse, need to eliminate body odors and perfumes and strong colognes that are offensive to the patient. It will help you establish a therapeutic rapport and increase the client's comfort. Body odors are interpreted as poor self-hygiene and communicate to the client that cleanliness and medical asepsis are not important to you. This makes clients reluctant to accept you as their nurse and to allow you to treat them. Clients have the right to refuse care from individuals they feel do not act in their best interests. The smell of smoke in the nurse's clothing is offensive to most patients. Some clients actually have an allergic response to "second-hand" smoke.

Clients frequently emit disagreeable odors because of their illnesses, treatments, or body responses. You need to be prepared psychologically so that you do not react negatively, either verbally or nonverbally, to these odors. When odor is present, clients who are alert also smell the odor and are embarrassed. You can best help the patient by accepting the odor as part of the process of illness and by communicating that you recognize that the situation is distressing to him or her.

▼▼▼
Verbal Communication

How you deliver a message is as important as what you say. Nurses use oral communications mainly when interacting with clients. However, written communications (reading, writing, computer) are also valuable skills when you research a topic for information, help clients understand a teaching plan, or document your data collection and the care given. In today's world, you need computer skills to obtain information and document observations and nursing care.

The greatest advantage of oral communication is its speed. This speed is valuable when time is important (Adler, 1991, p. 300). Emergency situations demand quick responses by care givers. Oral communication requires the attention of the person you are communicating with. A written communication may not be read by the person it was intended for. Thus, your chances of being recognized are greater with oral communication. The advantage of written communication is that it is a permanent record of your ideas. Listeners may forget a portion of your oral message, but with the written document they have a record to refer to. When you leave a message on another person's voice mail or answering machine there is a recorded message. Written records prevent distortion of your ideas. Written messages can be planned and designed in regard to content and tone. You can plan oral messages to some extent, but your verbal messages are usually spontaneous because you can only guess at what the other person will say (Adler, 1991, p. 301). You can learn some verbal communication techniques that will help you respond effectively and therapeutically.

The ability to use language skills accurately in the form of speaking, reading, and writing is essential to the business of giving care and is as important as nonverbal communication skills. You need to assess your skills in these areas and make the necessary improvements. The following discussions include suggestions for improvement.

▽▽▽
Speaking

Careful thought should be given to what you say and how you say it. Generally, avoid set speeches because they are impersonal and are not individualized. Set speeches may be appropriate when you are instructing clients about tests or routine procedures, to ensure accuracy and completeness. Address adults by title such as Doctor, Mr., or Mrs., unless the person asks you to do otherwise.

The manner of delivery of the communication is important in conveying its quality, acceptance, and understanding. Voices vary in quality, tone, rhythm,

and stress. Control a loud, raspy, or whiny voice. Avoid slurring your words; speak clearly and distinctly. The following are seven keys to effective speaking:

1. Speak with enthusiasm by varying tone, rhythm, and loudness.
2. Enunciate. Pronounce vowels and consonants clearly. Some medical terms sound very similar.
3. Use inflection to amplify the meaning of your message.
4. Avoid words that antagonize. For example, the word contaminated to a lay person may mean dirty or filthy, whereas to the nurse it means unsterile or lacking medical asepsis.
5. Use short, simple sentences.
6. Adjust the volume, rate, and speed of voice to the situation. If the receiver is knowledgeable about the situation, you can go faster.
7. Keep the door open for feedback. Allow the receiver time to ask questions.

Evaluate your speaking skills through the use of a recording device such as a tape recorder or video recorder. A videotape will reveal your nonverbal communication skills as well as your verbal skills.

▽▽▽
Reading

Reading is one of the most important tools in your present and future education. In your practice as a nurse, you will need to be able to understand with accuracy and sometimes with quickness the information in clients' records, textbooks, professional journals, and on computers. You will be taking your licensure examination (NCLEX-PN) on the computer. Textbooks and professional journals are frequently used in the care-giving setting to help answer questions and to solve problems. The literature contains the information required to remain updated on issues in everyday practice. Today's technology allows you to scan the Internet for information using a computer and a telephone modem.

Reading is a skill that requires practice to improve speed and comprehension. Your speed will slow down when you read technical materials and literature that contains unfamiliar or complex terms. Your rate of reading also depends on the number of pauses your eyes make. If you read one word at a time, your speed will be slower than if you read in whole phrases. It is usually easy to increase reading speed, but it is more difficult to improve comprehension.

Developing a good vocabulary is essential. The tools you should use include medical and general dictionaries and glossaries. Note the pronunciation as well as the meaning of the word and state the meaning in your own words. Note prefixes and suffixes of medical terms. You can determine the meanings of new or unfamiliar words that use similar or familiar prefixes and suffixes. Use the language-development centers at your school or college in your community if you have reading problems. Reading skills can be improved by learning and practicing proven techniques (Meltzer and Palau, 1993, p.1).

▽▽▽
Writing

Writing skills are essential for the student and the graduate practical nurse. You will be taking notes in class and during meetings and reports. You will constantly be making notes in clients' records or entering information on the computer. Many acute care facilities use computers as a communication tool. Writing and spelling skills are essential when processing requisition forms or other communication forms. Considering the importance of communicating accurately in health care settings, the message or information must be correct, concise, and legible.

A written communication that is accurate and legible usually relays the message better than a verbal communication only. You do need to select the correct words to communicate the message accurately. This requires a knowledge of medical terminology as well as a knowledge of the situation.

Your observations and nursing interventions will be recorded on a legal document that becomes the client's record. Be specific about your documentation. Use only accepted or standard abbreviations. Your ability to communicate to others the client's condition and response is vital to his or her well-being. Medications, treatments, and nursing care orders are based on accurate communications between professionals. Record and report only information that is relative to recovery or treatment.

▼▼▼
Developing a Therapeutic Relationship

▽▽▽
Determine the Purpose of Communication

Social conversation can be used to begin a more purposeful conversation, but it should be limited. Social conversation does not usually lead to the information-sharing needed by the nurse and client. Social conversation can, however, help to establish rapport with a new client.

Gathering information is an essential everyday activity of the nurse. When clients enter the health care setting or the nurse enters the client's home to give care, the nurse conducts an interview to formulate a health history. Past and present illnesses, the events leading to present needs, and the specific details of the presenting complaint or need are recorded. This information will be used during the entire treatment phase to help direct the medical and nursing orders. Thus, accuracy is of utmost importance. This is when the nurse–client relationship begins. First impressions are important to the development of this relationship.

The nurse shares information and ideas when teaching the client about the illness, treatment, and plan of care. The client many times participates by contributing information or ideas about how the plan might best work. You share feelings about the client by displaying warmth, support, and caring. A trusting relationship is developed by demonstrating that you care about and respect the client and that you feel he or she is important. Techniques that you can use to share observations about the perceived feelings of the client are discussed later in this chapter.

▽▽▽
Factors Influencing Communication

The nurse who understands the factors that might help or hinder the communication process will be a better communicator. Several factors influence the communication process and apply to three categories: the environment, the nurse, and the client. Age will influence the vocabulary you use. A child has limited language skills compared with an adult. You will need to use language based on the client's age and understanding. "Talking down" to a person of any age demonstrates disrespect and destroys rapport. The sex of your client can influence the type of information that your client or you will feel comfortable discussing. A female client may feel more comfortable discussing intimate and sexual topics with a female nurse, and males tend to discuss such matters more openly with a male nurse. Some clients may feel uncomfortable in discussing the topic of sex with anyone. You need to consider this and create an accepting, comfortable situation.

Privacy, quiet, and comfort are essential to providing an environment and situation that are conducive to effective and therapeutic communication. Avoid teaching and lengthy conversations when the environment is full of interruptions. When the client is too fatigued or is experiencing pain or anxiety, delay the interaction until the client is able to communicate more effectively.

The intelligence and educational level of the client have to be considered when communicating. Use vocabulary and terminology that are understandable to the client and avoid "talking down" to any client. A person's age, occupation, and interests often give clues to the amount of information he or she has on a particular topic. A person in a health occupation probably is knowledgeable about illness and treatment.

Other factors that influence communication are mental or sensory impairments, the attitudes and values of the nurse and the client, and past experiences with illness. Often a client is not capable of engaging effectively in the communication process or developing a rapport because of a mental, hearing, speech, or touch disorder. The attitudes of the nurse about sex, race, role

identification, and illness can affect the communication process. Acceptance of others is essential to effective communication.

Communication provides the means by which people establish a sense of bonding or connection with one another. It permits sharing of information, signals, or messages in the form of ideas and feelings. It is a process by which you affect another through verbal and nonverbal language.

The diverse backgrounds of clients and nurses frequently present barriers to the communication needed to provide the most effective care. The client who does not understand what is happening may feel misunderstood, alienated, helpless, or angry, and may be noncompliant or withdrawn. The healing process may be impaired. As the nurse in this situation, you may feel helpless and frustrated in knowing how to provide adequate care. You should have a thorough awareness of racial, cultural, and social factors that may affect communication with people from cultures other than your own (Giger, 1991, p. 8).

Culture influences how feelings are expressed and what verbal and nonverbal expressions are appropriate (Giger, 1991, p. 8). Americans tend to use touch less and to be less open about feelings and the demonstration of feelings than people of some other cultures. Keep in mind that there are cultures within cultures. It is important not to stereotype individuals based on apparent differences. Although you should keep in mind common cultural patterns, it is essential to approach your client as an individual with a unique cultural heritage (Giger, 1991, p. 9).

The same words often have different meanings for different individuals within and between cultural groups. Slang words or phrases are notorious for creating misunderstanding. Common English words have different meanings in different cultural groups. The phrases "I will deal with it" and "That is cool" have several meanings. Avoid using medical terms when speaking to a client who has only a partial understanding of the language you speak. Abbreviations should be avoided. You can use a dictionary that has both the client's and your language in it. Several medical dictionaries have sections that give common medical statements and questions in several languages.

Keep in mind that when you try to speak a language

other than your own you may still be misunderstood or not understood because your accent is different. When needed, language interpreters are valuable assistants. Family members sometimes can act as interpreters.

A person's dialect or accent may make it difficult to understand him or her even if the same language is being spoken. We all have accents to someone who speaks a different language or who lives in a different part of the country or world. Listen carefully and be certain others understand you. Some people speak very fast. Ask them to speak more slowly so that you can ensure your understanding. If you yourself speak fast, practice slowing down.

Language barriers are obvious problems in effective communication. Nonverbal communication skills are especially important in these cases. Members of the family or a bilingual health care worker can provide assistance. Lack of communication can lead to frustration on the part of the client and the nurse. It can also lead to ineffective, unsafe care.

Honesty and Empathy

Honesty and empathy are essential to the development of effective relationships. These qualities demonstrate caring and support. Empathy is identification with and understanding of another's situation, feelings, and motives. To elaborate, empathy is the ability to recognize and to some extent share the emotions and states of mind of another and to understand the meaning and significance of that person's behavior. It is an essential quality for effective communication.

Empathy involves striving to understand what the other person is feeling and experiencing. It is difficult to put yourself in the same situation when you are not experiencing the same pain and anxiety that the client is. You will not be able to empathize with all clients because of your limited personal experiences with illness and treatment.

It is possible to expand empathetic skills by the use of imagination. Imagine yourself having the same experience of pain, frustration, anxiety, and concern about the effects of the illness on your life and family. Be careful not to drain your physical and emotional energies by identifying too closely with the situation because this will prevent you from being helpful to the

client when he or she needs your strength and support. With empathy there is a momentary entry into the world of another while the self is abandoned. However, the empathizer never loses sight of his or her separateness and is always aware that the feelings of the other are not his or her own (Pike, 1990, p. 235).

Listening skills are essential to communicate empathetically. You have to get an accurate picture of the other person's situation. This requires active listening (empathy), which lets the speaker know that you know how he or she is feeling and why. The goal of empathy is to aid in the establishment of rapport in order to secure a helpful relationship. It is the intention of the sender and the perception of the receiver that are beneficial (Smith, 1992, p. 95).

Caring

Caring is having a positive regard for another person. It is basic to a helping relationship. Nurses show caring by accepting clients as they are and respecting them as individuals. When clients feel cared for they feel secure, even though they may be in threatening or anxiety-producing situations. Caring also promotes trust (Potter and Perry, 1995, p. 213). Accepting clients as they are may be difficult at times depending on the particular illness involved or the problems it presents. For example, it may be difficult to accept clients with criminal records, those with Alzheimer's disease, or those who are socially dysfunctional.

Trust

Trust is an essential component of caring. Trust is reliance on someone without doubt or question. Confidentiality and dependability are essential to the development of a trusting relationship. Trust makes communication more effective as individuals become more open and can express their thoughts and feelings. The therapeutic nurse–client relationship is greatly enhanced by the trust in the nurse that may develop in the client.

Responsibility

It is important to take responsibility for what you say. It is also important to listen to what others say. Native

Americans sometimes use a "talking stick," which is passed around to remind others to listen. The stick reminds the speaker of the responsibility to speak from the heart (Silha, 1995, p. 4). Therapeutic relationships require the care giver to listen to the client and the family and to respond responsibly in a caring, empathic way. You have the responsibility to ensure that what you say is accurate and reliable.

Listening

To hear is only part of listening. The ability to hear certainly affects your listening skills. Hearing is the process whereby sound waves reach the eardrum and cause vibrations that are transmitted to the brain. Listening occurs when the brain reconstructs these impulses and gives them meaning (Adler, 1991, p. 91). Listening is the interpretation of the sound. Many times we hear but do not listen. Sometimes the best way to help people with problems is to listen to them (Adler, 1991, p. 91).

The client's problems and feelings are the center of the nurse–client communication. You must develop listening skills to help the client. Listening is essential in establishing a therapeutic relationship. Most people communicate openly if they believe they have an attentive, caring listener who does not impose his or her beliefs and values and does not give unwanted and unneeded advice. Listen to the tone in which the words are conveyed. Listening skills can be developed.

At times we are all selective listeners. If the topic does not interest us we frequently tune out. If we are involved in doing a procedure, sometimes we are not really listening. Our concentration is focused on doing the procedure correctly. We all have a self-tape that runs all the time. It takes discipline to learn to shut it down. To be an effective listener you need to be totally involved in the moment; you are not thinking about what you are going to do or say next (Grossman, 1995, p. 10).

Active listening demands that you focus on what the other person is saying and feeling. Listen for the who, what, where, when, how, and why of the conversation. Listen for ideas. Good listening requires an open and accepting attitude. The client must know that you are interested and that you care before he or she will share personal, perhaps embarrassing, information. To communicate interest and caring you can start with eye contact, sitting down, and an alert body posture. The nurse is usually standing while providing care; you do not want to communicate that you are in a hurry. Sitting down implies that you are willing to take the time to listen. It also communicates equal status. Sit facing the client rather than on the side, again indicating interest in the person. Sit within a comfortable distance. Being close may intimidate the client. For personal interaction and when discussing personal information, the range is approximately 1½ to 4 feet, or near enough to shake hands. It also prevents people who should not hear from overhearing the conversation. An intimate interaction distance is 3 to 18 inches, and a social interaction distance is 4 to 12 feet.

Do not begin or continue significant conversations while hanging onto the door or door frame. Provide for privacy by shutting the door or moving to a private area whenever possible. Be certain that the client is comfortable. It is difficult to communicate clearly when in pain or in need of bowel or bladder elimination.

Try not to write a great deal during the interview. Writing communicates inattention and interferes with the client's spontaneity and your ability to listen. If you need to take notes, take brief ones. Be attentive, concentrate, and show interest in what the client is saying so that you understand fully what is being communicated. Ask the client to express his or her perception of the problem. For example, what brought the client to the hospital?

Active listening requires a willingness to devote time and energy to the process. The nurse must use an extensive knowledge base. You must first listen before you can respond appropriately. Nursing students frequently feel ill at ease and useless when they are talking to clients because they do not feel as if they are "doing" something for the client. Listening is one aspect of observation and a means of developing a confidential relationship.

While you are listening you may express agreement with a smile or nod of the head and respond to cues, but do not interrupt. Ask questions when the client is finished to clarify or solicit more information. Try not to probe into areas that the client does not wish to share. Being an attentive listener and allowing clients to talk helps to relieve anxiety.

One suggested activity to increase one's listening ability is to practice with fellow students or friends. The task is to be able to repeat verbatim what the first person has said before you are permitted to say something and to continue until all persons have had a chance to say something. This activity forces you to listen attentively. Your friend or fellow student can tell you if you are accurate. Record your interactions with clients and evaluate their effectiveness.

Territoriality

Territoriality is the geographic area that we assume is ours. Examples are: our room, house, and neighborhood (Adler, 1991, p. 142). Nurses have to recognize that the client's territory exists and must be sensitive to the need for privacy. Knocking before entering a client's room and getting permission to enter communicates sensitivity to the need for privacy.

Personal space is related to territoriality. It is the distance a person feels comfortable with when relating to another person. Nurses frequently invade this space when providing nursing care. A trusting relationship needs to be developed before the nurse is permitted into this space. A child instinctively rejects someone with whom they have not developed a trusting relationship. Clients sometimes refuse care that involves invasion of their personal space. Permission needs to be sought and obtained prior to providing care. Clients give permission for treatment and care on admission. However, verbal permission needs to be sought to provide specific treatment and care.

Intonation

The tone of the nurse's voice can have a dramatic effect on the meaning of a message. Depending on intonation, the phrase "How are you?" can express enthusiasm, concern, indifference, and even annoyance. A nurse's emotions can directly affect the tone of voice. Often this is unconscious, and the words send one message while the voice tone conveys something different.

Clients may question a nurse's credibility and caring if there is a discrepancy between the message and the tone of voice used in sending the message. The nurse must be aware of any emotions that send messages that negatively affect the development of a helping relationship.

The nurse should be aware that voice tone and pitch communicate the client's emotional and physical states such as fear, anger, grief, and energy level. The voice of a rested, healthy person has clarity, inflection, and variations, whereas a fatigued, ill person sometimes has a weak, monotonous, unclear voice. Sensitivity to voice tone, facial expression, and other nonverbal cues enhances the nurse's assessment skills.

Humor

When used appropriately, humor can be therapeutic. It can decrease anxiety and tension, build relationships, and make very difficult situations bearable. You must carefully assess the client and the situation to determine whether humor is appropriate. When people are from different cultures, humor can be detrimental to the relationship if it is misunderstood (Giger, 1991, p. 22)

When used for a specific purpose, humor can cut through overly intense situations. Humor is most effective when rapport is well established and a level of trust exists between the nurse and the client (Arnold, 1995, p. 223). One physical effect resulting from laughter, which hopefully results from the use of humor, is the production of β-endorphins, which lift the spirit and enhance physical healing. The depression that frequently accompanies illness can be avoided or lessened when humor is used. Humor can reduce tension and aggression. You need to assess the situation so that humor is not used at the wrong time. A frustrated client who is out of control or in severe pain may react negatively to humor.

Sarcasm ridicules, is not humorous, and has a destructive effect on your relationship with clients. Jokes that are offensive to cultural or religious groups or are sexually explicit are not acceptable. Jokes of this nature are detrimental to caring relationships and diminish your effectiveness and professionalism.

▼▼▼
Techniques That Encourage Therapeutic Communication

Some communication techniques are designed to encourage communication. These techniques include broad opening statements, open-ended questions or statements, reflecting, selective reflecting, general leads, and silence.

Broad opening statements or questions allow the client to select the direction of the conversation and the opportunity to express what his or her concerns are. Examples:

Nurse: How are things going?

Nurse: How are things today?

Nurse: Tell me about yourself.

Open-ended questions and statements are identical to broad opening statements. You may hear or read both terms. Both terms allow the client to expand or elaborate on a topic he or she selects.

Reflecting leads the client to consider fully and to expand on his or her remark. It is a form of feedback or response that encourages the speaker to continue talking about a subject. It may include all or part of the speaker's statement. The following statements are examples:

Client: I was awake all night because I was so nervous.

Nurse: You were nervous? *or* You were awake all night?

Be careful not to overuse this technique because it may sound as if you are parroting or echoing the client, and that could be annoying.

Selective reflecting encourages further exploration of a part of the patient's statement. Although similar to reflecting, the nurse selects the part of the statement that seems most significant and repeats or restates it.

For example:

Client: This brace is giving me a bad time, I was awake all night.

Nurse: The brace is giving you a problem?

Client: I can't go home, not like this.

Nurse: You think you can't go home?

General leads are one- or two-word responses by the nurse that encourage the client to continue. Such words include go on, and then, yes, and oh.

Silence slows the pace of the conversation and gives the client time to reflect on what has been said. This usually encourages further conversation. It allows the nurse time to observe the client for nonverbal cues. You will need to practice feeling at ease during silence.

Other communication techniques are designed to ensure mutual understanding and include clarifying and validating.

Clarifying helps to make meanings clear and to avoid misunderstanding. Sometimes it is difficult to identify another person's feelings or to understand what is intended. When you speak to another person, there are at least six messages involved in the conversation: what I mean to say, what I actually say, what he hears, what he thinks he hears, what he says, and what I think he says. You must recognize these different messages and attempt to clarify them. Examples of clarifying are:

Nurse: I am not sure I understand.

Nurse: I am not sure I follow.

Nurse: Is this what you are saying?

Validating means checking to see whether a client's need has or has not been met. Evaluation statements are attempts to validate. Examples are:

Nurse: How are you feeling after your pain medication?

Nurse: Has your nausea subsided since I gave you the injection?

Nurse: How did you sleep last night?

Still other communication techniques are designed to encourage expressions of thoughts and feelings.

These techniques are sharing observations, acknowledging thoughts and feelings, and verbalizing implied thoughts and feelings. These are clarification techniques.

Sharing observations tells the client that you have noted his or her response (physical or emotional) and are concerned and interested. Examples are:

Nurse: You look like you have pain.

Nurse: I noticed you tossing and turning.

Nurse: I see that you are eating more today.

Acknowledging thoughts and feelings communicates to the client that you understand and accept his or her feelings. Examples are:

Nurse: This must be difficult for you.

Nurse: It must be difficult to be on bed rest.

Verbalizing implied thoughts and feelings helps the nurse to verify impressions and helps the client to recognize or explore his or her feelings. Examples are:

Client: What is the point in talking about it?

Nurse: Do you think I won't understand?

Client: One thing after another, always something going wrong.

Nurse: Are you concerned about your progress?

Giving information means sharing information with clients about their illness, hospitalization, nursing care, and treatment. *Direct questioning and exploring* are used to obtain information from the client. Exploring is a means of seeking information to obtain details about a situation.

Techniques Used to Encourage Communication

Identify the technique being used:

_d_ 1. *Nurse:* You seem restless since your doctor was here.

_h_ 2. *Client:* Why is this happening?
   Nurse: I am not certain I understand. Are you referring to your wound?

_b_ 3. *Nurse:* How are things right now?

_i_ 4. *Client:* This IV sure is bothering me.
   Nurse: Bothering you?

_e_ 5. *Client:* Things are a real mess today.
   Nurse: Oh?

_c_ 6. *Client:* My mother should be here.
   Nurse: Your mother?

_f_ 7. *Nurse:* When was your last bowel movement?

_a_ 8. *Nurse:* Are you more comfortable since your brace was adjusted?

_g_ 9. *Client:* My husband has been too attentive lately.
   Nurse: Do you think he is overly concerned or anxious about you?

a. Validating
b. Broad opening statement or open-ended question
c. Reflecting
d. Sharing observations
e. General lead

f. Obtaining information or direct questioning
g. Verbalizing implied thoughts and feelings
h. Clarifying
i. Selective reflecting

Answers: 1. d, 2. h, 3. b, 4. i, 5. e, 6. c, 7. f, 8. a, 9. g

▼▼▼
Blocks to Therapeutic Communication

Responses, questions, or statements that hinder the flow of conversation and the development of a therapeutic relationship with the client should be avoided. The nurse must be aware of the blocks and attempt to avoid them by using therapeutic communication techniques. Blocks include reassuring clichés, stereotyped comments, questions that require a yes or no answer, probing, leading questions, giving advice, belittling, changing the subject, and hostility.

Reassuring clichés are trite or pat answers and tend to minimize the significance of the client's feelings and convey a lack of understanding or interest. Examples are:

Nurse: Everything will be okay.

Nurse: You will be just fine.

Nurse: Things always work out for the best.

Nurse: Don't worry, it will be all right.

Comments such as these convey the impression that the nurse is denying that the client has a problem. The client is interested in his or her own feelings and problems and not in how everyone else feels. Clichés give false reassurance—maybe everything is not going to be all right.

Stereotyped comments lead the client to respond in a like manner, thus keeping the conversation at a superficial level. Important information is not sought or given about the client's condition or concerns. This tends to convey to the client that you are not listening or not interested and are answering automatically. Examples are

Client: I am concerned about tomorrow.

Nurse: Everyone is afraid of surgery.

Nurse: Everyone feels that way.

These comments may communicate to the client that his or her concerns are not unique and are not important.

Closed questions or questions that can be answered by one word, such as yes or no, should not be used when you are seeking information that is more complex. For example, do not ask, "Did you take your medication?" when you want to know whether the client is having any difficulty taking the medication or having any side effects. Do not ask, "Did you have a good day?" when you want specific information about the nature of the client's comfort or discomfort.

Probing may cause clients to become resentful. They will usually respond by avoiding conversation with you. Probing may be interpreted by the patient as an invasion of privacy. As the nurse, you are given private, privileged information. Use the therapeutic techniques to encourage conversation. Explain why you need certain information and do not seek information that you do not need. For example:

Nurse: Now, let's find out what the real problem is.

Nurse: Is that all you are going to tell me?

Nurse: Tell me why you feel that way.

Requesting an explanation could be viewed as probing. Often the person does not know the answer and, if he or she does, may resent your asking. It makes the client uncomfortable when he or she has to explain feelings or actions.

Leading questions suggest a response that the nurse wants to hear. Leading questions tend to produce answers that may please the nurse but are unlikely to encourage the client to respond without feeling intimidated. Consider the following two examples:

Nurse: You are not going to smoke that cigar, are you?

Nurse: You have been well cared for by your nurses, haven't you?

Giving advice indicates that the nurse knows what is best for the client and is imposing her own values and judgments rather than seeking and acknowledging the client's rights to his or her own feelings. It tends to encourage dependency. Advice should be given by the nurse when requested. Examples of giving inappropriate advice are:

Nurse: You should take up golf. It is good exercise and will take your mind off your worries.

Nurse: You should not worry about that. It only increases your blood pressure.

Belittling the patient's feelings or actions encourages resentment. It implies that the client's feelings are not unusual or important and are not accepted. It conveys that something must be wrong with the client for having these feelings or concerns. Examples are:

Client: I cannot believe I still have this pain.

Nurse: Most people have more pain than you have.

Nurse: You are acting like a baby. Keep your chin up.

Nurse: Most clients do better than you are doing at this point.

Disagreeing with the patient and *expressing disapproval* produce the same responses as belittling.

Changing the subject quickly stops a conversation. It takes the lead away from the client, thereby blocking attempts to discuss his or her feelings or concerns. Furthermore, it prevents the client from asking questions and causes frustration. The nurse frequently uses this block unconsciously when she or he is not knowledgeable about the topic and when the topic, such as

sex or chronic or terminal illness, is embarrassing or uncomfortable. Examples are:

Client: I understand that the operation I need is pretty serious.

Nurse: Yes. Would you like to eat now?

Client: When will I be able to get off bed rest? I am really tired of lying in bed.

Nurse: Soon. Let's talk about your medication now.

Hostility is obviously destructive to the client–nurse relationship. Anxious clients frequently react with anger or hostility. Nurses and other health care workers frequently bear the brunt of this anger from clients and families, and it is difficult not to feel defensive and hostile in return. A hostile comment from the nurse will hinder the nurse–client relationship. Hostile comments may infringe on a client's rights and may lead to legal problems. Threatening or abusive comments violate clients' legal rights. Examples of hostile comments are:

Nurse: You have no right to say that.

Nurse: Don't ever do that again.

Nurse: I will not bring your pain medication if you behave that way.

Blocks to Communication

Identify the block being used:

____ 1. *Nurse:* Of course you are going to be okay.

____ 2. *Nurse:* Did you have a good breakfast?

____ 3. *Nurse:* Let's talk about your sexual problem.

____ 4. *Nurse:* You should take up swimming; it will take your mind off your problem.

____ 5. *Nurse:* Everybody is afraid before surgery.

____ 6. *Nurse:* You have to expect some pain.

____ 7. *Client:* This lump is serious, isn't it?
   Nurse: Maybe. Do you want your bath now?

____ 8. *Nurse:* You are not going to get out of bed alone, are you?

b   9. *Nurse:* Don't you talk to me in that tone of voice.

a. Stereotyped comment
b. Hostility
c. Reassuring cliché
d. Probing
e. Changing the subject

f. Belittling
g. Closed question or question with one word answer
h. Giving advice
i. Leading question

Answers: 1. c, 2. g, 3. d, 4. h, 5. a, 6. f, 7. e, 8. i, 9. b

▼▼▼
Communications with Colleagues

Communication with other members of the health team is an important aspect of the nurse's role. Few nurses work independently, and most nurses work in a complex information-gathering and information-sharing system. Communication is essential to the accurate planning, coordination, delivery, and evaluation of care and documentation of that care. The planning and delivery of care is a coordinated effort by a team. The nurse works and communicates closely with a variety of health care workers other than nurses. These other health care workers include the physician, respiratory therapist, physical therapist, laboratory technologist, dietician, social worker, various types of technicians, and business office personnel.

The same principles of communication used in the nurse–client relationship apply when relating with other health team members. Listening to each other, respectfully relating to each other, empathy, and caring are all essential to the development of positive workplace and collegial relationships. Ultimately, the workplace atmosphere will have an effect on the nurse-client relationship (Arnold and Boggs, 1995, p. 514).

Networking or peer consultation and collaboration are valuable resources. It helps you obtain information or validates your nursing actions. Networking involves your peers who work with you in the same facility as well as those hundreds or thousands of miles away. You can network in your work setting, at professional meetings and conferences, by reading professional literature, and by using the Internet.

Communication takes place in many ways. The most frequent channels are face to face, telephone, and written messages, such as those on the client's record. It is essential to communicate effectively. Communication becomes more effective when people are aware of their effect on others and know how to avoid poor communication.

Think about how you would feel and respond if your supervisor or instructor said to you, "Make certain this medication is given on time; you've made enough mistakes already." You would probably not feel very good about yourself or the person who made the statement. Another statement that is not effective is, "You are not allowed to do that without checking with me first" or "You can't do anything right today." Think about how these messages could be delivered without destroying relationships.

An example of an effective interaction is as follows: "I see you are having difficulties with that procedure. Would you like help?" It is important to address others as your equal and with respect. When you feel uncomfortable after an interaction at home, at school, or as the nurse, evaluate the transaction to determine why it went poorly. You need to be able to "read between the lines." You or the person communicating with you may have used the negative parts of the child or parent personality. Analyze the following interactions and reconstruct them, if necessary, to get positive results.

You: I am feeling anxious, I don't think I can give this injection.

Your supervisor: In my opinion, you usually do things well.

You: I am sick and tired of all the work I have to do.

Your supervisor: If you don't do it, you will be fired.

You: I've had it, everybody is yelling at me today.

Your supervisor: How about taking a few minutes in the lounge to collect yourself and then let's talk about it.

▽▽▽
"I" Messages

"I" messages are used in assertive responses and therapeutically with patients in mental health settings. Assertiveness is covered in Chapter 11. "I" messages can and should be used when the client or a colleague is infringing on your personal rights, you are explaining how you see the situation, or you are asked for your opinion. Overuse of "I" messages focuses on the nurse, not the client, and gives the impression that the nurse is self-centered and is not interested in the client. Avoid overuse of "I" messages in social conversations for the same reasons.

▼▼▼
Communicating with Clients with Special Needs

▽▽▽
Older Adults

Older adults vary greatly in their capabilities, interests, and capacities for relationships. Some have reduced intellectual and physical functions, whereas others have a high level of physical and intellectual function (Arnold and Boggs, 1995, p. 434). Many communication and relationship problems can be avoided by recognizing that older adults are unique individuals with specific needs. Healthy older adults sometimes require more time to complete verbal responses or to remember events. Allowing a little more time for processing may be all that is required (Arnold and Boggs, 1995, p. 435).

Older adults frequently have communication problems owing to sensory or motor impairments. Sensory refers to the senses: sight, hearing, touch, taste, and smell. Motor refers to muscular function. Muscles used in speech are sometimes affected by some diseases. Many older adults adapt to these losses and can learn to communicate effectively. The nurse needs to use non-verbal and written communications when necessary and appropriate.

If a client has a hearing deficit, speak slowly and clearly, stand in front of the client to provide an opportunity for lip reading, talk toward the client's best ear, and reduce background noise (Potter and Perry, 1995). Be certain only one person is talking at a time. If the client has a hearing aid, be certain that the aid is clean, is inserted properly, and has a functioning battery. Adjust the volume of the aid to a comfortable level or help the client do so. Keep eyeglasses clean. This helps the client to see nonverbal cues (Potter and Perry, 1995, p. 224).

Sometimes the client's only means of communication is nonverbal messages. The nurse needs to be alert to the cues such clients are communicating. For example, a client with Alzheimer's disease may use an inanimate object such as a doll to communicate a need such as hunger, pain, or fatigue.

▽▽▽
Children

Communication with a child requires the nurse to develop a relationship with both the child and the parents. The nurse receives much information from the parents. To communicate effectively with children, the nurse must adjust to the developmental level of the child.

Young children communicate mainly through nonverbal messages. It is important to be honest with children. Explanations are always necessary when doing procedures and should be simple, short, and direct. Sometimes play is necessary to communicate at some age levels. Pictures, drawings, stuffed toys, and dolls are helpful to relate a message.

Crying is an important nonverbal communication used frequently by children. Children use crying to communicate a need or problem such as pain, hunger, or the need for comfort.

▼▼▼
Computer Communication

Computers have long been a part of our everyday lives. Computers entered the health care system during the

1950s. At first they were used primarily for financial purposes. As technology advanced, many departments in health care facilities became aware of the possibilities of the computer and began to use it as a tool to increase the effectiveness and efficiency of health care delivery. Today, many acute care facilities use automated nursing documentation or use computers in some form. Nurses now recognize the potential of computers to improve nursing care practice and delivery of high-quality patient care. Computer systems are available to help facilitate documentation of patient data, prepare care plans, monitor clients' progress, and facilitate scheduling of staff. Computers are used to manage diagnostic procedures such as scanning, radiologic studies, and clinical laboratory tests. The mundane, routine tasks are performed by the computer and the professional's skills are reserved for tasks that cannot be performed by computers or robots. Computers are helpful tools for nurses.

At first, computers were used for calculation of numbers. Today, they can measure pressures and temperatures as well as control sophisticated equipment such as chemical analyzers and computed axial tomography (CAT) scanners. Computers are also used as word processors or office automation equipment.

There are basically three types of computers:

1. Mainframe—the largest; controls and performs many functions.
2. Microcomputer—a small unit that links with the mainframe, permitting a large number of functions.
3. Personal computer—the smallest computer that has the fewest functions; presently used in the home and in office settings.

Nurses use the microcomputer or a personal computer in the nursing department. The same confidentiality in regard to the information entered and received by computer is required as when using the manual method of documentation. Nurses receive a computer code after they successfully complete a computer course, usually provided by the employing facility. The computer code allows nurses access to the computer system. This code is known only to the individual nurse and the person in charge of assigning codes. This code is secured and cannot be shared with anyone else. Any break in security is a basis for dismissal from the job.

The reason for the tight security is client safety and privacy, the legal protection of the nurse and the facility, and accountability. The facility must be confident that the person who entered the data regarding care is truly the person identified by the code.

The nurse does not need to know the mechanics of the computer but he or she should be computer literate. This means that you should understand some terms used and have a basic understanding of the way computers function. Two terms frequently used are *computer hardware* and *computer software*. The hardware is the machine itself. Computer hardware has four essential components: devices that (1) receive input, (2) process data, (3) store data, and (4) process output. The most common input device is the keyboard, which functions much like a typewriter with some modifications. Most systems use a mouse, a light pen, or a trackball to enter information on the computer screen. The central processing unit directs information to the appropriate area in the system and processes the data, such as calculations. Devices for storing data or information are called memory. The two types of memory that exist are permanent internal factory-installed memory or read-only memory (ROM) and temporary or random-access memory (RAM), which is generated by the user.

Computer software is the package of programmed instructions that direct and permit the computer to carry out functions. A programmer develops the program or set of instructions. The complexity of the particular set of instructions determines the capacity and function of the computer. A client-care documentation system is programmed considerably differently from a CAT scanner. However, the same computer can be programmed for multiple functions.

CD-ROM is a compact disc that stores words, pictures, and other information for computers that have a special drive. ROM means "read only memory," which means that you cannot record, only read the information (Silha, 1995, p. 6).

E-mail or *electronic mail* sends messages electronically through computerized bulletin boards or the Internet. The Internet is the decentralized global network designed by the U.S. Department of Defense that is now used as an "information superhighway" (Silha, 1995, p. 6).

A *modem* is a machine that hooks your computer to telephone lines, enabling it to send and receive messages. The *fax*, short for facsimile, is a machine that transmits copies of pages over telephone lines. It is a fast and inexpensive way to communicate in writing (Silha, 1995, p. 6).

What does all this mean for the person entering nursing? Familiarity with computers helps you adapt to and understand how high-technology information systems can assist you. Computer-aided instruction is used in many schools of nursing to enhance your learning and to familiarize you with computer use. Refer to Chapter 8 for information about computer-assisted instruction.

▼▼▼ S U M M A R Y

▶ Effective communication between clients and nurses and between nurses and other health care workers is essential because it contributes to the quality of care and the client's well-being. The nurse must develop effective verbal and nonverbal skills to help the client meet his or her health care needs. It is essential for the nurse to understand the communication process and the barriers or factors that influence the process such as age, culture, past experiences, feelings, values, and emotions.

▶ Communication skills such as listening, nonverbal and verbal therapeutic techniques, and recognition of the effects of blocks all help the nurse to establish a rapport with the client. This rapport and these skills enable the nurse to conduct client interviews effectively, allowing the nurse to receive, give, clarify, or validate information and establish client-care goals. Understanding the effects of culture, the use of humor, and transactional analysis will further enhance the nurse's ability to communicate effectively with clients and colleagues.

▶ Process recordings of actual communications with clients and colleagues in clinical settings help the nurse to analyze interactions and the effectiveness of communication techniques. These recordings help the nurse recognize and identify blocks to communication. The nurse can then improve his or her communication skills by reconstructing ineffective responses, statements, and questions to a more effective form, which will help in similar future situations.

▶ Computer literacy and an understanding of the use of computers will further develop the nurse's communication skills. E-mail and the Internet help nurses communicate with their colleagues and keep up-to-date in nursing skills.

▼▼▼ R E F E R E N C E S

Adler R, Rodman G. *Understanding Human Communication,* 4th ed. Orlando: Holt, Rinehart, and Winston, 1991.

American Heritage College Dictionary, 3rd ed. Boston: Houghton-Mifflin, 1993.

Arnold E, Boggs K. *Interpersonal Communications: Professional Communication Skills for Nurses.* Philadelphia: W.B. Saunders, 1995.

Giger JL, Davidhizar R. *Transcultural Nursing: Assessment and Intervention.* St. Louis: C.V. Mosby, 1991.

Grossman J. Two intertwined arts: Listening and asking questions. Creative Living, Spring, 1995.

Meltzer M, Palau S. *Reading and Study Strategies for Nursing Students.* Philadelphia: W.B. Saunders, 1993.

Pike AW. On the nature and place of empathy in clinical nursing practice. J Prof Nurs 1990;6(4): 235–240.

Potter P, Perry A. *Basic Nursing Theory and Practice,* 3rd ed. St. Louis: C.V. Mosby, 1995.

Silha S. The network of conversations. Creative Living 1995; Spring, 4, 6.

Smith S. *Communications in Nursing,* 2nd ed. St. Louis: C.V. Mosby, 1992.

Cultural Uniqueness, Sensitivity, and Competence

CHAPTER 14

▼▼▼ OUTLINE

▼▼▼ KEY TERMS

acculturation
assimilation
assumption
biomedicine
cultural bias

cultural diversity
cultural pluralism
cultural sensitivity
cultural uniqueness
cultural universality

culture
customs
discrimination
ethnic groups
ethnocentrism

health beliefs

melting pot

naturalistic system

nonjudgmental

personalistic system

prejudice

repatterning

stereotype

world view

▼▼▼   O B J E C T I V E S

Upon completing this chapter you will be able to:

1. *Explain in your own words nine basic daily needs of all persons.*

2. *Define in your own words the following terms:*
   a. *Culture*
   b. *Cultural uniqueness*
   c. *Cultural diversity*
   d. *Ethnocentrism*
   e. *Cultural bias*
   f. *Cultural sensitivity*
   g. *Cultural competence*

3. *Explain the importance of the following in developing an ability to provide culturally competent care:*
   a. *Awareness of your own cultural self*
   b. *Attainment of knowledge about culturally diverse groups*
   c. *Negotiation of plans of care for culturally diverse clients*

4. *Explain in your own words the philosophy of individual worth as it applies to health care.*

5. *Describe your culture in the areas of*
   a. *Family*
   b. *Religion*
   c. *Communication*
   d. *Educational background*
   e. *Economic level*
   f. *Wellness and illness beliefs and practices*

6. *Describe specific differences between cultural groups in your geographic area that may have importance in client care situations.*

In the nineteenth century, waves of immigrants from throughout the world entered the United States. The United States was referred to as a melting pot. This term indicated that the immigrants had given up their native cultures and adopted the culture of the people already in the United States. In the 1990 U.S. census, a write-in blank for racial ancestry was provided on the census form. Americans reported nearly 300 "races," 600 Indian tribes, 70 Hispanic groups, and 75 combinations of multiracial ancestry (Morganthau, 1995, p. 65). Obviously, the concept of the melting pot has not occurred.

You have chosen a career that will give you an opportunity to meet people who are different from you! Some of these people will be your clients. Some will be your coworkers. Some will be of a different age. Some will belong to a different social class. Some will have disabilities. Some will have different health care beliefs about what causes them to get sick. Some will have different values. In addition to all these differences, some of your clients and coworkers will have different cultural backgrounds owing to ethnic group status. Regardless of cultural background, some differences will be the result of a growing diversity in individual and family life styles. It may come as a surprise when you discover that people think, feel, believe, act, and see the world differently from you and your family and friends.

Review the code of ethics of the National Association of Practical Nurse Education and Service (NAPNES) and the National Federation of Licensed Practical Nurses (NFLPN) (see Chapter 20). You will note that both organizations include statements that describe the need of the practical nurse to provide health care to all clients regardless of race, creed, cultural background, disease, or life style. This is an ethical expectation. Review your state's nurse practice act. You might find that failing or refusing to render nursing services to a client because of the client's race, color, sex, age, beliefs, national origin, or handicap is listed as unprofessional conduct. The ethical expectation now becomes a legal mandate. Leininger (1994) reports that some nurses face legal suits because of their ignorance of the culture of the client and resulting poor nursing judgment.

This chapter has three purposes. The first is to encourage you to identify how all persons, despite observed or assumed differences, are similar (**cultural universality**). The second is to encourage you to identify how all persons, despite similarities, are unique (**cultural uniqueness**). The third is to help you develop a **sensitivity** to **cultural diversity** among people. When in a health care situation, it is not enough to stop once you identify diversity and the differences it displays. Not only do practical nurses need to provide care for all persons, they need to provide culturally competent care. When differences are identified in a health care situation, the practical nurse should suggest adaptations to the plan of care so that the plan recognizes these differences. In doing so, the client will be encouraged to follow suggestions, avoid treatment failures, and return to health as quickly as possible. Practical nurses then will be able to say that they have truly met the clients' needs.

▼▼▼
What We Share in Common

Because of our genes, each individual the world over is different from every other person. The only exception is identical twins. Before you start to think about the differences among people, it is a good idea to think about what people share in common.

When you are among a group of your peers (for example, in class, eating lunch in the cafeteria, walking to the parking lot), take a few minutes to play the "what we have in common" culture game. Excluding sex, age, marital status, and culture group, try to find five items you share in common with *each* member of the group. This activity is especially helpful when the group includes classmates you perceive as "different" from you. Discuss the items you have in common in a class situation. Were you surprised by any items you share in common with other members of the group?

▽▽▽
Basic Daily Needs

All people share the same basic daily needs regardless of age, sex, economic status, life style, religion, country of origin, or culture. Chapter 9 discusses human needs as understood by the psychologist Abraham Maslow. Many years ago, Vivian Culver, a registered nurse (1974, pp. 375–376) listed nine essential daily needs of all persons. These needs have stood the test of time. They are a good place to start in learning to understand

that all people, regardless of background, share some things in common.

1. Personal care and hygiene
2. Sleep and rest
3. Nutrition and fluids
4. Elimination
5. Body alignment and activity
6. Environment
7. Emotional and spiritual support
8. Diversion and recreation
9. Mental hygiene

These nine basic daily needs can form the basis for planning client care. However, you need to understand the meaning of these basic needs for well persons, including yourself, before you can apply them to individuals in the clinical area. Once you gain understanding, the application of these needs to clients will be easier. As you read about the nine basic needs of all people, think about how you specifically meet each need in your own daily life. Could it be that some of your peers meet their daily basic needs in different ways than you meet your needs?

Personal Care and Hygiene

Clean hair, skin, nails, teeth, and clothing serve two general purposes: protection from illness and promotion of well-being. Skin constantly secretes sebum, the cold cream–like substance of the body, to keep the skin suppl`. Daily, epidermal skin cells (the outer layer of the skin) are shed as new cells push toward the outer layer. Skin eliminates fluid in the form of perspiration to help keep body temperature stable. Sebum and perspiration are odorless substances. Ever-present bacteria on the skin are responsible for the body odor we associate with the body's oils and perspiration. We meet personal care and hygiene needs by bathing, shampooing, handwashing, maintaining oral hygiene, and grooming. Do you prefer a shower or a bath or another method of cleansing your body? How often do you cleanse your body? During what part of the day do you cleanse your body? How often do you shampoo? What grooming products do you use to style your hair? How often do you visit the dentist?

Sleep and Rest

Sleep is needed to refresh ourselves. The actual number of hours of sleep required varies with the individual. Rest and periodic relaxation are just as important because they also help the body restore itself. How many hours of sleep do you get each night or day? Where do you rest or relax? What do you do to rest or relax?

Nutrition and Fluids

As you learned in Chapter 10, to stay healthy, we all need to eat a diet composed of a variety of foods. A minimum of six to eight glasses of water each day is recommended to help our body complete its many chemical reactions, transport nutrients, regulate temperature, and lubricate body parts. These six to eight glasses are in addition to the food and other beverages we eat and drink. How many calories do you consume each day? How many glasses of fluid do you drink each day? What fluids do you prefer to drink?

Elimination

Elimination of wastes from the body is primarily accomplished by the kidneys (in the form of urine) and the large intestine (in the form of feces). The skin is not as good at elimination as these organs, but it does eliminate some body wastes through perspiration. What do you consider to be "normal" time intervals for urinary and intestinal elimination?

Body Alignment and Activity

Body alignment, or the relationship of the body parts to one another, is better known as posture. When posture is "good," the body can be used in a comfortable manner without danger of injury. Good posture also enhances the functioning of the respiratory, gastrointestinal, and circulatory systems. You will not get tired as quickly if good posture is maintained. The function of these body systems can also be enhanced by exercising the body daily. Exercise also helps to maintain muscle tone. Have a peer evaluate your posture while sitting and while walking. How much exercise do you get each day? How do you get your exercise?

Environment

Environment refers to the space that surrounds us. Our environment changes many times during a day. Regardless of our specific environment, the most essential component of our surroundings is oxygen. After that environmental need has been met, the next most important need is safety. When oxygen and safety needs have been met, the individual can focus on changing his or her environment to accommodate comfort and personal taste. Describe your home environment. Do you feel safe in your environment?

Emotional and Spiritual Support

Our emotions greatly influence our health because the body and the mind are linked. This linking enables the body to influence the mind and the mind to influence the body. All emotions, including excitement, fear, anger, worry, grief, joy, surprise, and love, can influence our bodies positively or negatively. Spiritual and emotional needs are closely related, yet different. People meet their spiritual needs in a variety of ways that are unique to their personal beliefs (see Chapter 15). Also, see Emotions and Feelings and Their Expression later in this chapter.

Diversion and Recreation

We all need to turn aside (diversion) from our usual activities and refresh our bodies and minds with activities other than work (recreation). What is work to one person can be play to another. How much time do you spend studying each week? How many hours do you work outside school? What type of recreation do you engage in each week? How many hours do you devote to recreation each week?

Mental Hygiene

Mental hygiene involves the care and hygiene of the brain. Just as there are good health habits for the body, there are also good daily health habits for the mind. You need to strive to understand and accept yourself, be happy, work well with others, accept criticism, know your abilities and limitations, trust and respect others, and accept responsibility for yourself. Who is responsible for your success in the practical nursing program? What is your attitude toward constructive evaluation? What kind of a team member are you in the clinical area?

▼▼▼
Definition of Culture

Culture is a way of life. Culture is the total of the ever-changing ideas, thoughts, beliefs, values, communication, actions, attitudes, traditions, customs, and objects that a group of people possess and the ways they have of doing things. Culture also includes standards of behavior and sets of rules to live by. The generally accepted ways of doing things common to people who share the same culture are called **customs.**

▼▼▼
Characteristics of Culture

An important point about culture is that it is **learned behavior.** The culture of a group is passed on from generation to generation. From the moment you were born you began to learn about the culture of the group into which you were born. The process of learning your culture (the way your group does things) is called **acculturation.** You are socialized (acculturated) to the ways of the group. Right now you are being socialized into the career of practical nursing. You are learning how to think and act like a nurse. The result of acculturation is a world view that is generally shared by persons with the same cultural background. The world view, or similar ways of thinking and seeing, becomes the reality of the group. This reality fills every aspect of life. It is a cultural bias (a mental leaning) that is never proven or questioned. The worth of everything, either within or outside of the group, depends on whether it fits the world view of the cultural group. One's world

view can lead to ethnocentrism, prejudice, and discrimination.

▽▽▽
Danger: Ethnocentrism, Prejudice, and Discrimination

People who belong to the same cultural group may develop the attitude, through their world view, that their way of doing things is superior to that of groups with different cultures (ethnocentrism). The group uses their culture as the norm against which to measure and evaluate the customs and ways of others. When intolerance of another cultural group occurs, **prejudice** results. When rights and privileges are withheld from those of another cultural group, **discrimination** is the result.

▽▽▽
Avoiding False Assumptions

Nursing students sometimes think that somewhere there is a cookbook that will tell them how to care for people who are different from themselves. This type of approach can lead to stereotyping. A **stereotype** is an inaccurate generalization used to describe all members of a specific group without exception. Stereotypes ignore the ever-present individual variations that occur within every cultural group. When texts and articles present highly specific information about a cultural group, stereotypes may be perpetuated about that group because individual variations are ignored.

> During a seminar on business practices, the presenter, while talking about a specific business practice, singled out an engineer in the group who was of Japanese descent. He used the engineer as an example of someone who thinks differently from "Americans" because he is Asian. The engineer was a third-generation American and had no clue what the presenter was talking about.

Did you discover any stereotypes present in your

group of classmates when you played the "what we have in common" culture game?

Cultural Diversity

The process of giving up your own culture and adopting the culture of the dominant group is called **assimilation**. Culturally different groups do adopt some of the culture of the dominant group. Although assimilation does occur, members of the generations that follow the original immigrants usually retain some elements of their original culture.

The concept of the melting pot has been replaced by the concept of cultural diversity. The many differences in the elements of culture (**cultural pluralism**) in groups of people in the United States and Canadian society is called **cultural diversity**. Traditionally, groups that usually have been identified as culturally diverse are Asians, blacks, Hispanics, Native Americans, and whites. As a practical nurse, you need to define this concept more broadly. Defined more broadly, examples of culturally diverse groups include single parents, people who live in poverty, homosexuals, bisexuals, the wealthy, and people with disabilities.

The concept of race as a means of categorizing people by biologic traits has come under attack by scientists. These scientists suggest using ethnicity as a more accurate means of capturing the great diversity found in the 5 billion people in the world. Members of **ethnic groups** are a special type of cultural group composed of people who are members of the same race, religion, or nation, or speak the same language. They derive part of their identity through membership in the ethnic group. Examples of ethnic groups in the United States include Irish-Americans, African-Americans, Asian-Americans, German-Americans, Hispanics, Jews, Native Americans, Arab-Americans, Greek-Americans, and many more.

Importance of Cultural Diversity

As a practical nurse, you must be aware that cultural diversity is ever-present in the clinical situation. Failure to develop sensitivity to and competence in handling this diversity could lead to misunderstanding between the client and you. Stress can result. The plan of treatment for the client could fail. You could make false assumptions. You might label clients as difficult or uncooperative when their lack of cooperation with the plan of care could be related to a conflict with their personal health belief system. Less-than-adequate care could be experienced by clients when cultural diversity and the differences it represents are overlooked or misinterpreted.

Philosophy of Individual Worth and Celebration of Our Uniqueness

The philosophy of individual worth is the belief shared by all members of the health care team in the uniqueness and value of each human being who comes for care regardless of differences that may be observed or perceived in that individual. As a practical nurse, you need to realize that each individual has the right to live according to his personal beliefs and values *as long as they do not interfere with the rights of others.* Each individual deserves respect as a human being. Many factors are responsible for differences in clients. They may think and behave differently because of social class, religion, ethnic background, or personal choice. Regardless of these differences, all clients have the right to receive high-quality nursing care. As a practical nurse you cannot decrease the quality of the care you give because of differences you observe or perceive. Practical nurses need to guard against making judgments about people who are culturally different. This does not mean you must accept for yourself the differences you observe. It means being open-minded and nonjudgmental. It means taking the difference at face value, accepting people as they are, and giving high-quality care. Be aware of your own attitudes, beliefs, and values as they affect your ability to give care. If you do identify biases, see them for what they are. Become sensitive to cultural differences, and acknowledge that they exist. Gather knowledge about them so that you can work on trying to modify your biases and provide more culturally competent care.

▽▽▽
Learning About Cultural Diversity

How to Begin

Unless you understand your own culture, it will be difficult to understand the culture of others. For starters, you need to look inside yourself to learn about your own cultural beliefs, values, and world view and how they influence how you think and act. Some elements of your culture are obvious—for example, your language, arts, celebrated holidays, and how and what you eat. However, much of your culture is hidden. Elements such as aspects of communication, beliefs, attitudes, values, sex roles, use of space, concept of time, and family ties and dynamics are more difficult to perceive and discuss.

How Many Hats Do You Wear?
Or What Roles Do You Play?

Each of you fills many roles in your daily life. Sometimes you refer to this situation as wearing many hats. Some of these roles are played out individually, one at a time. Sometimes you play many roles at the same time. The exercises that follow will give you the opportunity to identify your personal cultural background.

Identifying The Roles You Play in Your Daily Life

The following categories describe the roles you play in several areas in your everyday life.

Category 1—Economic Status Role

Although standards are available to assign persons to each of the following economic classes, people generally place themselves in one of the following categories by how they perceive their economic status. Place a checkmark next to the economic class that best describes you. I am in the

_____ Lower economic class

✓ Middle economic class

_____ Upper economic class

Category 2—Political Role

Put a checkmark next to the word(s) that best describes the political role you play in society. I am

_____ Republican

_____ Democrat

✓ Independent

_____ Liberal

✓ Conservative

✓ Moderate

_____ Indifferent

_____ To the left of liberal

_____ To the right of conservative

Other _____

Category 3—Racial or Ethnic Role

Place a checkmark beside the racial or ethnic term that best describes you. Be sure to read the complete list before you choose. I am a (an)

_____ African-American

_____ American

_____ American-Indian

_____ Amerindian

_____ Anglo-Saxon

_____ Anglo

✓ Asian-American

✓ Asian

_____ Black

_____ Chicano

_____ Ethnic

_____ Gypsy

_____ Hispanic

_____ Indian

_____ Latin American

_____ Latvian-American

_____ Native American

___✔___ Oriental

_____ Spanish-speaking

_____ White

Other _____

Category 4—Social Role

Circle the social roles that best describe you.
I am (a)

Female, male
Married, single
Separated, divorced
Blended family
Wife, husband
Significant other
Mother, father
Daughter, son
Sister, brother
Stepmother, stepfather
Stepdaughter, stepson
Stepsister, stepbrother
Half-sister, half-brother
Godmother, godfather
Godchild
Grandmother, grandfather
Granddaughter, grandson
Aunt, uncle
Niece, nephew
Cousin
Other _____

Category 5—Work Role

Place a checkmark beside each work role you
play in your life.

_____ Blue-collar worker

_____ Business person

_____ Laborer

_____ Professional

_____ Service provider

___✔___ Skilled worker

___✔___ Student

_____ Technician

___✔___ Unemployed

_____ White-collar worker

Other _____

Summarize the hats you wear by listing the
items you have checked and circled in the categories below.

Category 1—Economic status role _____

_____

Category 2—Political role _____

_____

Category 3—Racial or ethnic role _____

_____

Category 4—Social role _____

_____

Category 5—Work role _____

_____

Make up a sentence using all the words you
listed in the five categories. This sentence describes you by the roles you play in your life.
Each student should write the sentence on a
piece of paper and put it in a paper bag. Someone can read each sentence, and the class can
guess who the sentence describes. (Adapted
from Randall-David, 1989.)

What Makes Me Unique?

During class time, take a few minutes to play
the What Makes Me Unique? culture game. The
class divides into small but equal-sized groups.
This activity is especially helpful when
classmates you perceive to be "the same as" you
are in the same group. Seek to find one item
that makes you unique from other members of

the group. This culture game was played by one of your authors with a group of people she had worked with for years and thought she knew inside out. What a surprise it was to find out that one person was a twin, another had worked with the lepers in Hawaii when she was very young, and another had a relative who was in a crowd scene in one of the Diehard movies. When discovering your uniqueness, it is not time to be humble. Let your uniqueness show. After your small-group work, share with the class the item that makes you unique.

▽▽▽
Areas of Cultural Diversity

Areas of cultural diversity that might ordinarily be taken for granted in client situations as well as everyday life include family, food preferences, religion, communication, educational background, economic level, and wellness and illness beliefs and practices. After reading the general information about each area, you will be given an opportunity to develop an awareness of your own cultural patterns in these areas by answering a group of statements or questions. Sharing this information with peers can be a good learning experience. Sharing will highlight the cultural diversity that exists in your nursing class, regardless of cultural background. See Table 14–1 for profiles of four culturally diverse groups.

Family Structure

No matter what culture is being discussed, the family is the basic unit of society. The role of the family is to have children, if desired or as they come, and to raise them to be contributing members of the group. Actual child-rearing practices vary from culture to culture. Families generally socialize the young to the culture of the group. They meet the physical and psychological needs of the young in culturally specific ways. Some cultures expect the nuclear family (mother, father, and children) to live in the same house. Others may expect the extended family (the

nuclear family plus the grandparents and other kinsmen) to do so. Some Vietnamese families are examples of extended families, with three or more generations living in the same house. In many of these families, ties are strong. Behaviors that enhance the family name are encouraged, for example, obedience to parents and those in authority.

The traditional nuclear family is being challenged by the single-parent family. According to the 1990 statistics of the U.S. Bureau of the Census, approximately 25% of all households in the United States were single-parent families. A parent may become a single parent on the death of a spouse, by electing not to marry at the time of pregnancy, or by divorce. Health care workers who have not been in the same situation may be unaware of and insensitive to the special way of life of this type of family. Respond to the following statements. Your responses will help you discover your own cultural patterns in regard to the family.

1. Describe your family structure (nuclear, extended, or alternative life style).

2. Describe the role of children, if any, in your family.

3. Discuss who gives permission for hospitalization in your family.

4. List factors that influence the decision of your family members to visit or not to visit the hospital when a member is ill.

5. Describe the effect that your hospitalization today at 4 PM for surgery tomorrow would have on you and your family.

Food Preferences

All cultures use food to provide needed nutrients. However, what they eat, when they eat, and how they eat differ vastly by cultural group. Knowledge of nutrition as a science differs by culture. It is interesting that the soil of some cultures, for example, Mexico, encouraged the growth of two complementary proteins (corn and beans) that became staples of that culture's diet. Specific foods in different cultures have different meanings. All cultures use food during celebrations. Through

Table 14–1
Cultural Diversity Profiles

These profiles reflect only one person's perspective of the culture discussed and are intended to be a general sketch of the culture.

	African Americans	Hmong	Latinos	Native Americans	Northeastern Wisconsinites
History/ Traditions	Origin: Africa. Elders pass on history and tradition and are held in high esteem.	Refugees from Vietnam.	Women carry on the family and religious traditions.	Traditions passed on through ceremonies.	Predominantly of German and Belgian origin. Home of the Oneida and Menominee Indians. Also home to Hmong, Hispanic, African-Americans, Arab-Americans.
Family Structure	Strong kinship bonds with extended family.	Immediate family plus father, mother, brothers, sisters, uncles, aunts, nieces, nephews considered one family.	Family not always defined by blood or marriage. Godparents are important part of family structure.	Biologic extended family. Also includes those who are not blood relatives.	Emphasis on extended family and large families. Newcomers may have problems being accepted. Emphasis on privacy.
Religion	Catholic, Episcopalian, Baptist, African Methodist Episcopal Church, Muslim, and Pentecostal.	Animism: worship of deceased ancestors. This worship helps to bless the living family.	Catholicism most common religion.	Spiritual rituals important. Religion and spirituality are different. In addition to practicing Indian spirituality, many belong to traditional Christian religions.	Traditionally Catholic and Lutheran but ecumenical in spirit. Live by motto Help thy neighbor. Green Bay Packers are a regional religion.

Table continued on following page

Food	Chicken, pork, fish. Prefer natural foods such as vegetables, fruits, nuts, beans, peppers, onions, greens, yams, corn bread.	Rice the main food—served at breakfast, lunch, and dinner.	Red meat, rice, vermicelli, pinto beans, tortillas, potatoes, tomatoes, chilies, onions, garlic, limes, oranges, bananas, mangoes. May not trim or drain off fat when cooking meat.	Each Indian ceremony is associated with a specific food that conveys a meaning. Bread, meat, fish, natural fruit, and potatoes are served. Soups are important. Sweets not a part of the traditional diet.	Chicken booyah, Belgian pie, bratwurst, beer, brandy, cherry bounce, kneecaps. Live in a state with one of the highest intakes of snacks in the United States (excess salt and fat intake).
Health Beliefs	Illness results from bad spirits, eating poisoned foods, angering the creator, or putting off the creator's warnings. May treat illnesses with home remedies. May wait until illness becomes too serious before seeking medical care. May visit a spiritualist.	Natural earth plants and roots used to cure a sick person. Shaman can be called on to sham a client.	Illness a consequence of behavior or the will of God. Therefore, a person is tempting fate by going to the doctor when there is nothing wrong. Sobadores work with complaints of stress, mood swings, or depression. The "bad spirit" in the body must be exorcised or massaged to bring body, mind, and spirit back in sync. May use herbs, roots, and ointments for body ailments. Curanderos have knowledge of homeopathic remedies.	Illness is seen as being out of balance or harmony. Spiritual well-being affects physical well-being.	Illness due to accident, germs, or may be a punishment from God. Folk remedies. Use traditional medicine.

Adapted from Reinhardt E. *Through the Eyes of Others—Intercultural Resource Directory for Health Care Professionals.* Minneapolis: University of Minnesota School of Public Health, 1995, pp. 5–6, 8–14.

generations of experience, different cultures have learned to use different foods to promote health and cure disease. To assist you in identifying your own cultural patterns in regard to food preferences, respond to the following statements or questions.

1. State your favorite food.

2. Identify one special occasion in which your cultural group participates. What foods, if any, are part of this celebration?

3. State your favorite "recipe" from your mother and from your grandmother. What special ingredients or techniques are used to make this food? Is there a written recipe?

4. List a food that is a comfort to you or makes you feel good. In what situation do you use this food?

Religious Beliefs

Religious beliefs are personal to the individual. Religion is an important aspect of culture. Religion can have different meanings in people's lives. For some, religion is a brief, momentary, and sporadic part of daily life. For others, it may influence every aspect of life and have a profound effect on personal outlook and on how one lives. Chapter 15 deals with religious differences. This aspect of life cannot be excluded from the present chapter. There is a close relationship between religious beliefs and the concept of wellness and illness in some groups. Practical nurses should be aware of their own religious beliefs, obligations, and attitudes. They should know whether these beliefs and attitudes influence the care that is given to clients. The questions that follow give you the opportunity to discover your own cultural patterns in regard to religion.

1. Do you have a religious affiliation? If so, state it.

2. What role does religion play in your life?

3. Is prayer helpful to you?

4. What is your source of strength and hope?

5. What rituals or religious practices are important to you?

6. What symbols or religious books are helpful to you?

7. What dietary inclusions or restrictions are part of your religious beliefs?

8. How does your religion view the source of and meaning of pain and suffering?

Concept of Time

Some persons follow clock time. An hour has a beginning and an end (after 60 minutes). People who follow clock time eat, sleep, work, and engage in recreational activities at definite times each day. Some persons live on linear time. Time for them is a straight line with no beginning and no end. People who follow linear time eat when they are hungry and sleep when they are tired. The questions that follow give you an opportunity to discover your own cultural patterns in regard to time.

1. What determines when it is time for you to eat or sleep?

2. Do you wear a watch if you are not in the clinical area?

3. Are you on time for appointments?

Communication

Chapter 13 introduced you to some types of communication and some barriers to the communication process. A major barrier to communication in health care is a different language spoken by the client or nurse. A person's language gives a view of reality that may differ from yours. For example, in English the clock runs, but in Spanish it walks. This illustrates the different concept of time between the two cultures. For a person with English as a first language, time could move quickly, and there may be a rush to get things done. For those with Spanish as a first language, time may move more slowly. The following is a list of areas of communication that may vary for people who are culturally different.

Forms of Greetings and Goodbyes.   You may greet your client and want to get right down to business, but the client might expect some light conversation before getting down to the matter at hand. In some cultural groups people take an hour to say good-bye, whereas in others people may get up and leave without saying anything.

Appropriateness of the Situation.   Some groups prefer people to sit, not stand, while they converse. In some groups the sharing of food is a good way to relate to others and get them to verbalize.

Confidentiality. All information the client gives the nurse is considered confidential. Some clients do not want their spouse questioned or informed about their problems of the reproductive organs because they fear the spouse may think they are less desirable sexually.

Emotions and Feelings and Their Expression. Emotions are universal, but the cues to those emotions vary considerably. A lack of awareness of this fact can cause unnecessary stress between the client and the nurse. In some cultural groups people cannot display affection in public, show disapproval or frustration, or vent anger. Some cannot take criticism. You may show dissatisfaction with other members of the health care team by approaching them directly, whereas some team members may show dissatisfaction with you by being polite to your face but then complaining about you to the rest of the staff.

Pain Expression. Pain has two parts, sensation and response. All individuals experience the same sensation of pain. However, one's culture influences the definition of pain and the response to the sensation. Pain is whatever the person says it is. It exists whenever the person says it does. One's culture provides guidelines for approved ways of expressing one's response to the pain sensation and ways to relieve the pain. Some cultures teach individuals that it is acceptable to cry, moan, and exhibit other behavior that calls attention to the pain. These behaviors may also be a cure for pain. Other cultures encourage uncomplaining acceptance of pain and passive behavior when pain is experienced (stoic behavior). Discuss some nursing situations in which these two different reactions to pain could have negative consequences if a practical nurse lacked knowledge of cultural differences in pain expression (for example, a woman in labor or a client having a heart attack).

Tempo of Conversation. You may tend to speak quickly and expect a quick response. The client may be accustomed to pausing and reflecting before giving a response.

The Meaning of Silence. Silence can mean anything from disapproval to warmth, but generally it does not indicate tension or lack of rapport. Silence can be difficult for some persons to tolerate. Resist the temptation to jump in at a pause in the conversation by forcing yourself to meditate or even by biting your tongue (hopefully, not literally).

Now develop an awareness of your own cultural patterns in communication by answering the following questions:

1. What facial or body habits are you aware of in yourself while you are talking?
2. How do you greet people and how do you say good-bye?
3. How do you express
   a. love?   f. dissatisfaction?
   b. hate?   g. humor?
   c. fear?   h. anger?
   d. excitement?   i. sadness?
   e. disappointment?   j. happiness?
4. Do you make eye contact when you talk to people?
5. Do you touch people while talking?
   a. If so, how do they react?
   b. How do you react when people touch you while they are talking to you?

See Table 14–2 for Hints for Using Interpreters.

Educational Background

Approximately 27 million persons in the United States have literacy skills below the fourth-grade level. These persons are called functionally illiterate. The functionally illiterate have trouble reading and understanding simple directions. Some adults have literacy skills below the eighth-grade level. Differences in educational background need to be taken into consideration when one is teaching clients. It has been estimated that one out of every three Americans has some difficulty with reading or writing. Adapt your explanations to the client's level of understanding. Responding to the following statements will help you to identify your own beliefs and practices in regard to education.

1. Calculate the number of years of education you have had.
2. State your ultimate educational goal.
3. Discuss the role education plays in your life.

Table 14–2
Hints for Using Interpreters

Interpreters provide an invaluable service when clients do not speak English or do not have sufficient experience with the English language to understand complex medical information. To decrease the possibility of difficulties in an interpreter situation, follow these suggestions.

1. The ideal interpreter should be trained in the health care field, proficient in the language of the client and the nurse, and understanding and respecting of the culture of the client.
2. If the ideal interpreter is not available, make sure that the individual chosen has training in medical terminology, understands the health matter that needs to be translated, and also understands the requirements for confidentiality, neutrality, and accuracy.
3. Use family members as interpreters cautiously. Clients of specific cultures may be embarrassed to discuss intimate matters with family members who are younger or older or of the opposite sex. Family members may censor information to protect the client or the family.
4. Make sure the interpreter is acceptable to the client.
5. Look and speak directly to the client.
6. Speak clearly and slowly in a normal voice. Use short units of speech.
7. Avoid slang and professional jargon.
8. Observe the nonverbal communication of the client.
9. Be patient. Remember that interpretation is difficult work.

Adapted from Reinhardt E. *Through the Eyes of Others—Intercultural Resource Directory for Health Care Professionals.* Minneapolis: University of Minnesota School of Public Health, 1995.

4. Describe your feelings toward a person who has less education than you have.

5. Describe your feelings toward a person who has more education than you have.

6. Describe your feelings if you were referred to your school's skills center.

7. Discuss the impact of your cultural background on your values and practices with regard to education.

8. Who in your family has graduated from high school, technical school, junior college, or college or university?

Economic Level

Economic level is frequently related to educational background. Sociologists use these two factors to determine the social class of individuals. You will meet clients who are very wealthy and clients who are at or near the poverty level. Others have midlevel incomes. A client's annual income determines the type of house he or she lives in, the neighborhood where he or she lives, the availability of food, and the ability to participate in certain types of preventive health care. Practical nurses have to take economic level into consideration when they make suggestions during client teaching and should adapt the suggestions accordingly. Identify your personal patterns in regard to economic level by responding to the following statements or questions.

1. Describe how your economic background affects your daily life in the following areas:
   a. Availability of food
   b. Availability of shelter
   c. Availability of clothing
   d. Amount and type of recreation
2. Discuss your feelings toward a person who has less money than you have.
3. Discuss your feelings toward a person who has more money than you have.
4. Describe how these feelings fit with those of your cultural group.
5. Discuss your ability to afford to go to a physician when you get sick.
6. If you work, do you have health insurance benefits?

Wellness and Illness Beliefs and Practices

Wellness and illness can have different meanings for persons who are culturally different. Wellness and illness are relative terms. What is good health to one person can be sickness to another. Wellness may not be a high-priority matter to some clients. Some clients believe that illness can be prevented; they practice elaborate rituals and engage special persons to carry out those rituals in an attempt to prevent disease. Some rituals may be used to cure disease. Other clients look at prevention as an attempt to control the future. They may consider this an impossible feat in the way they view their lives. Some people may think prevention is tempting fate or the gods; to follow through with prevention would be risky. Others wonder about the necessity of making a trip to a health care provider for preventive care, for example, immunizations. When disease does strike, some people blame pathogens (germs), others spirits, and others an imbalance in the body. Generally, death and dying bring out strong emotions in most people. Be aware that some cultures have special taboos and prohibitions when death occurs. Roles that family and friends carry out at the time of death may vary.

Some cultural groups attach a stigma to mental illness and psychiatrists. They may not attach the same stigma to impairments of physical health. Some groups may feel that the mental symptoms manifested are a healthy reaction to an emotional crisis. Some cultural groups believe that the mind and body are united and are not separate entities. These cultures may have traditional healers that are expert at healing both the mind and the body. Some people may seek out traditional healers to heal the mind while at the same time consulting Western medicine to heal the body.

In the area of nutrition, some groups believe that special foods or food combinations can prevent or cure illnesses. Others see no relationship between the diet and health. Individuals in some cultures are embarrassed when they have to discuss bodily functions or allow certain body parts to be examined. Others are not bothered by this. Hygiene practices vary according to beliefs, living conditions, personal resources, and physical characteristics. To assist you in identifying your own cultural patterns in regard to wellness beliefs and practices, respond to the following statements and questions.

1. Describe what it means to you to have good health.
2. What are some of your own practices or beliefs about staying well?

3. Describe what it means to you to be sick.
4. List some foods in your diet that you think help to prevent illness.
   a. How does eating these foods prevent illness?
   b. What are some foods you must avoid to prevent illness?
5. List some foods in your diet that help you recover when you are sick.
   a. What foods are they?
   b. What illnesses do they cure?
   c. How do they cure illness?
6. How do you care for your skin and hair?
7. Describe the customs you follow when there is a death in your family.
   a. Who makes the burial arrangements?
   b. Who should be present when the death occurs?
   c. Describe what you believe happens to a person after death.
   d. Do you have a get-together after the burial? If so, for whom?
   e. How does your family remember the dead?
8. Describe your attitude toward mental illness.
9. Describe what you think causes mental illness.
10. Who do you think should treat mental illness?

It is hoped that some of these exercises have started you thinking about the many ways you and your peers differ, regardless of which cultural group you belong to. And along with that awareness a tolerance may be developing for ways of doing things that may be different from yours. No particular way or world view is correct. *It merely is.*

▽▽▽
Increasing Your Knowledge of Culturally Diverse Clients

Before discussing how to increase your knowledge of specific cultures, it must be said that no one can be an expert on every culture in the world. Even "experts" of one culture are cautious about being labeled an expert. These people are aware of the ever-changing nature of cultures and of the important individual variations that occur within any cultural group. Experts are always cautious about stereotyping persons in any particular cultural group.

There are strategies that can help you increase your knowledge of different cultures. First, avoid applying the information you gain automatically to all individuals in that group. This may be called the cookbook method of learning about different cultures. To apply information in this way makes you guilty of stereotyping individuals—assuming that everyone in that cultural group is the same. You have already learned that classifying people as being the same just because they share the same religion, life style, or ethnic background is stereotyping. Leave room for personal variations within each cultural group about which you gather information.

Suggestions for Learning More About Culturally Diverse Groups

1. Identify the different cultural groups in your community.

2. Read about the different cultures to which you are personally exposed. The list of suggested readings on pages 218 to 219 can help you get started. Use the suggestions given in Chapter 8 to find additional information about specific cultural groups through your learning resource center.

3. A helpful class activity is to hear reports from peers about various cultural groups. Remember to think beyond the more traditional cultural groups based on ethnicity. Include the disabled, aged, single parents, different sexual life styles, and so on. And remember to allow for individual variations and the fact that cultures are always changing.

▼▼▼
Categories of Major Health Belief Systems

Anthropologists are scientists who study the physical and cultural characteristics of human groups. A helpful framework for generally discovering and understanding health belief systems has been developed by these scientists. They divide systems of health beliefs into three major systems—biomedicine, personalistic, and naturalistic. **Biomedicine** is the primary belief system of

the United States and is also called Western medicine. There is a movement in nursing education at all levels to transform curriculums so that they reflect multicultural concepts in nursing. However, it is possible that the curriculum of your school of practical nursing is set up to reflect biomedicine. The **personalistic system** is found among groups native to the Americas as well as those south of the Sahara and among the tribal peoples of Asia (Jackson, 1993; pp. 30 and 32). The **naturalistic system** of beliefs developed from the traditional medical practices of the ancient civilizations of China, India, and Greece. Variants of this belief system are found today in the Philippines and among low-income blacks and poor white southerners (Jackson, 1993; p. 37). Rarely does a group ascribe to all the beliefs in one system. You might see elements of each of the three systems at work in one individual. With this in mind, Table 14–3 compares these three health belief systems according to: (1) location of the belief system, (2) cause of the disease, (3) how the disease is diagnosed and treated, (4) who is responsible for curing the disease, and (5) how the disease is prevented.

▼▼▼
Developing Plans of Care for Culturally Diverse Clients

Jackson (1993) offers suggestions for discovering the health beliefs of clients along with guidelines to develop plans of care that incorporate those beliefs through a process of negotiation with the client. Jackson points out that discovering specific health beliefs is easier if the nurse is familiar with a specific culture, but this is not absolutely necessary. She suggests ways of negotiating a treatment plan when dealing with culturally diverse clients. The practical nurse can collaborate with the professional nurse to incorporate these beliefs into the client's plan of care.

1. **Discover the health beliefs of the individual.** Be respectful and open-minded when you question the client about the cause of the problem, when it started, its severity, its course, the problems it has caused in the client's life, and the treatment the client thinks will cure

Table 14–3
Categories of Major Health Beliefs

	Biomedicine	Personalistic	Naturalistic
Location of belief system	United States, Western countries	Native Americans, Africa south of the Sahara	Japan, China, Vietnam, Korea, Taiwan
Cause of disease	Abnormalities in structure and function of body organs by pathogens (germs), biochemical alterations, environmental factors	Sick person punished by a deity, ghost, god, evil spirit, witch, or angry ancestor; punishment may include poisoning, stealing of soul, witchcraft	Imbalance of body elements caused by excessive heat (yang) and cold (ying)
How disease is diagnosed	Physical exam, x-ray, identification of pathogens by lab studies	Agent is identified by magical powers, trances, and so on	Cause is identified as excess heat or cold
How disease is treated	Drugs, surgery, diet	Curing rituals, relief of symptoms by herbs	Restore body balance: "hot" illness treated by cold, "cold" illness treated by hot; also, acupuncture, coining, cupping
Who cures the disease?	Physician	Diviner, herbalist	Physician or herbalist
How disease is prevented	Avoidance of pathogens, preventive life styles including diet, exercise, moderation, safety, immunizations	Faithful obedience to rituals (e.g., wearing amulets), protective spells	Maintain balance of hot and cold in body, mind, and environment

Adapted with permission from the article "Understanding, eliciting and negotiating clients' multicultural health beliefs," from the April, 1993 issue of *The Nurse Practitioner*, © Springhouse Corporation.

the disease. Avoid assuming anything. When you are unsure of anything, ASK! In situations of cultural diversity, our clients are the teachers and we are the students.

2. **Negotiate treatment plans with the client.** Avoid trying to change clients' beliefs. This is an impossible feat. Cultural health practices are deeply ingrained. Tradition means more than your word, although you are a person representing a health profession. Instead, involve the client in making decisions

about his or her own care. Do so in a way that does not threaten the client's beliefs and practices or conflict with them. Explain from the biomedical point of view the cause of the disease, how the body is altered by the disease, the role of treatment, and the expected outcome. Then compare the client's belief system with that of biomedicine. All clients need to have this information to help ensure their cooperation with the plan of care. See Table 14–4 for an example of negotiating treatment plans with the client.

Table 14–4
Negotiating Treatment Plans with the Client

Situation

Nancy Thai, a Cambodian refugee, resides in Chicago with her husband and three children. She delivered an 8-pound boy early this morning at St. Mary's Hospital. The practical nurse who was assigned to Mrs. Thai on the day shift reported to the evening staff that the client was "uncooperative." Specifically, Mrs. Thai refused to eat and take her pills. In frustration, the nurse stated, "I just do not know what to do with her."

Cultural Health Beliefs in This Situation

Mrs. Thai's health beliefs include the belief that pregnancy and birth weaken the body. Also, blood loss during delivery is considered a ying (cold) condition. Mrs. Thai believes that for one month after delivery a mother must have a yang (hot) diet to restore strength, keep the stomach warm, counteract heat loss, prevent incontinence, and prevent itching at the site of the episiotomy. Among preferred foods are rice, pork, and chicken. Cold foods (for example, beef, salad, sour foods), as well as cold water, are bad for the stomach and the teeth.

Negotiating Treatment Plans

The nurse assigned to Mrs. Thai on the evening shift informed Mrs. Thai that the doctor had ordered pills to help prevent bleeding after delivery. After discussing this, Mrs. Thai agreed to take her pills with warm water. In a respectful manner, the evening nurse asked if Mrs. Thai did not like the hospital food. Mrs. Thai smiled and explained her need for a yang diet. The evening nurse said that she could arrange to have the dietary department send rice, chicken, or any other food Mrs. Thai would find helpful after childbirth. Mrs. Thai said her husband would bring rice and chicken from home. The nurse canceled Mrs. Thai's food but requested a pot of hot water, silverware, and napkins for her use.

3. **Preserve the beliefs and practices that are helpful to the client.** Starting in 1993, the Office of Alternative Medicine of the National Institutes of Health began to identify, study, and bring together the best healing practices of other cultures with those of Western medicine. Many of the beliefs and practices of non-Western systems of health beliefs have proved beneficial. Examples are acupuncture and accupressure. More are about to be approved. Other practices of your client may not yet have been researched or found effective. Collaborate with your professional nurse about these practices. If they seem to help the client and do no harm, include them in the plan of care, regardless of your ability to see the benefit of the practice. These practices have special significance and meaning to some individuals despite the fact that you may be unable to

see how or if they help. See Table 14–5 for an example of preserving the beliefs and practices that are helpful to the client.

4. **Repattern harmful practices.** Harmful practices prevalent in Western society include lack of exercise, smoking, and diets high in fat and refined sugar. In Burma, when a woman is pregnant, extreme dietary restrictions are imposed. In Cambodia, mud is placed on the umbilicus of newborns. All of these practices are dangerous. If followed, these practices could lead to high blood pressure, heart disease, obesity, poor fetal development and maternal toxemia, and tetanus in the newborn. Explain your reason for opposing the harmful practice and offer alternatives. See Table 14–6 for an example of repatterning harmful practices.

Table 14–5
Preserving the Beliefs and Practices That Are Helpful to the Client

Situation

Ted Washington, a 72-year-old black American, lives in a rural area of South Carolina. He was admitted to Brent Hospital with pneumonia and advanced osteoarthritis. An LPN, John, is his nurse. John cannot understand how anyone can get to such a state of ill-health without seeing a doctor. John is especially upset because Mr. Washington could have prevented much of his disability due to arthritis if he had followed a preventive program when he first developed symptoms of this disease.

Cultural Health Beliefs in This Situation

Mr. Washington has been poor during his entire life. As with any person experiencing poverty, his main concern in life has been the present and getting through his problems on a day-to-day basis. Mr. Washington's time orientation is the present, not the future, so preventive regimens have not been central to his way of thinking. Persons with similar backgrounds and situations delay care until the disease interferes with their ability to work or results in a disability. It cannot be said that Mr. Washington ignored his condition. He participated in self-treatment by using cultural health practices in the form of topical application of oils and ointments to his aching joints. These self-treatments helped Mr. Washington deal physically and psychologically with his condition. Mr. Washington looks at his disability as a punishment from God who let something get into his joints. His belief stems from the wellness and illness beliefs brought by African slaves. These beliefs center on wellness as a state experienced when one is in harmony with nature and illness as a state experienced when disharmony with nature occurs.

Preserving the Beliefs and Practices That Are Helpful to the Client

John supported Mr. Washington's application of oils and ointments. He applied backrub lotion to Mr. Washington's joints at bedtime. John made arrangements for a friend of Mr. Washington's to bring his ointment from home. After clarifying self-treatment with the client, John realized that such applications could give psychological comfort to the client as well as relieve pain. In the future, John will make it a point to ask all newly admitted clients about self-treatment for their diseases.

Table 14–6
Repatterning Harmful Practices

Situation

Over a two month period of time during the summer, a Chinese infant was seen in a New York clinic for diarrhea that did not respond to treatment. Stool cultures showed no unusual organisms. A change in formula did nothing to stop the diarrhea. During a home visit, the visiting nurse found a hot apartment with several bottles of home-prepared formula on the windowsill. Several other bottles were in the refrigerator.

Cultural Health Beliefs in This Situation

The child's mother explained that she had recently given birth. Because of this she had to avoid cold. In order to avoid exposure to the cold of the refrigerator, her husband would remove the bottles from the refrigerator that she needed during the day, before he left for work, and line them up on the windowsill.

Repatterning the Client's Harmful Practices

The visiting nurse explained that by being exposed to the heat of the day, the formula would grow germs that could cause diarrhea. She asked if there was a way that the bottles could be kept cold till needed. After some thought, the mother said she could put on a hat, coat, and gloves before removing bottles from the refrigerator. The nurse agreed with this plan. The baby had no further episodes of diarrhea.

Reproduced with permission from the article "Understanding, eliciting and negotiating clients' multicultural health beliefs," from the April, 1993 issue of *The Nurse Practitioner,* © Springhouse Corporation.

Table 14–7
Modifying the Environment to Accommodate Culturally Diverse Clients

The health care environment can be made more "welcoming" to culturally diverse clients. Many of these changes require little cost or time to implement. But the results can promote better health among culturally diverse clients.

1. Identify the various cultural groups that use the health care facility.
2. Post welcome signs in the languages of the groups you serve.
3. Arrange for messages on answering machines to include the languages of the clients you serve.
4. Place magazines in the waiting room that reflect the diversity of the clients you serve.
5. Play background music that reflects the diversity of the clients you serve.
6. Provide handouts, appointment cards, and client education materials in the languages of the clients you serve.
7. Decorate the environment (pictures, posters, objects, etc.) to reflect the diversity of the clients you serve.
8. Stock band-aids that do not match any specific skin tone. For example, Walt Disney characters and fluorescent colors.
9. In waiting areas, provide books, toys, and multicultural videos for children that promote acceptance of diversity. Barney and Sesame Street themes are especially effective.

Adapted from Reinhardt E. *Through the Eyes of Others—Intercultural Resource Directory for Health Care Professionals.* Minneapolis: University of Minnesota School of Public Health, 1995, pp. 19–20.

▼▼▼
Developing Cultural Competence in Health Care Situations

You have been given the opportunity to begin developing skills that will help you become a practical nurse who gives culturally competent care. You have been given the opportunity to identify your culture and its strengths and limitations. You can begin to see how your culture affects your thinking and behavior. Knowledge of the three major health belief systems increase your awareness of different world views about the cause, treatment, and prevention of disease. Awareness of ethnocentrism can help you gain respect for these health beliefs and practices even when they are different from yours. Your goal is to respond flexibly when your values and assumptions differ from those of your clients.

Follow Jackson's (1993) suggestions for negotiating client care with culturally diverse clients. Doing so will result in fewer dissatisfied clients and more compliance with the plan of care. Table 14–7 includes suggestions for the practical nurse working in a community with culturally diverse clients.

▼▼▼ S U M M A R Y

- ▶ A good place to start learning about how people are different is to remind yourself that all persons have similarities. The nine basic daily needs are shared by everyone. How individuals meet these needs varies with their culture, the learned ways they have of doing things.
- ▶ One guideline in health care is the philosophy of individual worth, the belief that all persons are unique and have value regardless of the way they view their world, and they deserve the best nursing care you can give.
- ▶ Awareness of cultural diversity is important for practical nurses so that they can avoid false assumptions and misunderstandings about the clients for whom they care. The first step in understanding other people's culture is to understand your own. It is important to be aware of your personal beliefs and practices in the areas of family, religion, communication, educational background, economic level, and wellness and illness beliefs and practices. Some ways to learn about cultural diversity include reading about different cultures, especially those found in your geographic area, and hearing reports from your peers who are culturally different. *Always allow for individual variations within specific groups.*
- ▶ Understanding your own culture, gaining knowledge about other peoples' culture, attaining sensitivity to cultural diversity, and adapting the plan of care to reflect the client's health and illness beliefs puts you well on the road to providing culturally competent nursing care.

▼▼▼ R E F E R E N C E S

Culver V. *Modern Bedside Care,* 8th ed. Philadelphia: W.B. Saunders, 1974, pp. 374–384.

Jackson L. Understanding, eliciting and negotiating clients' multicultural health beliefs. Nurse Practitioner 1993; 18(4): 30–32, 37–43.

Leininger M. Transcultural nursing education: A worldwide imperative. Nurs Health Care 1994; 15(5): 254–257.

Morganthau T. What color is black? Newsweek 1995; 125(7):63–65, 67–70, 72.

Randall-David E. *Strategies for Working with Culturally Diverse Clients.* Bethesda, MD: Association for the Care of Children's Health, 1989.

Reinhardt E. *Through the Eyes of Others—Intercultural Resource Directory for Health Care Professionals.* Minneapolis: Directory compiled by Hennepin Co. Medical Society, United Way *Success by 6* Intercultural Awareness Task Force, the Junior League of Minneapolis, and the University of Minnesota School of Public Health; 1995.

▼▼▼ *B I B L I O G R A P H Y*

AT&T Language Line Services. Call 1-800-752-6096 for over-the-phone interpretation of more than 140 languages, 24 hours a day, 7 days a week.

AbuGharbieh P. Culture Shock: Cultural norms influencing nursing in Jordan. Nursing Health Care 1993; 14(10):534–540.

Alvarez A. Mentoring undergraduate ethnic-minority students: A strategy for retention. J Nurs Educ 1993; 32(5):230–232.

Beeber L, et al. The challenge of diversity. J Psychosoc Nurs 1993; 31(8):23–29.

Beverly A. Transforming the nursing curriculum: Integrating concepts of gender, race, class, and ethnicity. DEAN'S Notes 1992; 13(4).

Bushy A. Ethnocultural sensitivity and measurement of consumer satisfaction. J Nurs Care Quality 1995; 9(2):16–25.

DeWit S. *Keane's Essentials of Medical-Surgical Nursing,* 3rd ed. Philadelphia: W.B. Saunders, 1992.

Diaz-Gilbert M. Caring for Culturally Diverse Clients. Nursing 93 1993; 56: 44–45.

Eliades DC, Suitor CW. *Celebrating Diversity: Approaching Families Through Their Food.* Arlington, VA: National Center for Education in Maternal and Child Health, 1994.

Foster G, *Medical Anthropology.* New York: John Wiley and Sons, 1978.

Giger J, Davidhizar R. *Transcultural Nursing: Assessment and Interventions.* St. Louis: Mosby–Year Book, 1991.

Hall E. *The Hidden Dimension.* New York: Peter Smith, 1992.

Hall E. *The Silent Language.* Westport, CT: Greenwood Press, 1990.

Hall E. *Understanding Cultural Differences: German, French, and American.* Yarmouth, ME: Intercultural Press, 1989.

Informed consent, cultural sensitivity, and respect for persons. JAMA 1995; 274(10):844–845.

Jezewski M. Culture brokering as a model for advocacy. Nurs Health Care 1993; 14(2):78–85.

Kuhni C. When cultures clash at the bedside. *RN* 1990; 53(1):23–26.

LaMarca K. Culturally competent cancer care? *Cancer Pain Update: Wisconsin Pain Initiative.* 1995; issue 37. Published in Madison, WI by the Wisconsin Cancer Pain Initiative.

Leininger M. *Transcultural Nursing.* New York: Nasson Publications, 1979.

Leininger M. *Transcultural Nursing: Concepts, Theory, Research, and Practice.* Columbus, OH: McGraw-Hill and Greyden Press, 1994.

Ludwig-Beymer P. The cultural aspects of pain. HT: The Magazine for Healthcare Travel Professionals 1995; 2(4):34–37.

Milliken M. *Understanding Human Behavior: A Guide for Health Workers.* Albany, NY: Delmar Publishers, 1993.

Promoting culturally competent nursing education (editorial). J Nurs Educ 1993; 32(5):195–197.

Pope-Davis D. Are nursing students multiculturally competent? An exploratory investigation. J Nurs Educ 1994; 33(1):31–33.

Rodriguez B. Understanding and integrating cultural awareness and related issues into specialized health curricula. Seminar at Northeast Wisconsin Technical College, Green Bay, Wisconsin, May 18, 1995.

Rooda L. Knowledge and attitudes of nurses toward culturally different clients: Implications for nursing education. J Nurs Educ 1993; 32(5):209–213.

Rosenbaum J. Teaching cultural sensitivity. J Nurs Educ 1995; 34(4):188–189.

Saylor C. Transformation: Nursing education and cultural diversity. Nurse Educator 1993; 18(1):26–28.

West E. The cultural bridge model. Nursing Outlook 1993; 41(5):229–234.

▼▼▼ S U G G E S T E D   R E A D I N G S

Amish

Randall-David E. *Strategies for Working with Culturally Diverse Clients.* Bethesda, MD: Association for the Care of Children's Health, 1992, Chap. 6.

African-Americans

Block B, Hunter M. Teaching physiological assessment of black persons. Nurse Educ 1981; 6(1):24–27.

Friedman M. Transcultural family nursing: Application to Latino and black families. Pediatr Nurs 1990; 5:214–222.

Grier M. Hair care for the black client. Am J Nurs 1976; 76(11):1781.

Morganthau T. What color is black? Newsweek 1995; 125(7):63–65, 67–70, 72.

Randall-David E. *Strategies for Working with Culturally Diverse Clients.* Bethesda, MD: Association for the Care of Children's Health, 1992, Chap. 6.

Asian-Americans

Kim M. Cultural influences on depression in Korean Americans. J Psychosoc Nurs 1995; 33(2):13–18.

Kobayashi S. Developmental process: Family caregiver's of demented Japanese. J Gerontolog Nurs. 1993; October:7–12.

McSweeney E. Cultural and pharmacologic considerations when caring for Chinese elders. J Gerontolog Nurs 1994; October:11–16.

Randall-David E. *Strategies for Working with Culturally Diverse Clients.* Bethesda, MD: Association for the Care of Children's Health, 1992, Chap. 6.

Filipino

Wilson S. The Filipino elder: Implications for nursing practice. J Gerontolog Nurs 1994; August:31–36.

Haitians

Randall-David E. *Strategies for Working with Culturally Diverse Clients.* Bethesda, MD: Association for the Care of Children's Health, 1992, Chap. 6.

Hispanics

Bond ML, Jones ME. *Short-term cultural immersion in Mexico.* Nurs Health Care 1994; 15(5):248–253.

Friedman M. Transcultural family nursing: Application to Latino and black families. Pediatr Nurs 1990; 5:214–222.

Randall-David E. *Strategies for Working with Culturally Diverse Clients.* Bethesda, MD: Association for the Care of Children's Health, 1992, Chap. 6.

Native Americans

Bell R. Prominence of women in Navajo healing beliefs and values. Nurs Health Care 1994; 15(5):232–240.

Crow K. Multiculturalism and pluralistic thought in nursing education: Native American world view and the nursing academic world view. J Nurs Educ 1993; 32(5):198–204.

Rowell R. Native American stereotypes and HIV/AIDS. *SIECUS Rep* 1990; 18(3):9–15.

The Family

Antai-Otong D. *Psychiatric Nursing: Biological and Behavioral Concepts.* Philadelphia: W.B. Saunders, 1995.

Betz C, et al. *Family-Centered Nursing Care of Children.* Philadelphia: W.B. Saunders, 1994.

Ignatavicius D, et al. *Medical-Surgical Nursing: A Nursing Process Approach.* Philadelphia: W.B. Saunders, 1995.

Varcarolis E. Blended families. *In* Varcarolis E. *Foundations of Psychiatric Mental Health Nursing, 2nd ed.* Philadelphia: W.B. Saunders, 1994.

Smith C, Maurer F. *Community Health Nursing: Theory and Practice.* Philadelphia: W.B. Saunders, 1995.

Wong D, Whaley L. *Whaley and Wong's Essentials of Pediatric Nursing,* 4th ed. St. Louis: Mosby–Year Book, 1993.

Single Parents

Betz C, et al. *Family-Centered Nursing Care of Children.* Philadelphia: W.B. Saunders, 1994.

Ignatavicius D, et al. *Medical-Surgical Nursing: A Nursing Process Approach.* Philadelphia: W.B. Saunders, 1995.

Wong D, Whaley L. *Whaley and Wong's Essentials of Pediatric Nursing,* 4th ed. St. Louis: Mosby–Year Book, 1993.

Homosexuals

Betz C, et al. *Family-Centered Nursing Care of Children.* Philadelphia: W.B. Saunders, 1994.

Ignatavicius D, et al. *Medical-Surgical Nursing: A Nursing Process Approach.* Philadelphia: W.B. Saunders, 1995.

Stevens P. Structural and interpersonal impact of heterosexual assumptions on lesbian health care clients. Nurs Res 1995; 44(1):25–30.

Varcarolis E. *Foundations of Psychiatric–Mental Health Nursing.* Philadelphia: W.B. Saunders, 1994.

Spiritual Caring, Spiritual Needs, and Religious Differences

▼▼▼ *O U T L I N E*

▼▼▼ *K E Y   T E R M S*

agnostic

atheist

emotional needs

empathy

pastoral care team

religious denomination

religious needs

rituals

spirit

spiritual care

spiritual dimension

spiritual distress

spiritual needs

symbols

▼▼▼ O B J E C T I V E S

Upon completing this chapter you will be able to:

1. *Identify the difference between the spiritual and emotional dimensions of individuals.*

2. *Discuss the practical nurse's role in providing spiritual care to the client and the family.*

3. *Discuss nursing interventions that can be used to meet the spiritual needs of clients.*

4. *List members of the health care team who can help provide spiritual care for clients.*

5. *Discuss your personal religious beliefs or the absence of them, and how these will influence nursing practice.*

6. *Discuss the general beliefs that account for the differences between various religions.*

7. *Describe specific nursing actions that can be used to meet the religious needs of clients.*

The spirit is the very essence of a person, the innermost part of a person. The spirit is a life force that penetrates a person's entire being. An individual's spiritual dimension is a very private and personal area. It includes the beliefs and value system that are the client's source of strength and hope. The spiritual self grows and matures throughout one's life.

▼▼▼ Spiritual Versus Emotional Dimension of the Individual

The spiritual dimension of a client's life requires the same emphasis that other daily needs receive. When spiritual needs of clients exist and are met, practical nurses can say they have directed care to the total person. Meeting the spiritual needs of clients through spiritual caring differs from providing emotional support. The spiritual dimension of a person gives insight into the meaning of life, suffering, and death. This dimension refers to the relationship of an individual to a higher being. Emotional needs include how people respond and deal with feelings of joy, anger, sadness, guilt, remorse, sorrow, and love, among others.

▼▼▼ Who Needs Spiritual Care?

Although all persons have a spiritual dimension, needs that arise in this area depend on a variety of situations and the individual's ability to cope with them. Crisis situations occur frequently in health care. An individual's beliefs and values can profoundly affect his or her response to these crises, the attitude toward treatment, and the rate of recovery. Illness, pain, and injury can intensify a person's spiritual needs. Be especially alert to the need for spiritual care in clients who are in pain, have an incurable disease, are dying, or who have experienced the death of a loved one. Clients who are facing an undesirable outcome of illness (such as an amputation) or have lost control of themselves also may need spiritual care. "When the body and mind are battered by time and use, the spirit, the very essence of the client remains" (Schoenbeck, 1994, p. 19).

▼▼▼ What Is Spiritual Care?

Florence Nightingale encouraged nurses to be instruments of spiritual caring. Avoid waiting for crisis situations to occur to be concerned about spiritual care. As a practical nurse, you have the responsibility to provide spiritual care to all clients. In addition, practical nurses should enhance the continued growth and maturity of the client's spiritual self in all client situations.

Perhaps the best place to start in providing spiritual care is to be comfortable with spiritual matters. Be aware of your own spirituality and the spirit that is the essence of you. Take a spiritual journey and get to know yourself. Have you ever thought about your philosophy of death? Do you have a relationship to a higher being? How do you cope? Who is your source of support? Who do you laugh with? Do you feel loved? Do you have someone to cry with? Have you ever said or heard others say "my spirit is broken"? What does this remark mean? Table 15–1 lists interventions that can be used by practical nurses when providing spiritual care.

▼▼▼
How Do I Meet the Spiritual Needs of My Clients?

Once you know your spiritual self, you will be better able to help others meet their spiritual needs. *When you acknowledge that your beliefs are effective for you but not necessarily for others,* you will be able to set your beliefs aside when helping clients meet their spiritual needs. Respect for the client's belief system can give strength, hope, and meaning to his life. Ask questions to help clients verbalize beliefs, fears, and concerns, such as, "What do you think is going to happen to you?" "Who is your source of support?" Show interest through supportive statements. Listen with an understanding attitude. Respond as naturally to spiritual concerns as

Table 15–1
Spiritual Care Interventions
1. Ask open-ended questions.
2. Actively listen to the client. Sit beside the client.
3. Be aware of nonverbal messages from the client.
4. Experience the feelings of the client but avoid adopting those feelings for yourself (empathy).
5. Expect to learn from clients.
6. Stay with the client after the person has received an unfavorable diagnosis.
7. When appropriate, offer to pray with clients.
8. After assessing the situation and when appropriate, offer to read scripture or other special readings to clients.
9. Assist the client to participate in religious rituals.
10. Protect the client's religious articles.

you do to physical needs. It is always a delicate matter to help clients face the reality of a terminal illness without abandoning hope. Encouraging the client's active involvement in his or her own care can help to uphold hope. When a client faces death, you can help to make his or her remaining days meaningful by attending to needs and approaching him or her in a supportive and empathetic manner. Feeling loved helps bring peace to the dying.

▼▼▼
The Pastoral Care Team

The pastoral care team is made up of ministers, priests, rabbis, sisters, and lay persons. All are educated to meet spiritual needs in addition to religious needs in a health care setting. The members of this team are allies with nurses in providing spiritual care. If a health care facility does not have a pastoral care team or a chaplain on the staff, a listing of religious representatives of area churches will be available. You can notify this department with a request to see a client. Whenever members of the pastoral care team come to your unit, inform them of the client's background and condition. Describe the interventions you have incorporated into the client's care to provide spiritual care. Remember that the pastoral care team does not relieve you of your responsibility to provide spiritual care.

▼▼▼
How the Client Meets Spiritual Needs

All clients have a spiritual self. Some clients help to meet their spiritual needs by belonging to a specific religious denomination. A religious denomination is an organized group of persons who share a philosophy that supports their particular concept of God. The different rituals and practices of a religion are stabilizing forces for the client. Rituals can bring the security of the past into a crisis situation. Concrete symbols, such as pictures, icons, herb packets, rosaries, statues, jewelry, and other objects can affirm the client's connection with God. Prayer is a spiritual practice of some individuals whether or not they are members of an organized religion. Prayer can put a client in touch with a personal God and sometimes can decrease anxiety as effectively as a drug. Illness sometimes interferes with the client's ability to pray. Honor requests to pray with a client. In other situations, carefully assess whether there is an unexpressed need for prayer.

The value of rituals and religious practices is determined by the faith of the client and not by scientific proof of their benefit. If a client expresses an interest in praying, ask what prayer he would like to say. Try to accommodate the request. When clients are not allowed to practice their religious rituals, practices, and responsibilities, they may feel guilty and uneasy. As a practical nurse, you need to develop an awareness of the general religious philosophy of the client's particular denomination. If membership is claimed in a specific denomination, be aware of the rituals and exercises that the client believes in and practices. Spiritual distress can be observed in clients who are unable to practice their religious rituals or who experience a conflict between their religious and spiritual beliefs and the prescribed health regimen.

Agnostics hold the belief that the existence of God can be neither proved nor disproved. Atheists do not believe that the supernatural exists, so they do not believe in God. Whereas Christians may find comfort and solace in their refuge in God, including passing into another life after death, the atheist does not have this belief to sustain him or her. It may be difficult for the nurse who believes in the supernatural to relate to a person with atheistic beliefs. The nurse may feel unsuccessful in meeting the total needs of the client who is an atheist because atheists do not believe in the supernatural. The nurse should encourage this client to express personal feelings about life, death, separation, and loss and not impose personal beliefs and values on the client.

▼▼▼
Religious Needs

Spiritual needs are not the same as religious needs. The religious self refers to the specific beliefs held by an individual in regard to a higher being.

The remainder of this chapter will present the beliefs and practices of various religions or groups found in the United States and Canada and their nursing implications. This information will serve as a reference to be used in meeting the religious needs of specific clients during your time as a student practical nurse and in your nursing career after you graduate. Although each religion has specific beliefs and practices, sometimes an individual will adapt them to fit his or her own circumstances. Do not assume that all Protestants, Catholics, Jews, for example, actually believe in all the aspects of their formal religion. Do not judge a client if there are variations in his or her beliefs. Clarify with the client whether health issues and decisions involve religious beliefs. The references at the end of the chapter can be used to learn more about a specific religion when such information is needed.

▼▼▼
Major Religions in the United States

▽▽▽
General Considerations

Tables 15–2 and 15–3 list features of the major non-Christian religions, Christian denominations, and groups found in the United States and Canada.

▽▽▽
The Bible

Many Christian clients will find comfort in reading or having someone read to them selected passages from the Bible. Treat the client's Bible with respect. In addition to believing it contains the inspired word of God, some persons have received their Bibles as gifts commemorating special occasions such as a wedding, graduation, confirmation, anniversary, or jubilee. Some Bibles list passages that can be used in specific client situations, such as pain, sorrow, sleeplessness, and so on.

Table 15–2
Major Non-Christian Religions

Religion	Special Features	Nursing Implications
Judaism	Observation of Sabbath	Provide time for rest, prayer, and/or study from sunset on Friday till after sunset on Saturday, if desired
		Provide yarmulke (skullcap) or prayer shawl, if desired. Inform family of need for these items
	Observation of dietary rules (Kosher). Clarify if client follows these dietary rules	Make arrangements for separate utensils for preparing and serving meat and milk dishes, if desired
		If separate dishes not available, these foods can be served in the original containers or on paper plates
		Meat may be consumed a few minutes after drinking milk, but six hours must pass after eating meat before drinking milk
		Do not serve pork, ham, Canadian bacon, eel, oysters, crab, lobster, shrimp, or eggs with blood spots
	The dying Jewish client	Family and friends may want to be with the client at all times
		Some Jews do not believe in autopsies, embalming, or cremation
		Some Jews may not want the nurse to touch the body of a deceased Jew and may request that the nurse notify the Burial Society for preparation of the body for burial
Islam	General beliefs	Some Muslims, members of the Islam religion, may desire to pray to Allah five times a day (after dawn, at noon, in mid-afternoon, after sunset, and at night). If client requests to face Mecca, the holy city of Islam, a bed or chair may be positioned in a southeast direction
		If a Muslim brings the Koran, the holy book of Islam, to the health care institution, do not touch it or place anything on top of it
		If a Muslim wears writings from the Koran on a black string around the neck, arm, or waist, these writings should be kept dry and should not be removed
		Rules of cleanliness may include eating with the right hand and cleansing self with the left hand after urinating and defecating
	Observation of dietary rules	Some Muslims might not eat pork and pork products, eel, oysters, crab, lobster, shrimp, and meats from animals that have not been bled to death by a Muslim
		Some Muslims might not drink alcoholic beverages
	Observation of female modesty	Some Muslim females prefer to be clothed from head to ankle. During a physical examination, they may prefer to undress one body part at a time

Table 15–3
Christian Denominations and Groups

Denomination/ Group	Special Features	Nursing Implications
Protestants	General practices to be clarified	Would client like to be visited by personal minister?
		Does client want Communion, anointing with oil, or time for bible reading?
		If client is an infant and condition is serious, do parents desire Baptism if child is not baptized?
		If client is dying, what are family's beliefs about death and dying?
Roman Catholics	General beliefs	If desired and condition allows, make arrangements for client to attend Mass. Ill Catholics are excused from this obligation on Sundays and holy days
		If desired, arrange for the sacrament of Reconciliation and provide privacy when the priest hears the client's confession
		If desired, arrange for the anointing of the sick, which offers hope and consolation and assists in physical, mental, and spiritual healing
	The dying Catholic client	Seriously ill Catholic clients may want to receive the Last Rites. Make arrangements for the priest to administer the sacrament of Reconciliation, the anointing of the sick, and Holy Communion
	Observation of dietary rules	When sick, a Catholic is excused from fasting (giving up food for a specified period of time) and abstaining (giving up meat at certain times)
	Desire for religious objects	Catholic clients may request that religious pictures and objects be kept at the bedside or on their persons. These are reminders of God's presence in their lives and are sources of consolation
Jehovah's Witnesses	General beliefs	Jehovah's Witnesses will refuse to receive blood products, including plasma. To receive such products is viewed as a violation of the law of God
Seventh Day Adventists	Observation of dietary rules	Adventists generally do not smoke or drink
		Some Adventist clients may avoid beverages with caffeine
		Many Adventists are vegetarians and use soybean products as a protein source. These dietary practices are not mandatory
	Observation of the Sabbath	Adventists observe the Sabbath from sunset on Friday to sunset on Saturday and do not pursue their jobs or worldly pleasures during this time
Mormons	General beliefs	Mormon clients may avoid tobacco, alcohol, coffee, and tea
Christian Scientists	General beliefs	Client may believe that sickness can be eliminated through prayer and spiritual understanding. Healing is considered an awakening to this belief
		Client may want to have a Christian Scientist practitioner contacted to give treatment through prayer
Amish	General beliefs and practices	The Amish do not believe in health insurance and social security and rely on mutual aid in time of need
		Clients may believe that sudden fright or blood loss may cause loss of the soul
		Female clients may not approve of cutting their hair

Table 15–4
Baptism Beliefs and Practices

Denomination/ Group	Age of Administration	Method	Comments
Assembly of God	Age of accountability	Immersion	The person should understand the meaning of Baptism
Bahá'i	—	—	No baptism
Baptist	Adult	Immersion	Not a means of salvation. Opposed to infant baptism. The person should understand the meaning of baptism
Christian Scientist	—	—	No baptism
Eastern Orthodox Churches	Infant	Immersion	Age of infant differs by group
Episcopalian	Infant	Sprinkle	Necessary for salvation
Jehovah's Witnesses	Adult	—	No infant baptism. Necessary for salvation
Lutheran	Infant or adult	Sprinkle or immersion	Infant baptism at 6 to 8 weeks
Methodist	Infant and adult	Sprinkle or immersion	An outward and visible sign of an inward and spiritual grace
Mormon	8 years or older	Immersion	Baptism causes remission of sins. Allows person to receive the gifts of the Holy Spirit. Required for salvation
Presbyterian	Infant	Usually sprinkling	—
Quakers	—	—	No baptism. At birth, infant's name recorded in official book
Roman Catholic	Infant or adult	Usually sprinkling, or immersion	Means of salvation and initiation into the community. Removes all sin. Person receives Holy Spirit
Seventh Day Adventists	Adult	Immersion	Opposed to infant baptism. Makes one a church member
United Church of Christ	Infant	Immersion	When baptized, become a church member

▽▽▽
Baptism

When a client who belongs to a religious group that believes that baptism is essential to salvation requests the sacrament, and death is imminent, the practical nurse may baptize him or her if the minister or priest has not yet arrived. When the dying client is an infant, baptism may be given if the religious beliefs of the parents include infant baptism. The procedure for baptism is as follows:

1. If the client is Protestant, have a witness present for the baptism if possible. This is not necessary for a Catholic client.

2. Allow water to flow over and contact the client's skin while saying the words: "[name, if known], I baptize you in the name of the Father, and of the Son, and of the Holy Spirit."

3. If the client is Catholic and it is uncertain whether baptism was received in the past, precede the above words with "If capable. . . ." These words indicate the client's desire for the sacrament if it has not been received before.

4. Report the baptism to the chaplain or pastoral care team and the family.

5. Record the baptism in the nurses' notes.

Table 15–4 summarizes the status of baptism in various religious denominations and groups in the United States and Canada.

▽▽▽
Communion

Various groups differ in their interpretation of the meaning of communion. Table 15–5 discusses the status of communion beliefs and practices for various denominations and groups in the United States and Canada.

Table 15–5
Communion Beliefs and Practices

Denomination/ Group	Do They Have This Practice?	Comments
Assembly of God	Yes	—
Baptist	Yes	A remembrance of Christ's death
Christian Scientists	No	—
Eastern Orthodox Churches	Yes	Belief same as Catholic
Episcopalian	Yes	Considered a sacrament
Lutherans	Yes	Considered a sacrament. Believe the presence of Christ is real
Methodists	Yes	Open to everyone including children
Presbyterian	Yes	Believe Christ is present in spirit
Quakers	No	—
Roman Catholic	Yes	Believe the bread and wine are the Body and Blood of Christ
Seventh Day Adventists	Yes	Practice washing of the feet in preparation
United Church of Christ	Yes	Considered a sacrament

▼▼▼   S U M M A R Y

▶ The practical nurse has a responsibility to care for the total person, including his physical, emotional, and spiritual needs. The spiritual self grows and matures throughout life. Practical nurses need to support this growth in clients. Spiritual needs of clients arise from their desire to find meaning in life, suffering, and death. Spiritual care is a part of all clients' care, not only in times of crisis. To meet the spiritual needs of clients, you need to be aware of the client's personal spiritual beliefs or the absence of them. Members of the health care team who assist the practical nurse in providing spiritual care to clients are the minister, priest, rabbi, chaplain, and pastoral care team. Many clients help meet their personal spiritual needs by their participation in an organized religion. Spiritual distress can occur when clients cannot fulfill the rituals and practices of their religion or when they experience conflict between their spiritual beliefs and their health regimen. For these reasons, you need to develop an awareness of religious differences and an understanding of the basic beliefs, rituals, and practices of the many religious denominations and sects that exist today. Although the majority of clients in the United States are Protestant, Catholic, Jewish, or Muslim, you will encounter other denominations and groups, including those who have no religious beliefs. By learning more about these groups, you will be able to accommodate their beliefs and practices and will be able to say you have met the needs of the total person.

▼▼▼ R E F E R E N C E S

Schoenbeck S. Called to care: Addressing the spiritual needs of clients. J. Pract Nurs 1994; 44:19–23.

▼▼▼ B I B L I O G R A P H Y

Berggren-Thomas P, Griggs M. Spirituality in aging: Spiritual need or spiritual journey? J Gerontol Nurs 1995; 21:5–10.
Carson V. *Spiritual Dimensions of Nursing Practice.* Philadelphia: W.B. Saunders, 1989.
DiMeo E. Rx for spiritual distress. RN 1991; 54(3):22–24.
Price J, Stevens H, LaBarre M. Spiritual caregiving in nursing practice. *Psychosocial Nurs* 1995; 33(12): 5–9.
When clients refuse blood. Emerg Med 1984; 16(18):65, 69.

Where You Are Going

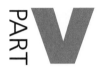

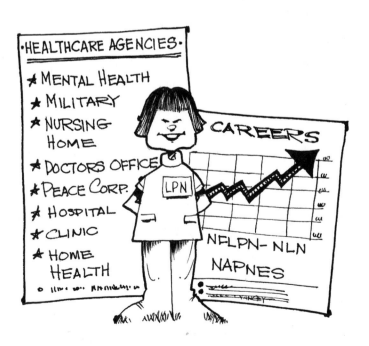

The Health Care System: Agencies, Financing, and Trends

▼▼▼   *K E Y   T E R M S*

acute care

alliances

capitation

catastrophic illness

charting by exception

continuous quality improvement

co-payments

cost containment

cost effectiveness

critical pathways

cross-trained

decentralized departments

deductibles

Diagnosis-Related Groups (DRGs)

downsizing (rightsizing)

fee-for-service

free-standing

group health insurance

Health Maintenance Organizations

incremental changes

Joint Commission on Accreditation of Health Care Organizations (JCAHO)

long-term (extended) care

managed care

Medicaid

Medicare

nurse extenders (multi-skilled workers, patient care extenders/externs, unlicensed assistive personnel)

official (government) health care agencies

patient-focused care

political activism

preexisting conditions

Preferred Provider Organization (PPO)

primary care

private health care agencies

private pay

restructuring

"seamless" system

service, quality, and cost of care

third-party payments

Total Quality Management (TQM)

universal coverage

voluntary health care agencies

wellness promotion

▼▼▼   *O B J E C T I V E S*

Upon completing this chapter you will be able to:

1. Compare public and private health care agencies according to the following criteria:
   a. Source of funding
   b. Services provided
   c. Examples of agencies in your geographic area
   d. Possible places of employment for practical nurses

2. Describe methods of financing health care costs:
   a. Personal payment (private pay)
   b. Private group and individual health insurance (nongovernmental)
   c. Government-sponsored health insurance plans
   d. Fee-for-service
   e. Capitation

3. Discuss trends affecting payment for health care:
   a. Need for cost containment

   b. Private health insurance limitationsMedicare and Medicaid regulations

4. Discuss how resulting government action and marketplace changes affect health care reform.

5. Discuss the effect of the following marketplace changes on health care agencies:
   a. Restructuring of the health care system
      1) Changes in staffing patterns
      2) Method of delivering health care
         a) Patient-focused care
         b) Managed care and Health Maintenance Organizations
         c) Health care alliances and regional alliances

6. Discuss how marketplace changes affect jobs for practical nurses.

7. Identify your reaction to change in your personal and professional life.

8. Develop a personal plan to help you adapt to change in the future.

9. Discuss additional trends that affect practical nursing:
   a. Aging of the population
   b. Shifts in nursing supply and demand

The United States health care system is complex. A large number of health care agencies and their personnel make up a system many people consider to be the finest in the world. Yet not all citizens have access to this fine system of health care.

The National League for Nursing's *Entry Level Competencies of Graduates of Educational Programs in Practical Nursing* (1994, p. 4) includes the following competency requirement for graduates of educational programs in practical nursing: "Political activism—is aware that the practical nurse, through political, economic, and societal activities, can affect nursing and health."

Practical nurses need to help shape health policy by educating the public and their state and federal legislators about issues in health care. To be politically active, the practical nurse needs to understand the many changes affecting health care. To understand these changes, the practical nurse needs knowledge of agencies that deliver health care services, the way these agencies are financed, and the issues and trends that affect the health care system. The purpose of this chapter is to provide information about health care agencies, financing issues, and trends. The various health care agencies described could also be a potential source of employment for practical nurses in health care, especially in the community.

▼▼▼
Public Versus Private Health Care Agencies

For ease of understanding, the various health care services in the United States can be grouped into two general categories: (1) services delivered by the *public* sector, and (2) those delivered by the *private* sector.

▽▽▽
Public Health Care Agencies

There are two types of **public health care agencies**—official and voluntary. **Official health care agencies** are government agencies that are supported by tax money and are accountable to the taxpayers and the government. The primary emphasis of government (official)

agencies is the delivery of programs of disease prevention and wellness promotion, but direct health care services are sometimes provided.

Voluntary health care agencies are supported by voluntary contributions and sometimes by a fee for service. Although they are tuned in to public opinion, voluntary agencies are accountable to their supporters, and their activities are determined by supporter interest, not legal mandate. The primary emphasis of these agencies is research and education. They may also offer direct health services to the client. Some official and voluntary health care agencies operate at the local, state, federal, and international levels.

▽▽▽
Private Health Care Agencies

You may be most familiar with **private health care agencies**. Entrance to the health care delivery system in the United States is generally gained through private health care agencies. Although some voluntary or nonprofit agencies are found in the private sector, private health care agencies are generally proprietary, or for-profit. They charge a fee for their services. Their primary emphasis has been on curing disease and illness, but recently a change in emphasis to include disease prevention and wellness promotion has occurred. Table 16–1 outlines the major differences between public and private health care agencies. As you read about public and private health care agencies, think of them as potential sources of employment for the practical nurse.

▽▽▽
Examples of Public Health Care Agencies

Official Government Agencies

Local.   The official health agency at the local level is the city or county health department. This agency is funded by local tax money as well as by subsidies from the state and federal levels of government. The local health department carries out state laws concerning community health. It also carries out nonmandated programs such as health promotion programs.

Table 16–1
A Comparison of Health Care Agencies in the Public and Private Sectors

	Public		Private
	Official (Government)	*Nonofficial (Voluntary)*	
Support	Tax money	Voluntary contributions and fees for service	Fees for service
Primary Service	Programs of disease prevention and wellness promotion	Research and education	Curing disease and illness
Additional Services	Sometimes direct service of health care	Offer direct health services	Disease prevention and wellness promotion
Accountability	Taxpayers and government	Supporters, boards, etc.	Owners
How Programs Determined	Mandated and nonmandated	Supporter interest	Defined goals of the organization

State. Each state has a state health department. This official health agency is funded by state tax money and sometimes receives money from the federal government.

Federal (National). The official health agency at the federal level in the United States is the Department of Health and Human Services (DHHS). It is funded by federal taxes and is headed by a person appointed by the President of the United States. This person advises the President in health matters. The division of the Department of Health and Human Services that is concerned primarily with health is the U.S. Public Health Service (USPHS). The six agencies that make up the USPHS are as follows:

▶ Food and Drug Administration (FDA)
▶ Centers for Disease Control and Prevention (CDC)
▶ National Institutes of Health (NIH)
▶ Health Services Administration (HSA)
▶ Health Resources Administration (HRA)
▶ Alcohol, Drug Abuse, and Mental Health Administration

International. Health activities take place at the international level through the World Health Organi-

zation (WHO), an agency of the United Nations. The WHO is located in Geneva, Switzerland. The major objective of the WHO is the highest possible level of health for people all over the world. This organization defines health as a state of complete physical, mental, and social well-being and not merely as the absence of disease or infirmity. The WHO is funded through fees paid by member nations of the United Nations.

▽▽▽
Examples of Voluntary Health Care Agencies

Voluntary or nonofficial health care agencies are so named because they are not for profit. The health services they provide are complementary to official health agencies and often meet the needs of persons with specific diseases (for example, heart disease) and certain segments of the population (for example, the handicapped). Although there are paid personnel working in voluntary health agencies, volunteers form a major part of their support system. Voluntary organizations are sites of volunteer service for practical nurses. A few examples of voluntary health agencies follow. Refer to your local telephone directory for additional names and numbers of voluntary health care agencies.

Community Hospitals

These nonprofit hospitals are operated by community associations or religious organizations. They provide short-term inpatient care for people with acute illnesses and injuries.

Visiting Nurse Association (VNA)

This public voluntary agency provides home nursing care for those with acute and chronic diseases. Staff of this agency visit mothers with newborns. Visiting nurses are engaged in health teaching. They frequently involve the family in the care of its own members. Visiting nurses assist with referrals for clients to other community services. Nurses with a bachelor of science in nursing are employed in public health agencies.

American Cancer Society (ACS)

This voluntary agency is a national organization with state and local units. It is involved in extensive cancer research and education of the public about cancer. ACS is a source of up-to-date information for health professionals in the prevention, diagnosis, and treatment of cancer. This association also assists clients with referrals and supplies as needed.

American Lung Association

This voluntary agency conducts research affecting people with respiratory and lung diseases. It provides educational materials for the general public and health care workers. The Christmas seals you receive each fall help to support this organization.

Alcoholics Anonymous (AA)

If assistance is desired, this voluntary agency provides rehabilitation help for alcoholics and their families.

ALS Society of America

This voluntary organization gathers information about clients with amyotrophic lateral sclerosis (Lou Gehrig's disease) for research purposes. It provides information about this rare disease to lay persons and health care

workers. This agency also gives client care tips to nursing personnel.

National Easter Seal Society

This voluntary organization conducts research into and provides information about cerebral palsy to the public and to health care workers.

National Multiple Sclerosis Society

This voluntary organization conducts on-going research with the aim of finding a cure for multiple sclerosis. It also provides education about this disease to clients, nursing students, and health care workers.

LaLeche League

This voluntary organization provides information and support for breastfeeding mothers. The League provides breast milk for infants who must have this form of nourishment but lack a source.

United Ostomy Association (UOA)

This voluntary organization provides education and support preoperatively and postoperatively for clients who are undergoing ostomy or urinary diversion procedures.

▽▽▽
Examples of Private Health Care Agencies

Private health care agencies also complement and supplement government agencies. Compared with public health services, the greatest changes in health care services have been noted in this area.

Family Practice Physicians

Primary care is a term used to describe the point at which an individual enters the health care system. Family practice physicians are a source of primary care. These physicians provide diagnosis and treatment. The client is billed a fee for the services. If further diagnostic evaluation is needed, the client is referred to a specialist.

Medical doctors function within the medical practice acts of their respective states.

Private Practice Nurses

Specializing in primary health care, advanced practice nurses (see Chapter 3) provide consulting and counseling services to groups of individuals. These nurses practice in all areas of health care. Private practice nurses fill an especially acute need in rural areas where physician services are sometimes difficult to obtain. These nurses function within the nurse practice acts of their respective states.

Proprietary Hospitals

For-profit hospitals are operated for the financial benefit (profit) of the owner of the hospital. The owner may be an individual, a partnership, or a corporation. By using good management techniques, the hospital can be run efficiently, and a profit can be realized. When clients are admitted to the hospital today, they are more acutely ill and require more skilled nursing care. This setting for health care is called acute care. Clients in acute care are now discharged sooner than they were in the past, which makes them seem "sicker" on discharge.

Ambulatory Services

The continual rise in cost of inpatient care has resulted in the rapid development of a variety of ambulatory services. As a consequence, the number of inpatient days and the length of stay in acute care facilities have decreased. Ambulatory services offer less expensive care because admission to an acute care facility is avoided. Examples of ambulatory services follow.

Outpatient Clinics. Outpatient clinics provide follow-up care to clients after hospitalization. These clinics manage disease on an ambulatory basis for those who do not need to be hospitalized. Outpatient clinics may be part of health care facilities or free standing. These clinics function by appointment only. They include specialty areas such as diabetes, neurology, allergy, and oncology. The number of specialized clinics

depends on the population of the area. A full-time staff is employed.

Ambulatory Care Facilities (Urgent Care Centers). Services are available in ambulatory care facilities for walk-in clients who do not have an appointment. These clinics make available primary health care as an alternative to care by a family physician or care offered in the more expensive emergency room. Ambulatory care clinics are used by persons who do not have a family physician. These clinics are also used by clients who desire quick service outside of regular office hours. The names given to ambulatory care services reflect the type of care they provide: convenience clinics, express care, quick care, and so on.

Ambulatory Surgery Centers (Outpatient Surgery). One-day surgical care centers perform surgery at a scheduled date and time. Clients are discharged when they have recovered from anesthesia and are considered to be in stable condition. This eliminates the need for and the monetary charge for being hospitalized overnight. These services are also known as outpatient surgery within an established hospital. Free-standing outpatient surgery centers provide outpatient surgery as their only service. By the year 2000, it is predicted that 80% of surgical procedures will be performed in this type of setting.

Free Clinics

Some communities have established free clinics as an alternative means of providing primary health care. These clinics are used by persons who cannot afford traditional health services or are reluctant to use more traditional services. The fee is minimal. The environment is as free of red tape as possible.

Long-Term (Extended) Care Facilities

Long-term care units offer care for clients who need more time to recover than the short term of hospitalization allows. These facilities offer nursing care with an emphasis on restoring individuals to their personal level of physical and emotional wellness and returning them to their homes and families. Extended care services may be offered by hospitals, separate facilities, or nursing homes.

Nursing Homes (Facilities)

Nursing homes are institutions that take responsibility for the care of persons who are disabled, terminally ill, homeless, or helpless when their families cannot or will not care for them at home. The aged and elderly are frequently nursing home residents. These health care agencies also serve chronically ill persons of all age groups.

Home Health Care Agencies

Home care agencies provide a variety of health services in the home, such as nursing, occupational therapy, and physical therapy. Some agencies also provide homemaker and companion services. Hospitals develop home care agencies as extensions of care. Private agencies offer services in an effort to keep people in their homes for treatment.

Adult Day Care Centers

Hospital-based and free-standing adult day care centers provide services for individuals who need supervision because of physical or safety needs, yet are not candidates for nursing home placement. Some clients and families prefer adult day care instead of nursing home placement.

Wellness Centers

Healthy People 2000: National Health Promotion and Disease Prevention Objectives (1991) is a document published by the U.S. Public Health Service. This document suggests preventive strategies to help avoid disease as well as promote wellness. An emphasis on promoting wellness continues to result in a multitude of services being offered in this area of health care. Not only have hospitals developed programs to detect disease in early stages, they have also developed programs to promote wellness. These programs include nutritional counseling, exercise programs, stress reduction, and weight control. The private sector con-

tinues to be active in the wellness area. People have developed an interest in exercise and fitness clubs, weight-reduction programs such as Weight Watchers, smoking cessation classes, stress control, and parenting classes.

> *Identify specific private health care agencies in your community. These agencies are a growing source of employment for practical nurses.*

▼▼▼
How Health Care Costs Are Financed

Knowledge of the methods by which health care costs are financed is necessary to help practical nurses understand the issue of health care reform. A knowledge of health care financing also leads to an appreciation of the value of health insurance as a fringe benefit of employment. The same persons who consider the United States' health care system to be the finest in the world may also say that the financial basis of this excellent system is illogical.

The traditional method of paying health care bills is the system called **fee-for-service**. In this method, the physician is paid a fee by the client for each service he or she provides to clients. Under the fee-for-service system, insurance companies reimburse the client for most diagnostic tests and treatments for illness ordered by physicians. The tests and treatments that could keep clients healthy or could catch illnesses in the early stages when they are less expensive to treat are often not reimbursed by insurance companies under the fee-for-service system. Insurance premiums soared under this type of fee system. Many unemployed individuals previously enrolled in group health insurance plans could not afford individual plans and became uninsured. To improve their margins of profit, insurance companies began charging **deductibles** (the amount the subscriber must pay before health insurance will begin to pay the bills) and **co-payments** (the percentage of the bill paid by the subscriber). The cost of health care continued to soar.

▼▼▼
Methods of Payment

▽▽▽
Personal Payment (Private Pay)

Paying the cost of health care directly by the client was the primary method of payment of health care costs prior to the 1940s. This method of payment is used by some clients today, but the cost of health care services discourages the use of this method by the average person.

▽▽▽
Government-Sponsored Health Insurance Plans

Medicare

Older persons generally find themselves ineligible for group insurance plans because they are not employed. Many are unable to afford private plans. This inability to get insurance occurs at the very time when individuals are likely to require more hospitalization and medical care because of their age. In 1965, a provision was added to the Social Security Act in the form of a federally sponsored and supervised health insurance plan that financed health care for all persons over age 65. **Part A** of the Medicare bill provides hospital benefits. Part A also applies to persons under age 65 who are permanently and totally disabled and to victims of end-stage renal disease. Coverage is also offered for posthospitalization convalescence in extended care facilities and home health services. The Health Care Financing Administration (HCFA) has proposed shifting home health services from Medicare Part A to Part B. Part A is available without cost to those who meet eligibility requirements, but it includes a deductible.

Part B of Medicare is similar to a major medical plan. Part B includes inpatient and outpatient physician services and a wide range of other related services for people over age 65. Part B is available for a monthly premium to those who are eligible for enrollment. Some persons over age 65 also carry private supplemental coverage in addition to Medicare to cover deductibles, coinsurance, and limited-coverage situations that exist in the federal program.

Diagnosis-Related Groups (DRGs)

Payment for Medicare is a major item in the federal budget. Approximately 35 cents of every federal dollar goes toward retirement benefits, including Social Security and Medicare. Because the federal deficit (caused by less money coming in than is going out to run all government programs) was consistently growing larger, the federal government was the first group to try to stop the skyrocketing cost of health care. On October 1, 1983, the HCFA adopted a system of paying hospitals a set fee for Medicare services by telling them in advance how much the hospitals would be reimbursed. Because the government announces to a hospital in advance what it will pay for health care costs, this system is called the **prospective payment system.** Prior to 1983, hospitals submitted a bill to the government for the total charges they incurred for Medicare clients and were reimbursed for this amount. This was called a **retrospective payment system.** Under the diagnosis-related group (DRG) system, hospitals have an incentive to treat clients and discharge them as quickly as possible. Hospitals receive a flat fee for each client regardless of the client's length of stay. If the hospital keeps the client longer than the government's fee will cover, and the client cannot be reclassified in the DRG system, the hospital has to make up the difference in costs. If the acute care facility can treat the Medicare client for less than the guaranteed reimbursement, the facility can keep the difference as profit.

Because Medicare clients are discharged sooner from hospitals than they were in the past (because of the DRG system of reimbursement), extended care units are frequently used to continue convalescence. These units need more skilled health care workers, such as practical nurses.

Medicaid (Medical Assistance)

The poor generally find themselves ineligible for private insurance coverage because they are unable to afford the cost of premiums. Another provision that was added to the Social Security Act in 1965 was the Medicaid program. This program expanded the financial assistance provided by the federal government to states and counties to pay for medical services for the eligible poor. The Medicaid system developed out of the welfare system that services low-income families. Medicaid also is a major item in the federal budget.

▽▽▽
Private Group and Individual (Nongovernment) Health Insurance

Group health insurance is a method of pooling individual contributions for a common group goal—protection from financial disaster due to health care bills. When insured, an individual is said to have third-party coverage, that is, a fiscal middleman. This fiscal middleman pays the individual's health care bills. Two examples of private group health insurance are as follows:

▶ Blue Cross and Blue Shield: Blue Cross covers hospital inpatient costs and Blue Shield covers inpatient physician costs. A major medical plan is available to include the cost of outpatient services. Individuals can purchase coverage from Blue Cross and Blue Shield, but the cost for individuals is higher than it is in group plans.
▶ Health policies offered through commercial or independent insurance companies: Many major insurance companies offer health insurance to individuals and groups.

▽▽▽
Issues and Trends

Need for Cost Containment

Today, the driving force in all public and private health care agencies is cost containment (the need to hold costs to within fixed limits) while remaining competitive in the health care marketplace. In 1960, health care was a $27 billion dollar a year industry. In 1996, the yearly cost of health care exceeded 1 trillion dollars.

> **What Is a Trillion Dollars?**
> *If you spent $1,000,000 an hour, 24 hours a day, 365 days a year, it would take you 171 years to spend 1.5 trillion dollars. The U.S. government spends 1.5 trillion dollars a year (Pintar, 1995).*

Pressure is being felt from the federal government, the insurance industry, and consumers to reduce the cost of health care while maintaining high-quality care and service. The practical nurse should remember that health care agencies are interested in streamlining their "bottom line" by reducing waste and inefficiency. Practical nurses who identify wasteful practices and inefficient routines in their work settings while maintaining quality may be saving their very jobs.

Private Health Insurance Issues

There are several concerns in the area of private health insurance as health care costs continue to rise. Some subscribers have been refused coverage for **preexisting conditions.** Examples of preexisting conditions include heart disease, diabetes, asthma, arthritis, and AIDS. Some subscribers have been refused coverage for **catastrophic illness.** Examples include cancer treatment and transplant surgery. Although government health care reform is focusing on Medicare and Medicaid, the issue of **guaranteed coverage** (the inability of an insurance company to drop a subscriber for any reason) has been addressed. In August 1996, Congress passed the Kennedy-Kassebaum health bill. This bill makes all health insurance portable from job to job. The bill also prevents persons from being dropped by insurance companies if they lose their job or have a preexisting condition. Other insurance issues to be addressed include (1) increasing amounts of coinsurance and deductibles, and (2) the rising cost of health insurance premiums.

The government's DRG system has encouraged private insurers to adopt cost-cutting measures. Some employers offering health insurance now require second opinions for surgery and clearance for hospitalizations and offer reduced premiums for selected wellness practices. Hospitalized clients with health insurance are discharged sooner than they expected to be discharged.

Clients who are privately insured face higher deductibles.

Government Health Insurance Issues

Medicare and Medicaid continue to be major issues at the state and federal levels because of the increasing cost of health care. There is continued debate about possible changes in future Medicare and Medicaid benefits. Higher monthly premiums and deductibles for Medicare are being considered. It is predicted by some that the Social Security trust fund will become depleted by the year 2002, whereas others dispute this calculation.

By August 1, 1996, Congress passed the Personal Responsibility and Work Opportunity Reconciliation Act of 1996 that ended the federal welfare system initiated by Franklin D. Roosevelt 60 years ago. Comprehensive Medicaid reform was not included in this welfare reform bill. Changes in Medicaid were made that affect eligibility for the program. However, each state has the option to modify this law according to strict guidelines.

> *What changes in legislation at the federal level and at your state level have affected Medicare and Medicaid since the third edition of* Success in Practical Nursing *was published? Review the resources listed in Chapter 8 for suggestions that can be used in obtaining up-to-date information for your nursing courses.*

▼▼▼
The Need for Health Care Reform

Despite the various methods of paying for health care services and the Kennedy-Kassebaum health bill, approximately 39 million Americans lack health insurance coverage. These numbers are growing. Two major ways to accomplish health care reform are (1) to enact comprehensive changes at the federal level and (2) to allow incremental changes in the marketplace. At the federal level, the 1993 health care reform debate included the issue of universal coverage, which is coverage of all Americans. Suggested ways of increasing

coverage of Americans include creating a system of national health insurance and mandating employers to provide health insurance benefits for all employees. Some persons opposed to universal coverage object to the idea of tax money being used to insure all Americans. Persons who favor universal coverage think it would be a more efficient and effective use of tax money that is already being used for health care but in an inefficient manner.

▽▽▽
Effect of Lack of Health Insurance Coverage

Lack of access to health care prevents individuals from seeking treatment when a health problem is developing. These individuals do seek treatment during the later stages of illness, usually at greater expense. For example, the most cost-effective means of diagnosing and treating a sinus infection would be an assessment by a family physician or nurse practitioner. However, this solution is not realistic if (1) you do not have a family physician or nurse practitioner, (2) your insurance company does not cover this type of office visit, or (3) you do not have the money to pay for a visit even if you do have a family physician or nurse practitioner. The individual with a sinus infection might seek treatment at the local emergency room when the problem reaches the stage when it can no longer be tolerated. Emergency room treatment is expensive for any condition. Such treatment is intended for seriously ill or injured persons and not for less serious illnesses.

> *If the client in the above scenario does not have health insurance or the ability to pay the emergency room fee, who pays the bill?*

▼▼▼
Response of the Marketplace to Proposed Health Care Reform

The Contract with America initiated by the one-hundred and third Congress after the November, 1994, elections contained issues that got Senators and Congressmen elected. These issues did not include comprehensive health care reform. There is an effort to reduce the federal deficit. Changes in health insurance for those with coverage has taken place. Because of these efforts, changes in health care are occurring.

Despite the lack of comprehensive health care reform on the national level, the marketplace continues to respond to the possibility of government health care reform as proposed in 1993. This method of solving health care problems is called the **incremental method.** In this method, changes occur here and there without affecting the system as a whole. Incremental changes can be beneficial in decreasing the rate of increase of health care costs. They can have a negative effect if they are initiated under the threat of comprehensive reform of health care. Incremental changes may disappear if the issue of comprehensive health care reform "disappears." The old rate of increase of health care costs could return. Incremental changes have not improved access to care for millions of uninsured persons. (See Private Health Insurance Issues, on p. 239.)

The force driving health care reform continues to be the escalating cost of health care. Today, the "person"

who pays for health care is calling the shots. **Capitation** is an alternative to the fee-for-service method of payment. Capitation involves a set monthly fee charged by the provider of health care services for each member of the insurance group for a specific set of services. At the end of the year, if any money is left over, the health care provider keeps it as a profit. Suddenly, if a provider of health care services can keep a member of the insurance group healthy, the provider will make a profit! Study Table 16–2 for a comparison of the fee-for-service and capitation methods of payment for health care services.

> *What are the positive and negative aspects of capitation?*

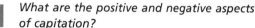

What Changes in Health Care Can Tell the Practical Nurse

Although there is currently no organized attempt at the federal level to achieve comprehensive health care reform, health care agencies and insurance companies

Table 16–2
Comparison of Methods of Payment for Health Care Services

	Fee-For-Service	Capitation
Services Covered	Each service claimed by the physician (e.g., diagnostic tests, treatments)	Services in group contract
Are Preventive Tests or Treatments Covered?	No	Yes. Wellness practices covered
Cost	Set fee per member of group	Set fee per member of group
Advantages	All tests and treatments for illness covered	Wellness encouraged. No deductibles and co-payments
Disadvantages	Emphasis on illness. Deductibles and co-payments keep patient from reporting illness in early stages	To realize a profit, needed tests may not be ordered

have been initiating their own incremental changes to control the cost of health care.

The single word that describes health care in the United States now is **change**. The changes are dramatic, staggering, and continual. Some persons see the changes as chaos. Those who will survive see the changes as opportunities to improve the delivery of health care (**service**), increase the **quality** of that care, and decrease the **cost** of care.

▼▼▼
Restructuring of the Health Care System

A major change taking place in health care services today is the restructuring of the health care system in response to escalating costs. Strategies designed to decrease the cost of health care require a radical shift in viewing how health care services are delivered, especially for those used to doing things the old way. These strategies require a "new lens" in the nurse's eye. They do not reflect business as usual. And the word business is used intentionally. Practical nurses need to look at health care services from a business point of view. Business principles are running health care services. Service, quality, and cost control are attributes of health care that need to be understood and brought to all clinical situations by the practical nurse.

▽▽▽
Changes in Staffing Patterns for Delivery of Health Care

The number of hospital inpatient days continues to decline. Fewer inpatients spend less time in the hospital. More clients receive care in **ambulatory service** (**outpatient**) settings. Hospitals continue to engage in **downsizing** (some hospitals call it rightsizing) both staff and services. This translates into fewer health care workers, including nurses, being hired. Regional nurse layoffs continue. When staff resign or retire, some of their positions are not filled. The responsibilities of these staff persons are assumed by other staff. Services are scaled down to essential services. Duplication of services is avoided.

One survival strategy for acute care facilities is the use of unlicensed assistive personnel (UAPs) (see Chapter 3 for a review). These workers are known as nurse extenders, multiskilled workers, patient-care extenders, patient-care assistants, and externs. They can be found as patient care team members in all patient care units. Business managers have found that many services and skills of highly educated persons can be delivered by less trained personnel without sacrificing quality. These skills include those performed by the practical nurse. Nurses contend that the quality of care has been decreased by using UAPs. Results of research studies on the effect of downsizing and the use of unlicensed personnel on the quality of care are mixed. Nurses assign not only routine and repetitive tasks to these staff persons but also technical tasks. In doing so, nurses take on new responsibilities and focus on the tasks that, by law, only the licensed nurse can perform. See Chapter 20.

Current staff are being **cross-trained** to perform specific tasks of other health care team members. Examples of this role shifting include nurses drawing blood and respiratory therapists bathing and feeding clients.

▽▽▽
Methods of Delivering Health Care

Patient-Focused Care

The most dramatic change in the way health care is delivered has been a shift toward **patient-focused care**. Delivery of health care through separate (centralized) departments in acute care facilities was inefficient. The client had to travel to different departments to be admitted and often to be diagnosed and treated. Separate departments discouraged the professional relationships necessary to deliver health care effectively. In patient-focused care, service departments, including equipment and supplies, are decentralized. Health care providers in this method of health care delivery are located in client care units instead of being scattered throughout the agency. Functions once performed by centralized departments are shifted to the unit level. Instead of asking the client to go to different departments for diagnostic tests and treatments, the client stays on the unit. The professional nurse is the coordinator of the team and is accountable for all client care under this system.

Procedures are simplified and made more efficient. One example is the charting method called charting by exception (CBE). In this charting system, normal events are charted merely by placing a check mark on a flowsheet. Only abnormal events or changes are charted in narrative form.

Another example of efficient health care is the use of critical pathways (CPs), also called care maps and care guides. CPs are plans of care that show a sequence of care that is to be delivered within a definite time frame. Critical pathways also include potential problems and expected outcomes. They form a picture of the expected course of recovery for the client that all members of the health care team can follow. This method helps the client reach discharge in the fastest time possible. See Figure 16–1 for an example of a CP for a client experiencing nausea and vomiting during chemotherapy for cancer.

Managed Care—Health Maintenance Organizations (HMOs)

Managed care is a health care delivery system developed to provide health care with cost controls. An example of managed care is the **health maintenance organization** (HMO). Regardless of how many services the HMO provides, it is paid an annual fee to maintain the health of each of its members (capitation). The HMO discourages physicians from ordering excessive diagnostic studies and treatments and encourages prevention of disease by the practice of preventive medicine. The healthier clients are kept, the fewer treatments the HMO needs to deliver and the larger the profit margin for the HMO.

For a fee, clients seek medical care at the first sign of symptoms. This is the time when health care is least expensive to deliver. In an HMO, the client may not have the option of choosing his physician each time treatment is needed. Depending on the HMO, a member may go outside the HMO to see a desired physician with a **point of service** (POS) option. With the POS option, the member pays an extra fee.

The National Committee for Quality Assurance (NCQA) provides objective nationwide assessment of HMOs. This group issues report cards similar to *Consumer Reports* guides so that potential subscribers can evaluate an HMO before they join it. Kaiser Permanente has been operating in California since the 1940s and is the largest HMO in the United States.

Preferred provider organizations (PPOs) are similar to HMOs. Whereas HMOs are located in buildings that are used solely for HMO business, and all physicians working in the HMO are hired specifically for the HMO, family physicians may be hired as members of a PPO. These physicians remain in the same office in which their practice is located and continue to belong to the same physician group. Part of their day is spent treating clients in their own general practice. However, part of the day is spent treating clients who are enrolled in the PPO under the rules of the PPO. Think of airline travel today. The person sitting next to you probably paid a different ticket price for the same service you paid for. The same may be true for the client sitting next to you in the waiting room of the family physician who has added a PPO service to his practice.

Health Care Alliances and Regional Alliances

Changes in the delivery of health care in the community involve new partnerships (alliances) among hospitals, clinics, labs, health care systems, and physicians. By joining together or networking, these alliances can coordinate the delivery of care and contain costs via partnerships among providers. This system is a way to deliver health care services in a climate of shrinking resources. All members of an alliance can buy supplies in quantity. They can share a computer system. Duplication of services and equipment is avoided. Client records can be more readily available on referral to another health care provider within the **network**. For this reason, alliances are called "seamless" systems. Alliances allow small rural hospitals to continue to exist in a competitive market. Public–private partnerships continue to emerge. For example, public health agencies contract for services from private community nursing agencies. Such services control costs and continue to deliver quality care.

1 - 7-3
2 - 3-11
3 - 11-7

LAST ☐ Chemotherapy Date ___
☐ Radiation Date ___

CARE NEED	DAY 1 ADMIT DAY date ___	DAY 2 date ___	DAY 3 date ___	DAY 4 date ___
ASSESSMENTS/ TREATMENTS	Postural BP on admission & prn Weight documented I&O Baseline vital signs documented Vital signs q shift and prn Review old chart Previous admit for n/v/d date: ___ Safety/fall assessment	AM weight I&O Vital signs q shift - stable Evaluate lab results	AM weight I&O Vital signs ONLY 7-3 and 3-11 if stable	
FLUIDS/ NUTRITIONS	Start IV hydration @ admit 1000cc D₅½NS 20 KCL @ 100 IV antiemetics Adjust IV fluids based on lab results within 8° of admit Clear liquids as tolerated	IV fluids continue Start PO or PR antiemetics q 8° around- the-clock Cont. IV antiemetics for BREAKTHROUGH Clear liquids-intake: 7-3 500; 3-11 400; 11-7 100 Advance to full liquid dinner or as tolerated	DC or HL IV by noon Antiemetics AC and HS PO only Advance to regular diet for lunch Fluid intake: 7-3 600; 3-11 500; 11-7 100	
LAB/ DIAGNOSTICS	CBC-if not available from MD office SMA 20-SMA 7 stat	SMA-7		
ACTIVITY	Up to BR Ambulate in room 1x day/evenings	Up to BR Ambulate ½ length of hallway TID	Ambulate full length of hallway TID	
SELF-CARE	Mouth care Face/hand washing Feeding	Mouth care Self bath @ bedside Feeding	Mouth care Shower	
DISCHARGE PLANNING	Evaluate home care support Refer to Social Services if: Social Work intervention needed	Document discharge plan: Social Services or Nursing	Finalize home care needs	Discharge by 11:00 AM
TEACHING	___ Assess current knowledge of antiemetics; document on kardex	___ Medication instruction ___ Dietary consult evaluate need for diet counseling	___ Review/reinforce med instruction ___ Review/reinforce diet instruction	___ Verbalizes understanding of meds for home care and diet
RN	D E N Initial Signature	D E N Initial Signature	D E N Initial Signature	D E N Initial Signature

Good Samaritan Hospital
A division of Good Samaritan Community Healthcare
407-14th Ave. SE, PO Box 1247, Puyallup, WA 98371-0192 (206) 848-6661

Oncology
Clinical Pathway

Nausea/Vomiting/Dehydration

Figure 16–1

Oncology clinical pathway. Nausea, vomiting, and dehydration in clients with cancer (Karen Graybeal, MS, RN: Cynthia Marion, RN, OCN; Margaret Brown, MN, RN, OCN; Patty Patch, RN, OCN; Deanna Kruckenberg, RN, OCN; courtesy of Good Samaritan Hospital, Puyallup, WA. In Ignatavicius DD, Workman ML, Mishler MA, *Medical-Surgical Nursing: A Nursing Process Approach.* 2nd ed. Philadelphia: W.B. Saunders, 1995, p. 576.)

From Quality Assurance to Quality Improvement

The emphasis on quality assurance is being replaced by an emphasis on continuous quality improvement (CQI) and total quality management (TQM). Quality assurance stressed the identification of care that needed to be given to clients and evaluation of the results of that care. Quality improvement stresses the need to search continually for new ways to improve the process of client care, prevent errors, and identify and fix problems. This makes the search for approaches to nursing problems a never-ending quest. Total quality management is the method by which CQI is carried out.

A major way of improving the process of client care has been the formulation of nursing care plans by the RN, assisted by the practical nurse. The Joint Commission on Accreditation of Healthcare Organizations (JCAHO) has removed the requirement for a separate nursing care plan for each client. However, JCAHO encourages quality improvement. Whatever method replaces the nursing care plan in health care situations, practical nurses still have a responsibility to assist the RN with problem-solving in client care situations.

As we approach the year 2000, practical nurses need to define their role as more than the list of nursing tasks they perform. These nursing tasks are also being performed by less trained, unlicensed persons on the health care team. Practical nurses need to define their role in light of their assisting role in the nursing process. Practical nurses are effective in noting new client problems and collaborating with RNs in setting client goals, performing nursing interventions, and evaluating the results of planning. It is this problem-solving and critical thinking aspect of nursing that makes practical nurses valuable members of the health care team.

▼▼▼ Impact of Restructuring the Health Care System on Jobs for Practical Nurses

Each change made in health care services places new demands and restrictions on health care careers. Opportunities also arise from the changes being made in health care. The change of focus from inpatient to outpatient care provides an opportunity for practical nurses to seek employment in the community in ambulatory service settings such as outpatient clinics, urgent care centers, and outpatient surgery centers. The impact of **downsizing and changes in staffing patterns** results in greater reliance on practical nurses functioning in their expanded role within the legal scope of practice of their state nurse practice act. The impact of **patient-focused care** on acute health care involves viewing the RN as primarily the coordinator of care. The practical nurse is needed to perform assigned tasks that UAPs cannot legally perform.

The area of **managed care** has provided job opportunities for practical nurses in insurance companies. Practical nurses are trained to review medical claims and develop alternative plans of treatment to meet the medical needs of clients in a more cost-effective manner. **Alliances (networks)** are also creating new job opportunities for practical nurses in the community in physicians' offices. Other community sources of employment for practical nurses are the practices of private practice nurses, wellness centers, dialysis centers, group homes, extended care units, nursing homes, home health agencies, adult day care centers, Red Cross, Alzheimer units, and companion services. Some practical nurses are also starting their own business ventures in health-related areas in the community.

> *Identify alliances or networks that have occurred in your area of the country.*
>
> *Identify health-related businesses owned and operated by practical nurses in your community.*
>
> *Identify health-related areas of need in your community for which practical nurses could develop a business.*

▼▼▼ Dealing with Change

If you have had no prior experience in health care before entering the practical nursing program, you may not be aware of the changes taking place in the workplace. If you have had prior experience in the health care field, some of the changes you now observe in health care services may be obvious and others may be more subtle. Even new workers in a health career will see changes as their program of study progresses. How do you react to changes in your life? Whether changes occur in your personal life or career, it is important for you to remember that you have choices. Shuman (1995) describes how you can be a victim, a survivor, or a navigator of change.

Victims look at change in a negative way. Victims fear the worst will happen because of the proposed change and feel helpless in the situation. Victims do not willingly participate in the change process, allowing change to control them. Survivors resist change but go along for the ride. Survivors claim the change will never work, and if their prediction comes true they will be heard to say "I told you so." Navigators of change feel in control of the situation. They feel confident and excited about the possibility of being part of the solution to a problem. Navigators believe they have some control over change rather than being controlled by the change. When change is in the wind, are you a victim, a survivor, or a navigator?

Practical nurses need to present themselves in clinical situations as invaluable to the health care agency. Be self-directed, motivated, positive, and a problem-solver in your daily work. Avoid being known as the staff person who always asks what needs to be done next. Identify what needs to be done and do it. Respond flexibly to changes that are presented. Identify tasks or protocols that could be done more efficiently. Use the critical thinking skills that were encouraged in nursing school to devise innovative suggestions to make these areas more efficient. Be a role model for practical nurses. The nineties have been identified as the "Whiney Nineties." Do not believe it! Whining, groaning, and moaning have no place in today's health care system.

▼▼▼
What Additional Trends Can Tell the Practical Nurse

Other trends also have an impact in the area of job possibilities in practical nursing. Although it is impos-

sible to predict the future, these trends generally affect your career in the present and will continue to influence the direction of your career in the future.

▽▽▽
Changes in the Nature of the Population

The population of the United States and Canada continues to grow older. By the year 2030, it has been estimated that there will be approximately 65 million persons over age 65 in the United States.

At the turn of the twentieth century, a major cause of death was infection, especially pneumonia and communicable diseases. Environmental health measures, the development of vaccines for immunizations, and programs to immunize children against childhood diseases helped to decrease the death rate from communicable disease. As the new century approaches, the world sees a new threat from infectious diseases. Strains of bacteria, especially *Streptococcus,* have become immune to many of the antibiotics medicine has in its arsenal to destroy pathogens. Despite this alarming trend, antibiotics that still cure infectious diseases have helped generally to reduce the death rate.

Persons still die from pneumonia, but today, heart disease, stroke, and cancer are major causes of premature death. Because of increased health education some people are avoiding these diseases. Because of advances in technology and medical science, these killer diseases are being diagnosed in the early stages more often. People with AIDS and HIV infection need health education to keep functioning to their highest capacity, and they need complex nursing care in the terminal stage of their disease.

In living longer, people are more prone to develop degenerative diseases such as arthritis. The emphasis on personal wellness in the areas of physical fitness, nutrition, and the control of stress is helping some people live not only longer but better.

Our population is getting older, but this does not mean that all people in the older age group become invalids or become dependent on others. The increase in the elderly population does mean that an increasing percentage of people depend on others for assistance in meeting one or more of their daily needs.

▽▽▽
Shifts in Nursing Supply and Demand

The nineties have seen nursing re-emerge as an attractive career option. Although employment possibilities are positive, an *acute* shortage of nurses does not exist at this time. The health care industry continues to change the way that health care services are delivered. Hospital growth continues to be slow but will account for one-third of the job growth in the health care arena (Nursing Data Source 1994, p. 5). Demand for nurses, including practical nurses, in acute care situations continues to decline. In hospitals in some regions, the area of subacute care is a site of jobs for practical nurses. Job opportunities for practical nurses are increasing in the community.

▽▽▽
Health Care Manpower Needs Challenged

Because of the tremendous shift to managed care in the 1990s and its emphasis on efficient operation, manpower needs in health care have been questioned by groups outside of health care. In November, 1995, a report entitled Critical Challenges: Revitalizing the Health Professions for the Twenty-First Century was released. This report was a study by the Pew Health Professions Commission on the role of health care professions in the emerging health care system. Valuable recommendations in this report include a strong focus on primary and preventive care, an increased commitment to cultural diversity and sensitivity, and a stronger presence of nursing education in community-based sites. The study forecast surpluses of nurses for the United States in the years ahead based on the predicted closing of half the hospitals in the United States (Marullo, 1996, p. 2). The Pew Health Commission recommended closing 10% to 20% of nursing education programs in the United States. Reactions to the projected manpower needs of this study are mixed. The present health care system is being challenged by different groups in United States society. The effects of studies such as these have yet to be realized.

▽▽▽
Current Trends in Practical Nursing Graduates

Traditionally, all levels of nursing have been attractive career choices for women. Currently, the number of men realizing the attractiveness of nursing as a career continues to climb. In 1993, men accounted for 11.1% of practical nursing graduates (Nursing Data Source, 1994, p. 53). In 1993, blacks accounted for 17.4% of the total graduates from practical nursing programs, Hispanics for 5.1%, Asians 2.5%, and Native Americans 0.8% (Practical Nursing's Role in a Community-Based Health Care System, 1994, p. 6). Nursing education programs have been successful in attracting older adult students, including college graduates. These adults are choosing nursing as a first or a second career because they know that a job in nursing, with benefits, is likely after graduation. This more mature type of student may lend more stability to the health care organization work forces. These nurses generally tend to be better established in the community and less mobile. Nursing schools continue to try to attract this type of student. The number of practical nursing programs in the United States is increasing slightly after a period of decline in the 1980s.

▼▼▼ *S U M M A R Y*

▶ Health care services are delivered in the public and private sectors. Public health care agencies are classified as official and voluntary. Official public health care agencies are supported by taxes. Voluntary health care agencies are supported by contributions. Private health care agencies are generally proprietary or for-profit. In addition to providing direct care, both public and private health care agencies are interested in preventing disease and promoting wellness. Some public and private health care agencies are potential places of employment for the practical nurse.

▶ The cost of health care has dramatically increased in past years. Cost is the driving force for change in the health care system. Traditional fee-for-service as a means of financing health care is being replaced by capitation. Insurance plans, both private and government-sponsored, are the major third-party payment systems in existence today.

▶ Major welfare reform has occurred. Persons with health insurance have guaranteed coverage and cannot be dropped for preexisting conditions. The millions without health insurance remain uncovered. Comprehensive health care reform has not occurred.

▶ Trends and incremental changes in health care include the restructuring of the health care system (patient-focused care and managed care or HMOs) and changes in staffing patterns (downsizing, UAPs, and cross-training). The community is a growing site of employment for practical nurses. Today's practical nurses need to be self-directed, motivated, and positive critical thinkers as well as problem-solvers who welcome the challenge of change. They need to remain flexible in the health care setting. Change is a way of life in the health care system today.

▼▼▼ R E F E R E N C E S

Entry Level Competencies of Graduates of Educational Programs in Practical Nursing. New York: NLN Council of Practical Nursing Programs, 1994.

Healthy People 2000: National Health Promotion and Disease Prevention. Washington DC: U. S. Public Health Service, 1991.

Healthy People 2000: Midcourse Review and 1995 Revisions. Washington DC: U.S. Public Health Service, 1995.

Marullo G. Pew Health Profession Commission recommendations still need work (editorial). Nursing*matters* (WI edition) 1996;7(1):2.

Nursing Data Source, 1994. Vol. III: Focus on Practical/Vocational Nursing. New York: NLN Division of Nursing, 1994.

Pintar L. What does Medicare cover? Do I need supplemental insurance? What about gaps in my insurance? Professional Development Seminar, Northeast Wisconsin Technical College, Green Bay, WI, December 22, 1995.

Practical nursing's role in a community-based health care system. Prism: NLN Research and Policy 1994; 2(4):1–8.

Shuman J. Navigating the white waters of change. Am J Nurs 1995; 95 (pt 1 of 2):15–17.

▼▼▼ B I B L I O G R A P H Y

Alter, J. Washington washes its hands. *Newsweek* 1996; 128 (7):42–44.

Baer E. Money managers are unraveling the tapestry of nursing. Am J Nurs 1994; 94(1):38–40.

Chornick N, Yocum C, Jacobsen J. *Job Analysis: Newly Licensed Practical/Vocational Nurses 1994.* Chicago: National Council of State Boards of Nursing, 1995.

Davidhizer R. Health care reform: What every practical nurse should know. J Pract Nurs 1995; 45:49, 52–55.

Ernst D. Total quality management in the hospital setting. J Nurs Care Qual 1994; 9:1–8.

Farley V. *Nurses: Pulling Together to Make a Difference.* Orange, CA: Innovative Nursing Consultants, 1995.

Hastings K. Health care reform: We need it but do we have the national will to shape our future? Nurse Practitioner 1995; 20(1):52–54, 56–57.

Ignatavicius D, Hausman D. *Clinical Pathways for Collaborative Practice.* Philadelphia: W.B. Saunders, 1995.

Manion J. Understanding the seven stages of change. Am J Nurs 1995; 95(4):41–43.

Mattera, M. A new shortage? (Editor's Memo). *R.N.* 1996, 59(8):7.

Neumann T. Speaker. Consultant of Wisconsin Board of Nursing. Update on legal matters in the state of Wisconsin. Fall Conference of Wisconsin Association of Licensed Practical Nurses. Chula Vista Resort, Wisconsin Dells, Wisconsin, November 3, 1995.

Nornhold P. Hospital restructuring: How to cope with the changes. *Nursing94* 1994; 24(8):46–49.

Panel: Too many doctors; trim medical schools. Green Bay Press Gazette. November 16, 1995; 80(142): section A, p. 3.

Pew Health Professions Commission. Reforming Health Care Workforce Regulation: Policy Considerations for the 21st Century. December 1995.

Porter-O'Grady T. Working with consultants on a redesign. Am J Nurs 1994;94(10):32–35, 37.

Practical Nursing's Role in a Community-Based Health Care System. Prism: NLN Research and Policy 1994; 2(4):1, 8.

Rosen A. Continuous quality improvement: Principles and techniques. J Pract Nurs. 1994; 44:24–35.

Sedgwick J. Welcome to the world of managed care. Self 1995; 195–201.

Trustees report Medicare fund is severely "out of balance."AARP Bull 1995; 36(5):3.

Turner S. Marketing yourself in the '90s. Am J Nurs 1995; 95(1):13–14.

The Wave of the Future. *HT: The Magazine for Healthcare Travel Professionals.* 1995; 2(5):23–25, 46–47.

Career Mobility and Vocational Organizations

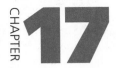

CHAPTER 17

▼▼▼ O U T L I N E

▼▼▼ K E Y T E R M S

career ladder   progression programs   vocational organizations

▼▼▼ O B J E C T I V E S

Upon completing this chapter you
will be able to:
1. Identify areas of LPN employment available in your community at present.

2. Discuss educational mobility
   available to practical nurses.
3. Discuss the purpose of
   a. NFLPN
   b. NAPNES
   c. HOSA

d. NLN
e. Alumni associations
f. State LPN or LVN associations
4. Name a journal written especially for practical nurses.

Introductory courses in nursing are meant to excite you about the process of nursing education, the careers available in practical nursing, the vocational organization support groups, and how you can be a part of it all. The formal educational process opens up new doors of knowledge and skill as well as responsibility for you. Many of the things you see and learn throughout your course of study will create a sense of awe and excitement in you. Careers in practical nursing are varied. Some of you have already made career decisions in advance, such as serving in the Peace Corps, working in a skilled care facility, or perhaps entering the military services. Both usual and atypical careers await you as a practical nurse.

Some schools also introduce student practical nurses to the state affiliate of the National Federation of Licensed Practical Nurses (NFLPN) or the National Association of Practical Nurse Education and Service (NAPNES) by allowing you to attend the state association of Licensed Practical Nurses convention. State conventions may include programming especially for student practical nurses. Some state and local associations offer a student membership rate as an inducement to join the association prior to graduation. Keep in mind that practical nursing organizations and organizations that include practical nurses are your support groups. The members understand practical nursing—the joys and the challenges that you experience. Participation in your professional organization is encouraged to keep you up to date on issues that affect practical nursing. Remember—no voice, no vote!

▼▼▼
Career Mobility

▽▽▽
Employment Opportunities

The 1994 Job Analysis Newly Licensed Practical/Vocational Nurses (Chornick et al, 1995, p.1) revealed the following from a study of 1872 entry level LPNs:

> The majority of participants (22.1%) worked in hospital based medical-surgical units or in skilled care facilities (38.3%). A majority reported that they were assigned to work a shift

other than "days." They primarily cared for adult and elderly clients with acute, chronic or terminal illness. Participants reported that the majority of their time was spent in the provision of direct client care. However, 35.7% indicated that they had administrative responsibilities. While administrative responsibilities were not related to shift assignment, there was an interaction between having administrative responsibilities and the type of agency/institution in which they were employed. A greater percentage of participants who were employed in nursing homes (54.0%) reported having administrative responsibilities than any other group.

The previous study was undertaken during 1991. Since that time there has been a greater shift into long-term care employment. Entry level LPNs and LVNs continue to work mostly with adult and elderly clients who are chronically ill. The study also shows that new LPNs work with clients of all ages including maternity clients and those who are well. They provide nursing care in acute, long-term, ambulatory, and home care settings.

Nursing education programs continue to evolve to meet the changing needs of the health care system. The National League for Nursing (NLN) Research and Policy Prism (1994, p. 1) discusses the need for graduates of all nursing education programs to be educated for a community-based health care system. Licenced practical and vocational nurses are already working in community-based settings such as home care, clinics, public health agencies, and school and student health services. These settings, plus ambulatory care settings, worksites, and community gathering places are suggested as other options that can provide community-based opportunities. The annual meeting of the NLN Council of Practical Nursing Programs in 1994 approved three new competency statements to address this issue. They were added to the 1989 edition of *Entry Level Competencies of Graduates of Educational Programs in Practical Nursing*. The first two statements were listed under the category of Management/Supervision:

1. Assumes responsibility for managing his/her actions when providing nursing care for individuals and groups of clients.

2. Is accountable for nursing care delegated to unlicensed health care providers.

3. The third statement was listed under Political Activism: Is aware that the practical nurse, through political, economic, and societal activities, can affect nursing and health.

Nursing continues to be a "hot" career. The total number of active licenses for LPNs, LVNs, and RNs has continued to increase since the drop in LPNs and LVNs during 1990. The total number of LPNs and LVNs in 1994 was 912,585 compared to 2,892,720 RNs (Yocum and White, 1995, p. 22). With the move to reduce soaring medical costs, nurses continue to be a cost-effective way of delivering health care.

Extended Care Facilities

The growing number of persons aged 65 and over has a positive impact on the availability of jobs for practical nurses. The Omnibus Budget Reconciliation Act (OBRA) of 1987 mandates that as of October 1, 1990, all Skilled Nursing Facilities (SNF) and Intermediate Care Facilities (ICF) provide 24-hour licensed practical nurse care 7 days a week, with at least one RN employed 7 days a week, 8 hours a day. Although this requirement can be waived if personnel are unavailable, if you enjoy longer-term contact with people, this employment option is certainly available and may be the area for you.

The nursing home population is made up of residents who are (1) completing recovery from surgery or trauma and are too well for the hospital but not well enough to go home; (2) elderly people who are unable to care for themselves because of medical or psychological impairment; (3) mentally retarded people who are unable to live independently or in group homes; (4) young to middle-aged victims of chronic debilitating disease or accidents; and (5) young chronically mentally ill persons who need continuing supervision and are not candidates for independent living or halfway houses.

The special qualities needed for this kind of nursing include patience, ability to see below the surface, willingness to listen, maturity, ability to determine priorities, ability to set limits, interest in working with people with disabilities, willingness to work with other health care givers, communication skills, acute observation skills of physical change, and a sense of security in regard to your own value system. Practical nurses who work in nursing homes are challenged to assist in providing a homelike atmosphere while dealing with the immediate, long-term, and terminal health problems of the residents.

The level of responsibility is great in that the LPN frequently works in a charge nurse role, and although supervision is available from an RN, at some times during the day supervision may be general, meaning at the other end of the telephone. Consequently, a solid knowledge and skill base is essential to know when to seek help and from whom.

The charge nurse role also means that the practical nurse is responsible for managing care given by other LPNs, aides, and orderlies. (Refer to Chapter 19 for more specific details.)

As the LPN in a nursing home facility, much of your work ultimately relates to assisting the residents to attain or maintain whatever capabilities they have in all areas of health. Through your efforts residents who are recuperating from surgery or trauma can realize their goal of discharge. For other residents, your role includes supporting them through the final step of the growth process—a dignified death.

Home Health Care

Because of shorter hospital stays, the home health care industry is flourishing. The actual care given is under the supervision of an RN, who makes the initial assessment and the nursing diagnosis and develops the plan of care. The postdischarge (subacute) level of care fits in well with the LPN's basic education, thereby making the LPN or LVN invaluable in implementing the plan of care. The LPN's background allows additions to the continuing data collection and evaluation of the plan of care. Because of difficulty in receiving payment from nonprivate sources, some home health agencies use LPNs for private-pay clients only. Others employ LPNs as home health aides to avoid the restrictions. This is an unfortunate practice because the pay is lower and you are always held to the requirements of your highest license in legal situations.

Helpful qualities for home health nurses include (1) flexibility—you will have to improvise in the home yet practice sound nursing principles; (2) communications skills—you will be working in the client's domain. You have to both understand the client's expression of needs and make sure that you express yourself clearly (and tactfully); (3) self-confidence—an air of insecurity or uncertainty will be picked up by the client, resulting in a lack of confidence in the LPN on the client's part. This does not imply that you should fake it. Rather, you must have knowledge and basic nursing skills that enable you to perform tasks efficiently. Do not ask for unnecessary reassurance when performing basic skills. Question what you do not know, but do it away from the client unless an emergency exists; (4) sensitivity to physical and emotional changes—once the initial assessment is completed by the RN, it will be up to you to be alert to any changes of which the RN must be made aware. The RN must be able to depend on your observational skills for safety's sake; (5) ability to deal with emergencies—staying calm and following the agency protocol is essential; (6) nonjudgmental attitude—a must, because you work right in the client's home. Remember at all times that you are providing a service. If you are comfortable with your own values, different values are not personally threatening.

Mental Health Nursing

Mental health nursing includes both community mental health centers and group homes for the recovering mentally ill. Many community mental health centers are staffed primarily with LPN and nursing assistants, with RNs in a supervisory role. Yet many practical nursing programs have dropped the mental health nursing theory class and related clinical experience. Concepts are integrated loosely into other areas of study.

In this area of work, LPNs are involved in performing treatments, administering medications, and tending to activities of daily living. Furthermore, LPNs perform a significant role in developing a therapeutic relationship with the client and following through with the appropriate interventions according to the client's care plan.

Helpful qualities include (1) an ability to deal with stress; (2) empathetic rather than sympathetic approach to clients; (3) good communication skills; (4) nonjudgmental attitude; (5) sound mental health; (6) alertness to physical and emotional changes in clients; (7) ability to set client-centered limits; (8) ability to differentiate between personal and client goals; (9) willingness to function as a team member; and (10) ability to not get involved in promises of client secrets, which may be damaging therapeutically.

Fortunately, some mental health facilities offer orientation and continuing inservice programs. If this is an area of interest for you, the authors recommend Bauer and Hill's *Essentials of Mental Health Planning and Interventions*. This book is written for all psychiatric health care providers and is useful both as a basic textbook and as a continuing reference book.

Military Services

As a practical nurse, if you volunteer for military service in the reserves or active duty, you will have to take basic training. If you are interested, contact recruiters for all branches of the military services. Compare the differences to determine which branch best fits your needs.

Desirable qualities for military service nursing include (1) interest in teamwork; (2) a strong ego; (3) ability to cope with changing situations; (4) emotional stability; (5) good communication skills; and (6) self-direction. Certainly, a desire for a challenging career and an ability to adjust quickly to new situations are handy prerequisites for this kind of nursing.

Hospital Nursing

The acute care experience in most practical nursing programs is found in the medical and surgical units of hospitals. This is an area of employment when available.

If you do consider specialty areas, they should be areas in which you have had both theory classes and clinical experience. Areas with complex nursing duties mean that additional postgraduate education and experience are required.

Refer to the nurse practice act for your state to see how performance of nursing acts beyond basic nursing care is handled. These acts are referred to as the expanded role of the practical nurse or performance of acts in complex client situations. See Chapter 19.

Desirable qualities in hospital nursing include (1) attention to detail in performing technical skills; (2) organizational skills; (3) data collection (assessment) skills; (4) strong ego; (5) ability to cope with stressful situations; (6) teamwork; (7) flexibility; (8) ability to prioritize; and (9) ability to think critically and solve problems.

The anticipated pay scale is approximately two-thirds that of the RN pay scale. Other benefits vary according to agency policy.

Outpatient Clinics and Doctors' Offices

Outpatient clinics and doctors' offices continue to provide jobs for many LPNs. Most clinics and offices are open Monday to Friday. The day begins later and consequently runs a little later. Assigned work varies. It generally includes checking supplies, greeting the client, taking vital signs, weighing the client, limited data collection (assessment) about the purpose for being there, giving the client directions on preparing for the examination, assisting the doctor with the examination, and performing additional duties delegated by the physician. If you are working as a private nurse for a physician, you can also expect to accompany the physician on hospital rounds, assisting with examinations as needed. Because the clientele remains essentially the same, these nurses develop a rapport with the clients, which is an asset to both the client and the physician.

Desirable qualities include (1) good communication skills, (2) attention to detail, (3) enjoyment of routine, (4) organizational skills, and (5) self-sufficiency because work expectations will vary with the number and type of clientele.

Other Job Opportunities

Other job opportunities to consider are

▶ VISTA or the Peace Corps
▶ Industrial nursing: Some LPNs have found excel-

lent support in this area and work under the general supervision of a doctor
▶ Veterans Administration hospitals and homes for retired veterans
▶ Hospices—care of terminally ill clients in institutional settings or in their homes
▶ Insurance companies: Companies provide in-depth orientation for the work required and some prefer to hire practical nurses on graduation
▶ Veterinary clinics: An opportunity to combine your love of nursing with a love of animals. In some states you may work as an assistant to the veterinarian in the care and treatment of animals. Other states, such as California, require a special training program and a passing grade in a state test to assist veterinarians
▶ Hospital equipment supply salesperson: Some pharmacies, for example, select LPNs to staff this particular area. One such nurse has become the colostomy care expert in her city and gives seminars on the topic to agencies, clients, and health professionals. She enjoys the backing of the drugstore management and a pharmaceutical company.
▶ Coroner's nurse: A former student practical nurse doing this work commented, "I never saw myself as doing this, but it is so interesting. I've learned a lot about myself, people, pain, compassion. The doctor I work with is a born teacher."

▽▽▽
Continuing Education

Historically, practical nurses have a reputation for being apathetic in pursuing continuing education classes. This is difficult to believe because many LPNs have gone on to learn complex nursing skills after graduation. Continuing education classes are available in many formats and through many agencies. Often the agency you work for is willing to pick up part or all of the fee if the education benefits the agency. Some agency courses are free and are part of continuing service within the agency. Continuing education includes the following:

Orientation to the Facility

This provides an opportunity to learn about variations in routine plus a review of selected previously learned information and skills if you have been out of nursing for awhile.

In-Service

In-service training is information chosen to meet specific needs within a facility. Attendance at some in-service programs such as a yearly update on blood-borne pathogens is required. You can offer employers suggestions for content. Usually a specified amount of time is required for in-service programs, such as one hour per month or three times per year, according to the agency policy. Depending on the credentials of the instructor, continuing education credits may be available.

Workshops

Workshops present information and an opportunity to practice what is being taught. Workshops provide excellent opportunities to learn new skills. The length varies according to the content. Some agencies pay the workshop fee or expenses if the topic is specific to and enhances your nursing skills. Workshops are also a major source of continuing education credits required by many states as a part of relicensure.

Continuing Education Classes

These are sometimes called *field services* in the vocational system. Classes are often taught on complex nursing skills such as intravenous therapy, physical assessment, LPN or LVN charge nurse, mental health concepts, nursing process for LPNs, and so on. Actually, many vocational schools and community colleges will provide any course you are interested in if you request it and there are enough people available to make up the required minimum enrollment. Many of these classes provide continuing education credits as opposed to course credit. You receive a certificate if you have completed course work satisfactorily. One of the most valuable benefits of continuing education classes is the opportunity to get together with other working LPNs. You discover similarities in challenges and satisfactions. Ideas are shared on how to deal with difficult situations in the work setting. It is a good idea to keep a running record of all in-service programs, seminars, and workshops offered, including dates, credits, and topics, for future reference. Ask for these records to be included in your file at your place of employment as well as copies for yourself.

▽▽▽
Moving Up

If you are an LPN who says "I want to be an LPN. I have no desire to be an RN," good for you. You have obviously given careful consideration to your personal goals. Satisfaction in nursing both for you and the clients you care for is closely related to clear-cut goals. If you decided that you want to be an LPN, chances are that you will be satisfied with your choice and will provide satisfactory care to your clients. If, however, someone else decided that you should be a nurse, chances are that you will never be entirely satisfied with the choice. This lack of satisfaction will be mirrored in the care you give to clients. The same process is true in regard to making a decision to become an RN. If you do not want to become an RN, avoid letting anyone push you into it. Only when a goal is truly your own will you be motivated to do your best both in the educational process and in the care of clients.

If, however, you want to enter an RN program, it is important to know what is available educationally. A major problem in developing upward-mobility programs for LPNs is the belief held by some educators that a practical nursing course is terminal in nature; that state boards of nursing will not permit such programs, nor will credit be given by professional nursing programs. Although the same reasoning continues to be held in some parts of the country, other directors of nursing have successfully negotiated with state boards of nursing to develop progressive LPN-to-RN programs. Contact your state board of nursing for a list of available professional nursing programs within your state.

Educational Mobility for Nurses

In *Career Ladder* the author states, "I believe that historically the Helene Fuld School of Nursing at the Hospital of Joint Diseases and Medical Center (New York City) is the first program to demonstrate the belief that practical nursing is indeed a part of the nursing profession, and that a curriculum can be constructed that effectively articulates with one that prepares for registered nurse licensure with minimal repetition" (Ahl, 1975, p. 143). The program, initially a 15-month course trimmed down to 47 weeks, was initiated in 1964. Justine Hannan, hospital Director of Nursing, worked with the Board of Nursing within New York State's Education Department, and by 1968 the department granted full registration to the program. By 1970, it was accredited by the NLN. "The school has had an impact on the quality of nursing in its home hospital, and has sent graduates into dozens of other health care facilities throughout New York and fifteen other states. It has willingly shared its experience with educators who have made inquiries about its work, and has demonstrated that career ladder education is both valid and appropriate for a large number of persons who have the aptitude and commitment to such a goal" (Ahl, 1975, p. 150).

Career-ladder programs are carefully planned to avoid duplication of content. "The curriculum is not a Practical Nursing curriculum for the first year and an Associate Degree Nursing curriculum for the second. It is a totally new curriculum designed in terms of essential learnings for beginning nursing competencies. It allows the student to be a competent Practical Nurse practitioner at the end of one year of study and a competent Registered Nurse practitioner at the end of an additional year" (Story, 1974, p. 2).

A unique program approved by the Minnesota Board of Nursing is available through seven northern Minnesota technical, community, and four-year colleges involved in the Itasca Nursing Education Consortium (INEC). It was developed in 1982 to help the student move through the upper levels of nursing education. Students may enter the practical nursing program at four of the schools and participate as a full-

or part-time student. On completion of the program the graduate practical nurse becomes eligible to apply to take the NCLEX-PN.

The second year is available at two community colleges. INEC LPNs who are admitted to the second year are granted 23 credits. Students take a three-credit nursing transition course. Students must receive a C or higher in all nursing courses and must maintain a 2.00 cumulative grade point average. A total of 96 nursing credits and at least 45 liberal arts electives are required to receive an associate degree. The graduate becomes eligible to apply to take the NCLEX-RN.

The nursing associate degree (ADN) RN may choose to continue her education to receive a baccalaureate in nursing. This degree is available through two four-year colleges that are members of the Consortium.

Similar programs exist in other areas of the country. Your state board of nursing is an excellent resource of information about these programs.

ADN Advanced Standing for LPNs

An innovative "progression to the nursing associate degree" program has evolved at the Northeast Wisconsin Technical College in Wisconsin. The program is available for Wisconsin LPNs. Individuals from other states who wish to apply without obtaining a Wisconsin license may request individual assessments. Graduation from an approved practical nursing program is required.

All participants are required to take general education courses in the first year of the program and the "Intro AD Nursing" course (two credits) prior to entering the second-year courses.

Requirements vary according to whether graduation from a practical nursing program took place within five years or six or more years ago. If the former, no proficiency testing is required. Advanced standing credit is granted on successful completion of Nursing Process II and III courses. Non-nursing credits may be transferred from colleges or vocational programs for all applicants. Wisconsin LPNs who apply six or more years after graduation require no proficiency testing if within the last three years they have (1) accumulated LPN work experience of 1000 hours in a licensed health care agency or facility, or (2) taken an approved refresher course. Applicants who do not meet these requirements must be tested (the NLN Mobility and LPN Gap test). Advanced standing is granted on successful completion of Nursing Process VI and VII courses. A total of 54 credits of nursing and non-nursing courses are required to complete the associate degree nursing curriculum.

No-Credit RN Programs

There continue to be RN programs that do not recognize the worth of an LPN education. These programs insist that LPNs start from the beginning and repeat all previously covered theory and skills courses, including basic nursing skills. The bottom line is that a number of programs are available throughout the country that can be used by the LPN to become an RN—if that is what is right for that nurse.

There are two resources for locating approved nursing programs. First, there are the state boards of nursing (see listing in Appendix A). Request a list of board-approved professional nursing programs preparing for registered nurse licensure. Second, a list of all nursing programs in the United States is available from the NLN in the publication called State Approved Schools of Nursing, which lists addresses, telephone numbers, and types of programs available. It is available in some libraries, or call (212) 989-9393, extension 138 to order.

▼▼▼
Nursing Organizations

If you want a voice in nursing, your vocation, join your vocational organization(s). The narrative below will be limited to discussions of those organizations that include or are composed of LPN members. Additional information can be obtained by writing to the organization headquarters.

NFLPN
1418 Aversboro Road
Garner, NC 27529
Telephone (919)779-0046

The NFLPN (National Federation of Licensed Prac-

tical Nurses, Inc.) is the policy-making body for LPNs and LVNs. NFLPN is made up of LPNs, student practical nurses, and associate members. It was formed by LPNs who wanted an organization to work for and speak on behalf of them. Membership includes a magazine called the *American Journal of Practical Nursing*. The organization (1) keeps its members involved with matters of interest to practical nursing, (2) makes health, accident, malpractice, and personal liability insurance plans available to its members, (3) works for LPN representation on boards of nursing, (4) provides a voice in nursing legislation on a national level, (5) encourages agencies to provide continuing education for practical nurses, (6) provides a statement of functions and qualifications of LPNs, (7) works with other health organizations to promote quality patient care, and (8) provides CEU opportunities.

NAPNES
1400 Spring St.
Suite 310
Silver Spring, MD 20910
Telephone (301)588-2491

NAPNES (National Association for Practical Nurse Education and Service) is a multidisciplinary organization that is involved with practical nurses, on both a student and a graduate level. It was the first organization formed to promote practical nursing schools and continuing education for LPNs. The membership fee includes a subscription to *The Journal of Practical Nursing,* the official magazine of NAPNES. Membership is open to anyone concerned with the advancement of practical nursing.

HOSA
6309 N. O'Connor St.
Suite 215 LB117
Irving, TX 75039

HOSA (Health Occupations Students of America) is a national vocational organization for students of health occupations. The national motto, "The hands of youth hold the health of tomorrow," reflects the purpose of the organization: better understanding of health-related issues, cooperation with other students of health occupations, and strengthening of leadership and citizenship abilities in preparing for the health care of tomorrow.

NLN
350 Hudson St.
New York, NY 10014
Telephone (212)989-9393

The NLN (National League for Nursing) is involved with all types of nursing: consultation; accreditation of nursing education programs; professional testing services; surveys on admissions, enrollments, graduation, studies on nursing education, and service; information source on trends in nursing; and conventions, meetings, workshops, and continuing education. NLN membership is open to all nurses and others concerned with health care. The membership fee includes a subscription to its journal, Nursing and Health Care.

Alumni Association
Your school

Practical nursing alumni associations provides a familiar, proud connection for classes past and those to come—you share a common bond. Activities vary from social gatherings welcoming a new class or celebrating graduation to those with educational intent and content. If your school does not have an alumni association, consider getting together with peers to start one. Seek help from your faculty.

Your state LPN association

Check with your state board of nursing for an address.

▼▼▼ *S U M M A R Y*

▶ Career opportunities to a large extent depend on where you live, the current trends in nursing, and your ability or willingness to go after the job you want. Career mobility on the other hand, depends on your personal goal in regard to nursing. If additional education is a goal, continuing education classes in various forms are available to you. RN completion programs vary considerably with regard to admission requirements, prerequisites, and length of program. Inquiries can be made directly to your state board of nursing or the NLN to assist you in locating an approved program that suits your needs.

▶ Valuable support groups exist in the form of nursing organizations. Student membership is available in the NFLPN, and state conventions frequently sponsor a student day. NAPNES continues to fight for the rights of practical nurses and supports continuation of the vocation. HOSA provides a balance of social and educational activities. The NLN focuses on nursing needs at all levels of nursing and provides broad services for nurses in all areas. Seek out your state LPN association to gain a voice in your vocation. Your alumni association will always provide a touch of home.

▼▼▼ *R E F E R E N C E S*

Ahl ME. *In* Lenburg C (ed). *Open Learning and Career Mobility in Nursing.* St Louis: CV Mosby, 1975.

Bauer B, Hill S. *Essentials of Mental Health Planning and Interventions.* Philadelphia: WB Saunders, 1985.

Chornick N, Yocum C, Jacobson J. *Job Analysis Newly Licensed Practical/Vocational Nurses 1994.* Chicago: National Council of State Boards of Nursing, 1995.

Entry Level Competencies of Educational Programs in Practical Nursing. New York: NLN Council of Practical Nursing Programs, 1989.

Minnesota Board of Nursing, Education Section. *Resources for Selecting a Nursing Program.* St. Paul; Minnesota Board of Nursing, 1995.

Northeast Wisconsin Technical College, Green Bay. ADN Advanced-Standing for LPNs. Fall 1995.

NLN Research and Policy. Practical nursing's role in a community-based health care system. Prism: NLN Research of National League for Nursing, 1994; 2:1–8.

Nursing Data Source 1994. *Focus on Practical/Vocational Nursing,* Vol. 3. New York: National League for Nursing, 1994.

Practical Nurses NWTC, Green Bay, WI, July 1995.

Ronchetti C. INEC Consortium Program, Lake Superior College, Duluth, MN: 1995.

Story D. *Career Mobility.* St Louis: CV Mosby, 1974.

Yocum C, White E. 1994 licensure and examination statistics. Chicago: National Council of State Boards of Nursing, 1995.

Developing Leadership Skills

CHAPTER **18**

▼▼▼ *O U T L I N E*

▼▼▼ *K E Y   T E R M S*

continuum

Howlett hierarchy

leadership

management

Maslow's hierarchy

organizational chart

situational leadership

▼▼▼ OBJECTIVES

Upon completing this chapter you will be able to:

1. *Describe the expanded role of the practical nurse as described in your state's nurse practice act.*

2. *Explain the difference between leadership and management.*

3. *Identify your personal leadership style.*

4. *Explain the following leadership styles in your own words:*
   a. *Autocratic*
   b. *Democratic*
   c. *Laissez-faire*

5. *Identify ways to attain competence in the three general areas in which knowledge is needed to be an effective leader:*

   a. *Occupational skills*
   b. *Organizational skills*
   c. *Human relationship skills*

6. *Describe how Maslow's hierarchy of needs acts as a motivator of human behavior.*

7. *Describe how the Howlett hierarchy of work motivators can help the practical nurse leader motivate subordinates.*

Polly Practical, LPN, Charge Nurse on the day shift, comes on duty in a frenzy. The staff shudders as she rearranges her uniform and papers. They murmur to each other, "Another day with Attila the Hun." Polly barks out the assignments after report. She reminds the staff (1) not to dawdle in their cares, (2) to have everything done by 10 AM, (3) to stay out of her way when she gives her meds, and (4) to give a thorough end-of-shift report because Polly has a headache and will be unable personally to check up on the residents that day.

Ann Assistant, NA, asks why everything has to be done by 10 AM. Polly takes off in a whirlwind of prose and assorted dramatics. Polly never answers Ann's question. This is unfortunate. The reason for getting cares done by 10 AM that particular day is because Doc Severinsen and his entire orchestra will be visiting the nursing home. Had Ann and the other nursing assistants known the reason for the command, they would have worked twice as hard to complete their cares in time for the residents' favorite entertainers.

Because of the manner in which Polly conducts herself as a charge nurse, it could be said that Polly may be a manager, but she is not a leader.

▼▼▼ The Practical Nurse as First-Line Leader

Have you ever experienced an employment situation similar to the one described with Polly Practical?

Perhaps you have received directions as a nursing assistant or in another job capacity and did not like the way in which you were approached by your supervisor.

Nurses at all levels manage client care. Some nurses are also leaders. Licensed practical and licensed vocational nurses have proved themselves to be effective in charge nurse positions. If you can manage client care *and* be a leader, you will be more effective in your expanded role in practical nursing.

Practical nurses need to develop leadership and management skills so that they can direct and supervise others in a manner that will meet the goals of the employing agency effectively. In your one-year program in practical nursing, you have started to build a strong, solid base in these skills. The purpose of Chapters 18 and 19 is to help you continue to develop skills in leading and managing. These skills will be used in future jobs when you function in an expanded role in a first-line manager position.

▼▼▼ The Expanded Role of Practical Nursing

The following is an excerpt from Chapter 441 of the Wisconsin State Statutes. It provides one state's law regarding the use of practical nurses as first-line managers.

N6.04 Standards of Practice (3) ASSUMPTION OF CHARGE NURSE POSITION IN NURSING

HOMES. In assuming the position of charge nurse in a nursing home as defined in s. 50.04 (2) (9b), Stats., an L.P.N. shall:

(a) Follow written protocols and procedures developed and approved by an R.N.;

(b) Manage and direct the nursing care and other activities of L.P.N.s and nursing support personnel under the general supervision of an R.N., and,

(c) Accept the charge nurse position only if prepared to competently perform this assignment based on his or her nursing education, including education, training, or experience or active involvement in education and training for responsibilities not included in the basic L.P.N. curriculum. (WI State Statutes, Chapter 441, N6.04, May 1990)

It is important for you to review the nurse practice act of your state. This law legally defines the exact role and boundaries for practical nurses. Also, review the National Federation of Licensed Practical Nurses (NFLPN) Specialized Nursing Practice Standards (found in Chapter 20 [Table 20–3]) for more guidelines to the expanded role of practical nurses.

One example of the expanded role of the practical nurse is the first-line manager position. In these situations, the practical nurse has the responsibility of assigning the care given by nursing assistants and other personnel. The practical nurse directs, guides, and supervises these health care workers as they attempt to meet the goals of the agency of employment. One agency that commonly uses the practical nurse as a first-line manager is the nursing home or long-term-care unit. The most recent job analysis of entry-level practical nurses by the National Council of State Boards of Nursing occurred in 1994. This survey showed that 57.9% of all practical nurses who reported administrative responsibilities on the job named those responsibilities as their primary position. And a greater proportion of these practical nurses worked in nursing homes (Chornick et al, 1995, p. 19). To carry out the first-line

manager role, you will need the abilities of a leader and a manager.

▽▽▽
How You Are Already Preparing for a Leadership or Management Role

The topic of leadership and management for the practical nurse is a vast one. The references and annotated bibliography (a bibliography that tells you the main points of the books listed and how the books may benefit you) at the end of this chapter provide valuable guidelines to this topic.

All practical nurses are managers in the sense that they consistently need to direct, handle, and organize care for assigned clients. It is worthwhile for you to review the ways in which your one-year program helps to prepare you for a management position.

The one-year practical nursing program encourages development of the following skills necessary for functioning successfully as a first-line manager:

1. Basic nursing skills, including the nursing process
2. Time management techniques for home and clinical time
3. Ability to learn new information, including use of resources for learning
4. Use of positive self-talk and thinking
5. Assertive behavior
6. Communication skills
7. Legal aspects of health care
8. Ethical aspects of health care
9. Problem solving and critical thinking
10. Stress management

You have received frequent verbal and written evaluations of your behaviors both in class and in the clinical area. This experience with evaluation will help prepare you for the need to evaluate others in your job as charge nurse.

"Learning leadership and management," as you can see, is much more than taking one course that turns you into a leader. Leadership is a process (continual development) that includes many skills and is something that evolves over time. This chapter will focus on leadership in practical nursing and will help you to think specifically about a leadership role.

▼▼▼
The Difference Between Leadership and Management

Management is the organization of all care required for clients in a health care setting for a specific period of time. The focus of management is planning and directing care to meet client goals. The tools needed for management could be written in a step-by-step manner and given to you to follow. Following the directions for using the management skills would possibly get the job done in an efficient manner.

Leadership is the manner in which the leader gets along with coworkers and gets the job done. The focus of leadership is to produce changes in the workplace that will meet the goals of the employing agency. The leader needs to influence others in the work setting so that they will want to implement the desired change. Directions for leadership skills can also be written, but it is through experience that leadership skills are really learned. The practical nurse who has the skills of a manager *and* a leader will get the job done in the most efficient and effective manner. And coworkers will enjoy the experience that much more! Your goal will be to develop the skills of leadership and management.

Leaders cannot be appointed. Leadership is an informal role that is given to the person by a group of workers. Leaders have developed the following skills and characteristics:

1. Leaders see change as a challenge and an opportunity to improve the quality of client care.

2. Leaders form visions that make complex things simple and obscure things clear.

3. Leaders transform the way things are done in the present into a more successful way for the future.

4. Leaders are respected by their followers.

5. Leaders in nursing are deeply involved in their discipline.

6. Leaders in nursing have demonstrated their knowledge of nursing.

7. Leaders are emotionally healthy.

8. Leaders manage well the stress in their personal and professional lives. Leaders have devised creative coping skills.

9. Leaders listen well to what others are saying about problems. Problems in today's health care systems are complex.

10. Leaders empower followers to follow the vision of the leader.

11. Leaders never stop learning and growing.

12. Leaders are willing to take risks and learn from mistakes.

13. Leaders have confidence in themselves.

14. Leaders do not seek to be loved. Leaders do seek to be fair.

15. Leaders are paid to *think!*

▼▼▼
The Organizational Chart

The organizational chart is a picture of the hierarchy of responsibility in an employment situation. In the **traditional organizational chart,** individuals lower on the chart report to those directly above them on the chart. See Figure 18–1 to visualize where the practical nurse fits into the organizational chart as a first-line leader in a traditional organization. As shown in Figure 18-1, the practical nurse reports to the nurse manager, who is a registered nurse. Nursing assistants report to the practical nurse. To whom does the director of nursing (DON) report?

Because of changes in the structure of organizations, some organizational charts have become more horizontal in appearance. See Figure 18–2 for an example of a more **contemporary organizational** chart. This "flattening out" has eliminated some of the middle manager positions in organizations. As a result, the remaining middle managers have taken on more responsibilities and are spread thin. Middle managers in this system have more people reporting to them than in the past. These middle managers depend on the per-

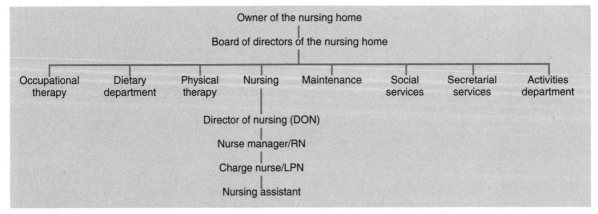

Figure 18–1
Sample traditional organizational chart for the role of the practical nurse in the nursing home/long-term care setting.

sons who report to them to think critically and solve problems. They expect to be contacted when their subordinates have tried and are unable to solve their own problems.

> *Organizational charts may differ by regions of the United States. Obtain organizational charts of specific agencies in your area. Clarify specific levels of responsibility as they apply to the practical nurse. Determine whether these charts reflect a traditional or more contemporary style of organization.*

▼▼▼
What Kind of Leader Are You?

There are several different ways to lead. What is your predominant leadership style? Each of the following statements in A Short Test of Leadership Style is an extreme. The responses are not positive or negative. One answer is no better than another answer. They just are. Make a check next to the statement(s) that *best* describe(s) the way you *might be* at work, not how you want to be.

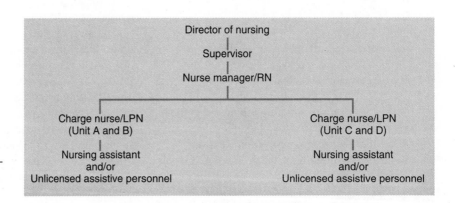

Figure 18–2
Sample contemporary organizational chart for the role of the practical nurse.

A Short Test of Leadership Style

1. My primary goal at work is to
   a. get the job done.
   b. get along with the people with whom I work.
   c. do the job correctly.
   d. hope the work I do is noticed.
2. My clinical coworkers would say I am
   a. domineering in my relationships.
   b. friendly and personable in my relationships.
   c. likely to attend to details of the client care plan.
   d. creative and energetic in giving care.
3. At work, I feel that I have to be
   a. in control of the client situation.
   b. liked by my coworkers.
   c. correct in giving care.
   d. recognized and praised for my care.
4. When I communicate on the nursing unit:
   a. I am usually direct and to the point.
   b. I am more considerate of the person to whom I am talking rather than interested in strongly getting my point across.
   c. I usually give detailed information.
   d. I usually elaborate on the point at hand.
5. My coworkers would say I am a person who
   a. gets the job done regardless of what shift I work.
   b. is very likable and patient.
   c. is precise and accurate in giving nursing care.
   d. is optimistic and has good verbal skills.
6. Select the behavior your charge nurse might attribute to you while on your shift.
   a. *Sometimes* I alienate people.
   b. *Sometimes* I waste time and fall for excuses others may give.
   c. *Sometimes* I can be stubborn with coworkers.
   d. *Sometimes* I appear like a flake to my coworkers.
7. How do you react to a stressful incident on the nursing unit?
   a. I become arrogant, blaming other departments and yelling at coworkers.
   b. I am accommodating to the person in charge and passive in behavior.
   c. I become silent and withdraw from the situation.
   d. I talk faster and louder.
8. When I deal with my coworkers on the nursing unit regarding patient matters, I like them to
   a. get to the point and be businesslike in their behavior.
   b. be casual and sincere in their behavior.
   c. use the facts of the matter and go step by step when explaining a client-care situation.
   d. be enthusiastic about the situation and use demonstrations to explain their points.

Count up your A and C answers. These answers are more characteristic of a task-oriented person. This person in leadership terms is called an *autocratic* leader. Add up your B and D responses. These are more characteristic of a people-oriented person. In leadership terms, this person is called a *laissez-faire* leader. Your score can give you a rough estimate of the tendency of your leadership style.

▽▽▽
Leadership Styles

The literature abounds with examples of leadership styles. Figure 18–3 illustrates a continuum (a line with extreme opposites at each end) of leadership styles and Table 18–1 compares and contrasts the leadership styles found on this continuum.

Benefits and Disadvantages of Leadership Styles

To adopt one of the extreme columns in Table 18–1 (autocratic or laissez-faire) to be used consistently as a leadership style is unrealistic and could be disastrous. As you can see, there is room for an autocratic leadership style, for example, in times of emergency. A purely task-centered leadership style (autocratic style) thrives on power. It involves telling someone what to do with little regard for the employee as a person who may have ideas about how to reach the goals of the employer.

> *List below two additional examples of situations that might require the autocratic style of leadership.*
>
> 1. _____
>   _____
>
> 2. _____
>   _____

A purely people-oriented style (laissez-faire style) focuses on people's feelings but ignores the task at hand and allows employees to act without any direction. The goals of the employer may be compromised when the laissez-faire leadership style is used. At times, persons in leadership roles may feel the need to be liked by all subordinates and use this leadership style, but the task of accomplishing goals will be seriously compromised.

▽▽▽
Situational Leadership

A popular system of leadership is called *situational leadership.* Situational leadership involves varying your leadership style to meet the demands of the situation in the work environment. According to this system, the practical nurse needs to pick a leadership style that fits the work situation at hand.

▽▽▽
Using the Leadership Continuum as a Guide

The value of a continuum, as shown in Figure 18–3, is that as you move along the continuum from each extreme toward the center or midpoint, the two extremes begin to blend together. You use some of each style, depending on where you are on the continuum. A blend of the two extremes to some degree according to the appropriate work situation would be the leadership style needed at the moment.

The leadership model presented by Hersey and Weaver (1989, pp. 9–10) illustrates the use of the concept of situational leadership. These authors identify four main leadership styles as

   1. Sell

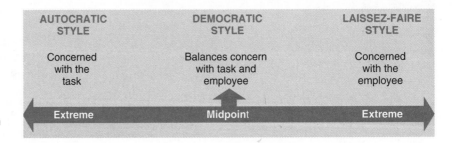

Figure 18–3
Extremes of leadership styles on a continuum.

Table 18–1
Comparing Autocratic, Democratic, and Laissez-faire Styles of Leadership

	Autocratic	Democratic	Laissez-faire
General description	Does not share responsibility and authority with employees	Shares responsibility and authority with employees	Gives away responsibility and authority to employees
Importance of agencies' policies	Emphasis on policies	Enforces policies but with concern for employees	Puts employees before policies
How leader gets the job done	Tells employees what tasks to do. Does not seek input from employees	Seeks input from employees and encourages problem solving	Tries to please everyone
What gets done	May reach goals	Because of involvement of employees, goals may be achieved with positive staff feelings	Maybe nothing
When style can be used	Crisis situations Code situations Emergencies	Daily nursing care situations Meetings Committees Review of care plans	When agency goals/policies are not a consideration

2. Tell
3. Participate
4. Delegate

Referring to Figure 18–3, *tell* would be the direct power approach used when the situation, such as an emergency, demands the autocratic style of leadership. *Delegate* allows subordinates who are self-directed and have proved their ability to function on their own to meet employer goals once the goals have been made clear. *Delegate* comes between the autocratic and democratic styles. *Sell* offers ideas and suggestions to subordinates (workers for whom you have responsibility) of the positive benefits of employer goals. The intention of *sell* is to persuade workers of the value of carrying out the goals. The staff then adopts the desirability of meeting the goals and will work hard to achieve them. *Sell* comes between the autocratic and the laissez-faire styles of leadership. *Participate* involves staff and leader working together to achieve identified goals. The leader offers various degrees of support or direction as needed by subordinates. This is an example of the democratic style of leadership.

▽▽▽
My Leadership Style Score

How did you score on the test of leadership style? Place an X on the continuum in Figure 18–3 to indicate where you are at this point in general leadership style tendencies. Remember, this score shows your tendency. If your X is far to the left or right, it may benefit you to be aware of this tendency and to avoid using this style consistently. Remember the continuum and the need to be flexible in your style. Balance task- and people-orientation as needed. Knowing what your predominant style of leadership is will help you to evaluate work situations and the style needed at that time. Some situations require a supportive style, whereas others require a more direct approach.

> *Using* A Short Test of Leadership Style *as a guide, have peers identify their general personal leadership style tendencies. Total up the number of autocratic styles compared with the number of laissez-faire styles. If peers are willing to share their results, offer feedback about the style of each class member as seen by other class members.*

▼▼▼
Specific Skills Needed for Leadership

To function well in your expanded role, you must be a good leader. The scenario at the beginning of this chapter is an example of what not to do as a nurse leader. It may be the sad fact that you can relate to the scenario because you have experienced Polly's style in your work environment. Much research about the business of leading others and the theories that go with leading is evident in the literature. To lead, research indicates that the leaders must have knowledge in three general areas:

1. Occupational skills
2. Organizational skills
3. Human relationship skills

The focus of your role as leader will be on tasks and people in an organization. Does the continuum of leadership styles come to mind? Developing the needed skills for your job is a responsibility you share with your employer.

▽▽▽
Occupational Skills for First-Line Practical Nursing Leaders

Solid nursing skills are necessary to be a good nursing leader. Visible expertise in nursing skills is a plus with your coworkers. This means the desire to see the client situation for yourself, assist in providing care, and demonstrate nursing skills to peers as needed. Your practical nursing program has started your skill development in this area. This is an area you will need to keep current and fresh.

▽▽▽
Organizational Skills for First-Line Practical Nursing Leaders

Survival skills and personal growth are essential ingredients for leaders. The emphasis on the personal and vocational issues course in your practical nursing program has given you an opportunity to learn and apply principles of assertiveness (see Chapter 11), time management (see Chapter 5), and methods of stress control (see Chapter 10). These skills are necessary parts of the development of any nursing leader.

▽▽▽
Human Relationship Skills for First-Line Practical Nursing Leaders

In addition to nursing and specific organizational skills, human relationship skills are necessary in your leadership role. Polly Practical *might* get the job done, but leaders with better human relationship skills will get the job done with finesse, style, and tact. Subordinates will like their leader's style a lot more and will be more effective in reaching the goals of the nursing unit. One of the nursing leader's most productive tools is the effective use of verbal and nonverbal communication. A review of the principles of communication described in Chapter 13 will benefit you.

▽▽▽
Additional Resources for Developing Organizational, Occupational, and Human Relationship Skills

There are various ways of adding organizational, occupational, and human relationship skills for leadership. Some of the following suggestions for additional learning offer continuing education credits.

1. Check with your local vocational or technical school for a practical nursing leadership course.

2. Ask your boss to consider in-service training on leadership techniques as well as updates on nursing skills. Consider cosponsoring such in-service training with the local technical college and making it available to a wide geographic area.

3. Form a network with other persons who fill first-line leadership positions. Be sure to go outside your institution as well as the discipline of nursing. You will find that the problems leaders have are very similar regardless of the discipline.

4. Attend seminars on leadership topics as well as nursing topics. Career Track is one example of companies that offer informative, interesting, fun, and affordable one-day seminars that could be beneficial to first-line leaders in nursing.

5. Read books and articles that offer hints for leaders. Be sure your nursing library is up to date. The annotated bibliography at the end of this chapter can help in this area. Some sources are new, and some have stood the test of time.

▼▼▼
Understanding Human Needs

As a leader, you will have the task of getting your subordinates to meet the goals set by your employer.

Getting persons to do what needs to be done is a complex task. Understanding human needs will help you get started.

All persons have needs that must be filled to meet goals. Individuals engage in various activities to fill needs. The activities are called behaviors and can be observed. Abraham Maslow, a psychologist, presented a pyramid of human needs that can assist the learner in understanding the ranking of human needs (Fig. 18–4). Meeting each level of needs on the pyramid acts as a motivator for meeting higher levels of needs. For example, before individuals can meet safety and security needs, they must have satisfied their physiologic needs. See Chapter 9 for a review.

▽▽▽
Adapting Maslow's Hierarchy

Maslow's hierarchy of needs can be adapted to help the first-line practical nursing leader understand the motivation of subordinates in a health care setting (Fig. 18–5).

In the pyramid shown in Figure 18–5, the Howlett hierarchy of work motivators, the lower three levels are considered externally motivated needs. These motivators exist outside a person. They depend on the employer or anyone else outside of self. If these needs are

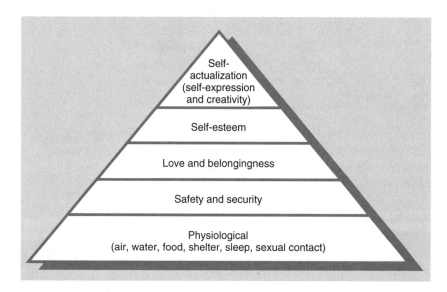

Figure 18–4
Maslow's hierarchy of needs.

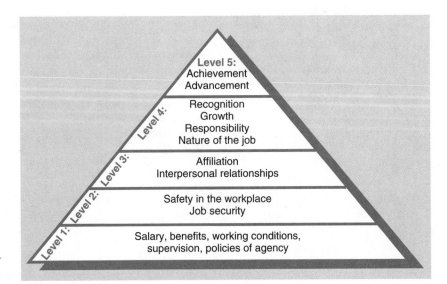

Figure 18–5
Howlett hierarchy of work motivators.

met, the person can proceed to the next higher level of the pyramid. If these needs are not met, a person will become dissatisfied with the work situation.

The upper two levels of the pyramid in Figure 18–5 represent internal motivators in the work environment. Internal motivators come from inside the individual. They result in individuals motivating themselves to reach goals.

Meeting needs on the Howlett hierarchy can motivate employees to behave in certain ways. It is a challenge for the leader to channel the motives of subordinates to meet the goals of the employer. As you read up the Howlett hierarchy shown in Figure 18-5, begin identifying behaviors that could be used to encourage meeting needs at each level. Also, decide whether the employer needs to initiate the behavior or whether the behavior could be initiated by the first-line practical nursing leader. As needs are met on one level, movement can then be encouraged to the next level of the Howlett hierarchy.

▼▼▼
Learning Exercise

Using the Howlett Hierarchy in Leadership Situations

The following activity gives you an opportunity to assume responsibility as a practical nursing leader. Examples of behaviors that encourage meeting needs at each level of the hierarchy are given.* The person responsible for the behavior is listed in parentheses. Space is provided for you to fill in additional suggested behaviors at each level to show how you can encourage meeting subordinates' needs at each level.

Level 1: Salary, benefits, working conditions, supervision, policies of agency

Examples:
Explanation of policies that affect employees (first-line PN leader)

Cafeteria-style benefits—pick and choose benefits (employer)

_____

_____

_____

Level 2: Safety in the workplace, job security

Provision of adequate equipment to carry out universal precautions (employer and first-line PN leader)
Establish policy for hostile clients (employer and first-line PN leader)

_____

_____

_____

Level 3: Affiliation, interpersonal relationships

Plan monthly potluck dinners, pizza lunches, get-togethers (first-line PN leader)

_____

_____

_____

Level 4: Recognition, growth, responsibility, nature of the job

Encourage attendance at continuing education seminars, in-service training, etc. (employer and first-line PN leader)
Recognition for working short-staffed (employer and first-line PN leader)

_____

_____

_____

Level 5: Achievement, advancement

Recognition of successful completion of class, seminar (employer and first-line PN leader)

_____

_____

_____

Share with your peers the behaviors you have listed to meet needs at the five levels of the Howlett hierarchy. Then give objective examples of how you can implement each of your suggested behaviors. For example, Level 5: recognizing successful completion of classes and seminars could be implemented by:

1. A written account in the facility's newsletter
2. Posting an announcement on a special section of the bulletin board
3. Personal note from the charge nurse

This learning activity can be fun. It allows the nurse to be creative in finding ways to give recognition.

---

*Appendix C: The Howlett Style of Nursing Leadership contains additional suggestions.

▼▼▼ S U M M A R Y

▶ When the state nurse practice act allows, practical nurses can be used as first-line leaders, especially in nursing homes as charge nurse. The practical nursing program itself offers students the opportunity to develop skills in nursing procedures, time management, assertiveness, and stress control. These are skills needed for everyday practice of nursing as well as leadership positions. Development of a leadership style is important in guiding staff to meet the goals of the health care organization.

▶ Established leadership styles range from the extremes of autocratic, which emphasizes the task, to laissez-faire, which emphasizes only concern for the employee. Situational leadership adapts the leadership style to the environment and the situation at hand. It is the suggested way of leading through the year 2000. Specific skill areas for nursing leadership include (1) occupational skills, (2) organizational skills, and (3) human relationship skills.

▶ No one chapter can teach you how to become a leader. In addition to training given by the institution, first-line practical nursing leaders need to educate and update themselves continually in the three specific skill areas noted. The references listed in the annotated bibliography at the end of this chapter can help you in your development as a first-line leader in nursing.

▼▼▼ R E F E R E N C E S

Chornick N, Yocum C, Jacobsen J. *Job Analysis: Newly Licensed Practical/Vocational Nurses 1994.* Chicago: National Council of State Boards of Nursing, 1995.

Hersey P, Weaver B. *Situational Leadership in Nursing.* Norwalk, CT: Appleton & Lange, 1989.

Howlett H. *The Howlett Theory of Management for Nursing Instructors* (unpublished paper), November 1989.

Wisconsin State Statutes. Chapter 441 N6.04. May 1990.

▼▼▼ B I B L I O G R A P H Y

Barker A. An emerging leadership paradigm. Nurs Health Care 1991; 12:204–207.

Blanchard K, et al. *The One Minute Manager Builds High Performance Teams.* New York: Morrow, 1991.

Blanchard K, Lorber R. *Putting the One Minute Manager to Work.* New York: Berkley Publishing, 1985.

Blanchard K, Johnson S. *The One Minute Manager.* New York: Berkley Publishing, 1983.

Chase L. Nurse manager competencies. Journal of Nursing Administration 1994; 24(45): 56–64.

Farley V. *Nurses: Pulling Together to Make a Difference.* Orange, CA: Innovative Nursing Consultants, 1995.

Farley V. Vision and Expertise: Nursing Education and the Future. Seminar presented April 24–25, 1995, Lake Geneva, WI.

Gable FG. *The Third Force: Abraham Maslow.* New York: Pocket Books, 1976.

Herzberg F. *The Motivation to Work.* New Brunswick, NJ: Transaction Publishers, 1993.

Rojas D. Leadership in a multicultural society: A case in role development. Nurs Health Care 1994; 15(5):258–261.

Wywialowski E. *Managing Client Care.* St. Louis: Mosby, 1993.

▼▼▼ *A N N O T A T E D   B I B L I O G R A P H Y*

Suggested References for Occupational Skills

Stone J, et al. *Clinical Gerontological Nursing: A Guide to Advanced Practice,* 2nd ed. Philadelphia: W.B. Saunders, 1991.

These authors provide a research-based reference text that can benefit nurses at all levels who care for elderly clients in all settings. Chapters cover assessment of all body systems as well as cognitive and functional assessment. Common clinical nursing problems are discussed as well as selected health problems.

Ignatavicius D, Varner Bayne M. *Medical-Surgical Nursing: A Nursing Process Approach.* Philadelphia: W.B. Saunders, 1995.

By means of a nursing process approach, this book emphasizes care of the seriously ill elderly patient throughout the text. Common assessment findings in elderly patients are highlighted. Each assessment chapter contains a Focus on the Elderly table that summarizes useful information.

Lammon C, et al. *Clinical Nursing Skills.* Philadelphia: W.B. Saunders, 1995.

This text presents nursing skills procedures with a rationale for actions. The book is intended to be used with a basic nursing textbook. This makes it a good review resource for nurses because fundamental information is not repeated. Each section of skills begins with principles and an overview of selected research studies for that skill and ends with home care variations.

Linton A, et al. *Introductory Nursing Care of Adults.* Philadelphia: W.B. Saunders, 1995.

This text addresses the evolving role and responsibilities of licensed practical nurses. Caring for the elderly is emphasized throughout. Disorders, treatments, and nursing care are presented in greater depth and detail to prepare LPNs for the complex care they will deliver. One chapter is specifically devoted to nursing in the long-term care setting.

Melonakos K, Michelson S. *Saunders Pocket Reference for Nurses.* Philadelphia: W.B. Saunders, 1995.

The authors provide nurses at all levels with an eclectic pocket reference that provides guidelines for common practice for adult clients of all ages with medical diagnoses. This reference guide contains great quantities of up-to-the-minute information and facts, as well as concise charts and tables. Information that is needed quickly can be easily accessed. Examples include assessment, psychosocial considerations, selected nursing diagnoses and interventions, lab testing, diagnostic procedures, nutrition therapy, infectious diseases, the client with cancer, and emergencies.

Murray R, Zentner J. *Nursing Assessment and Health Promotion Strategies Through the Lifespan,* 6th ed. Stamford, CT: Appleton & Lange, 1996.

Murray and Zentner present a usable text that discusses the total person (physical, mental, emotional, sociologic, cultural, and spiritual aspects). Emphasis is on assessment and health promotion through the entire lifespan. The chapters on the person in later maturity and death as the final developmental stage are particularly useful for nurses in the long-term–care setting.

Ringsven M, Bond D. *Gerontology and Leadership Skills for Nurses.* Albany, NY: Delmar, 1991.
This text is of value to the student and graduate practical nurse. Using a nursing process focus, both active and dependent elderly populations are discussed. In addition to discussion of physical and psychological conditions, community services and approaches to patient teaching are included. See listing in the next section on references for organizational skills.

Suggested References for Organizational Skills

(Note: All books listing Blanchard as an author are easy and fun to read and can be completed in a few hours. They offer excellent suggestions for leaders.)

Allen R. *Winnie-the-Pooh on Management.* New York: Dutton, 1994.
This readable book uses A. A. Milne's characters and stories to help lay the foundation of management skills. Winnie the Pooh, Eeyore, Christopher Robin, Piglet, and Tigger are used to illustrate how to set clear objectives, show strong leadership, gather accurate information, and communicate clearly.

Allen R, Allen S. *Winnie-the-Pooh on Problem Solving.* New York: Dutton, 1995.
This book returns to Pooh Corner for an effective yet simple discussion of problem-solving in a step-by-step manner. Personal, social, and business problems are tackled. So (as one advertisement for this book stated), whether you have your "head stuck in a honey pot" or a "sticky situation at work or home," this book will offer you all the advice you can "bear."

Blanchard K, Johnson S. *The One Minute Manager.* New York: Berkley Publishing, 1983.
In story form, the authors teach their three secrets of good management: setting goals, praising, and reprimanding. The aim is to get people to feel good about themselves. Then the quantity and quality of productivity in the workplace will be increased. These principles are also applicable to our daily lives.

Blanchard K, Lorber R. *Putting the One Minute Manager to Work.* New York: Berkley Publishing, 1985.
This sequel to The One Minute Manager *turns the three secrets of good management—setting goals, praising, and reprimanding—into skills for real-life situations.*

Blanchard K, Carew D, Parisi-Carew C. *The One Minute Manager Builds High Performing Teams.* New York: William Morrow, 1991.
The teamwork emphasis of this book will help increase any working group's productivity and satisfaction. The four stages that groups move through on their way to becoming high-performance teams are discussed as well as ideas on how to make groups more effective sooner while experiencing less stress.

Blanchard K, Zigarmi P, Zigarmi D. *Leadership and the One Minute Manager.* New York: William Morrow, 1985.
Situational leadership is described, and the hints given can help you become a flexible and successful leader. Suggestions are given to help you diagnose the work situation and can help you determine when to delegate, support, or direct subordinates.

Blanchard K, Oncken W, Burrows H. *The One Minute Manager Meets the Monkey.* New York: William Morrow, 1989.
Do you have the time at work to do all the things you want or need to do? If not, this book will help you decide if you are taking on problems at work that really belong to other people. The scenarios are funny, especially the manager who is loaded down by monkeys that have jumped from their owners' (the workers') backs to the manager's back. Oncken's Rules of Monkey Management will help you get the workers' monkeys off your back and become a more effective leader.

Fisher R, Ury W. *Getting to Yes: Negotiating Agreement Without Giving In.* New York: Viking Books, 1991.
This book discusses conflict and gives a "how-to" on reaching mutually acceptable agreement between opposing parties. Specific how-to advice is given for (1) separating people from the problem, (2) focusing on interests and not position, (3) creating options that are agreeable to all, and (4) negotiating with persons who do not play fair or by the rules. This book can be helpful at home as well as at work.

Peters T. *The Tom Peters Seminar: Crazy Times Call for Crazy Organizations.* New York: Vintage Books, 1994.
Peters' basic message is that organizational change is constant, rapid, and radical. We need to get rid of the word change in our vocabulary, replacing it with revolution or abandonment instead. To make organizations successful, he suggests putting a different lens in our eyes and learning to think and act differently in the everyday work world. This will prepare us for the coming Age of Imagination. Peters discusses decentralization of operations and empowerment of employees.

Ringsven M, Bond D. *Gerontology and Leadership Skills for Nurses.* Albany, NY: Delmar, 1991.
Includes a thorough, easy-to-read section on specific leadership skills for the first-line nurse manager. Very helpful for the practical/vocational nurse in a leadership position. See earlier listing in references for occupational skills.

Ritvo R, Litwin A, Butler L. *Managing in the Age of Change.* New York: Irwin Professional Publishing, 1995.
Discusses how to cope with the rapidity of change in business today. Discusses complex issues of hiring, budgeting, rewards, planning, and organizational downsizing. Especially helpful in developing critical skills that allow one to respond quickly and effectively to problems with minorities, persons with disabilities, and working mothers.

Suggested References for Human Relationship Skill Development, Including Personal Growth

Arnold E, Boggs K. *Interpersonal Relationships: Professional Communication Skills for Nurses.* Philadelphia: W.B. Saunders, 1995.
The author includes a chapter on communicating with older adults and communication strategies for long-term care settings. One chapter deals with communication with other health professionals and includes client advocacy, networking, conflict resolution, negotiating and collaborating with peers, responding to putdowns, barriers to interprofessional communication, leadership, and work groups.

Covey S. *Seven Habits of Highly Effective People: Restoring the Character Ethic.* New York: Simon and Schuster, 1989.
This book presents an ethical basis for human behavior. Covey presents a holistic integrated approach to solving personal and professional problems. Using Covey's seven habits, self-defeating habits at home and at work can be ended and success can occur.

Satir V. *The New Peoplemaking.* Mountain View, CA: Science and Behavior Books, 1988.
The editor's note to this book states that the author's "writings are like homemade bread. They are yeasty, hearty, and nourishing." This readable book by a family therapist offers suggestions for improving communication, increasing self-esteem, and getting along with others. Another book that benefits one's personal as well as career self. Just reading this book makes one feel good!

von Oech R. *A Whack on the Side of the Head.* New York: Warner Books, 1993.
Activities in the form of puzzles, games, exercises, and stories are presented to help break through mental blocks and unlock one's mind for creative thinking. Activities may be useful to help committees, the nursing team, and others develop problem-solving abilities by awakening the right side of the brain. This author also published Creative Whack Pack *(Stamford, CT: U.S. Systems Games, 1988), which offers the above activities on individual game cards.*

Management, Supervision, and Charge Nurse Skills for Practical Nurses

▼▼▼ O U T L I N E

▼▼▼ K E Y   T E R M S

assigning

change-of-shift report

delegating

nurse practice act

setting priorities

▼▼▼ *O B J E C T I V E S*

Upon completion of this chapter you will be able to:

1. *Using your state's nurse practice act, identify the following as they apply to the charge nurse position for practical nurses:*
   a. *requirements before assuming the charge nurse position*
   b. *site of employment as charge nurse*
   c. *scope of practice*

2. *Identify specific institutional policies and routines that the practical nurse should clarify when assuming a charge nurse position.*

3. *Describe elements that should be focused on when receiving and giving a change-of-shift report.*

4. *Discuss the assignment of tasks vs. the delegation of duties with regard to the following factors:*
   a. *your state's laws regarding the role of the practical nurse and the delegation of tasks in the charge nurse position*
   b. *differences between assigning tasks and delegating duties*
   c. *examples of tasks that may be assigned and duties that may be delegated*

   d. *legal aspects of assigning tasks and delegating duties*
   e. *items that should be included when assigning tasks and delegating duties*

5. *Discuss strategies for handling the following common workplace problems:*
   a. *chronic lateness for assigned shift*
   b. *excessive absences*
   c. *lack of job skills*

▼▼▼
Sample of a Job Description for Charge Nurse Position

```
Quality Care Nursing Home

Day Charge Nurse - LPN

Job Description
```

QUALIFICATIONS:

```
Licensed practical nurse with a current license to practice in the
state of Wisconsin under Chapter 441 N 6.04 (3). The LPN should have
a certificate of successful completion of an approved course in
Medication Administration.
```

STANDARDS:

```
The job of the charge nurse is to ensure that residents receive
nursing care, treatments, and medications that have been ordered by
their physician. The charge nurse shall help to coordinate patient
care services, e.g., physicians, dietician, activity therapist,
physical therapist, and social worker. The charge nurse shall assist
the Director of Nurses in the hiring, firing, and orientation of new
employees. The charge nurse shall adjust grievances, hours of
employment on his/her shift, evaluate work performance of nursing
assistants, and recommend to the Director of Nurses those employees
who merit wage increases according to review as per policy.
```

RESPONSIBLE FOR:

1. Knowledge of residents' condition at all times.
2. Assigning actual nursing care.
3. Providing nursing care according to physician's orders and in agreement with recognized nursing techniques and procedures, established standards of care as described in Wisconsin state statutes, and administrative policies of this extended care unit.
4. Recognizing symptoms, reporting residents' condition, including changes, and assisting with remedial measures for adverse developments.
5. Assisting physician in diagnostic and therapeutic measures.
6. Administering medications and treatments as prescribed.
7. Maintaining accurate and complete records of nursing assessments and interventions, including documentation on the residents' chart and kardex record.
8. Studying trends, techniques, and developments in nursing practice and evaluating their appropriateness to the work setting.
9. Efficiency of execution of work load, including neatness and orderliness.
10. Maintaining a safe and hazard-free environment.
11. Ensuring the residents' right to privacy.
12. Maintaining the dignity of residents.
13. Authorizing all actual work hours of employees prior to final review by the Director of Nurses.

DUTIES:

1. Observes and reports symptoms and conditions of residents.
2. Administers medications as prescribed by physicians. Assesses therapeutic response and side effects of same.
3. Takes and records vital signs when appropriate.
4. Maintains charts and kardexes including patients' condition and medications and treatments received.
5. Calls physician when necessary. Receives and records telephone orders.
6. Calls pharmacist for prescription drugs as needed.
7. Assists in maintaining a physical, social, and psychological environment for residents that is conducive to the best interests and welfare of residents.
8. Receives report at beginning of shift from off-going personnel and assigns duties to nursing assistants under the charge nurse's supervision.
9. Evaluates the completion of nursing assistant assignments in a safe and timely manner.
10. Provides report to oncoming shift.

11. Adjusts hours and wages of employees to reflect overtime and sick days. For each time period, reviews time cards and initials same for those employees assigned to the charge nurse. This duty will be completed prior to final review by the Director of Nurses.

12. Evaluates nursing assistants in the performance of their job description and reports same to Director of Nursing.

13. Attends supervisory staff meetings.

14. Handles grievances at the appropriate level.

15. Interprets state and federal guidelines to employees. Uses authority as charge nurse to ''follow code.''

16. Participates in:
    a. orientation of all new employees assigned to charge nurse.
    b. hiring, firing, disciplinary process of employees assigned to charge nurse.

▼▼▼
Where to Begin?

Note: Before continuing, review your state's nurse practice act for the law regulating assumption of the charge nurse position in your state. An example of one state's definition in the law of the charge nurse position for practical nurses is included below.

N6.04 Standards of Practice (3) ASSUMPTION OF CHARGE NURSE POSITION IN NURSING HOMES. In assuming the position of charge nurse in a nursing home as defined in s. 50.04 (2) (9b), Stats., an LPN shall:

(a) Follow written protocols and procedures developed and approved by an RN;

(b) Manage and direct the nursing care and other activities of LPNs and nursing support personnel under the general supervision of an RN, and,

(c) Accept the charge nurse position only if prepared to competently perform this assignment based on his or her nursing education, including education, training, or experience or active involvement in education and training for responsibilities not included in the basic LPN curriculum (WI State Statutes, Chapter 441, N6.04, May 1990).

The charge nurse job description for Quality Care Nursing Home might seem overwhelming at first. But it illustrates the reason why state laws require that first-line practical nurse managers have education, training, or experience beyond the basic practical nursing curriculum. It is impossible in one year to prepare health care workers to be able to function in this position immediately after graduation. After additional education, training, and experience, many practical nurses become first-line managers in extended care units and nursing homes. And they are doing an excellent job in that role.

You are probably thinking, "How long will it take for me to get to this point in my practical nursing career?" The answer to that question depends on the person asking it. The law of the state used above as an example specifically states that the charge nurse functions *in a nursing home* and under the general supervision of a registered nurse. In this particular state the practical nurse may not function as a charge nurse in a medical clinic or other facility. And in this state the practical nurse may not function under general supervision until he or she has passed the NCLEX-PN.

> *Be sure to check and keep up to date on your state's nurse practice act.*

This is an important point because some states are developing quick, creative ways to change legislation that affects all areas of state law. It would also be helpful to obtain job descriptions of practical nurse first-line manager positions from agencies with which you affiliated during the year.

The answer to the question about how long it will take you to get to this point in your practical nursing career depends on your state nurse practice act, any additional education you may have had, your motivation to learn the manager role, your ability to be a risk taker, and how you use your nursing experience. When questioned about their administrative responsibilities, 35.7% of practical nurses in the latest data gathered for content areas for NCLEX-PN stated that they had responsibilities as team leaders or unit managers (Chornick et al, 1995, p. 19).

No one book can provide you with a concise cookbook of how to function in the role of first-line manager as a practical nurse. This chapter discusses the following skills needed to function in the charge nurse role in an extended care unit or nursing home:

▶ Assigning client care
▶ Assessing residents
▶ Delegating tasks if allowed by your state's nurse practice act
▶ Reporting
▶ Handling common workplace problems of lateness, excessive absences, and lack of job skills

Development of management skills is an ongoing challenge, just as improving clinical skills is.

▼▼▼
A Checklist of Policies and Routines for the Charge Nurse

Not all of the areas included below are the responsibility of the charge nurse. But practical nurses functioning as charge nurses need to have information about all of the areas included so that they can carry out their management duties. Information about policies and routines that apply to the unlicensed personnel the charge nurse is responsible for is also needed.

▽▽▽
Personnel Policies

▶ Time sheets—location and interpretation
▶ Vacation, holiday, sick leave policy
▶ Special requests for time off, leave of absence

▶ Communication—reporting: on and off duty, sickness, and absence; memos, bulletin board
▶ Meal "hours," coffee breaks
▶ Smoking regulations
▶ Use of facility telephones
▶ Uniform regulations
▶ Job descriptions and duties of unlicensed personnel
▶ Organizational chart

▽▽▽
Records, Unit Routines, Federal and State Regulations

▶ Inspection protocols
▶ Current federal and state regulations
▶ General shift routine
▶ Duties of each of the three shifts
▶ Methods of reporting
▶ Procedure manual
▶ Facility policy manual
▶ Procedures specific to each division of the facility
▶ Nursing care plan system
▶ Routine for care planning conference
▶ Routine for physician's visits
▶ Location of reference books

▽▽▽
Unit Administration

▶ Admission, placement, transfer, and discharge of residents
▶ Care of clothing and valuables, including personal property list
▶ Routine for seriously ill residents
▶ Routine for death of a resident
▶ Autopsy permit
▶ Authorization procedure and forms for diagnostic tests and surgery
▶ Visiting hours
▶ Notary Public

▽▽▽
Safety Policies

▶ Siderails
▶ Restraints

▶ Fire regulations: reporting, evacuation plan, fire exits, location of fire extinguishers, preventive measures

▶ Use of oxygen

▶ Transportation of residents by cart, wheelchair

▶ Body mechanics

▽▽▽
Housekeeping, Maintenance, and Supplies

▶ Linen—how supplied, extra linen

▶ Care of contaminated linens and dressings

▶ Unit cleaning procedure and responsibilities

▶ How to obtain supplies: drugs, sterile supplies, personal care items, kitchen items

▶ Maintenance and repairs

▶ Conservation of supplies, linen, and equipment

▽▽▽
Equipment—How to Use and Where to Obtain

▶ Oxygen

▶ Suction equipment

▶ Therapeutic beds

▶ Respiratory therapy equipment and services

▽▽▽
Food Service for Residents

▶ Ordering diets and diet changes

▶ Tray service

▶ Unit food stock items

▶ Special nourishments

▶ Policy for feeding residents

▶ Policy for dining room

▽▽▽
Nursing Care Procedures, Assisting Physician

▶ Bathing, mouth care

▶ Bedmaking

▶ Temperature (devices used), pulse, and respiration

▶ Blood pressure

▶ Catheterization

▶ Enemas

▶ Suppositories, rectal and vaginal

▶ Recording intake and output

▶ Systems used for pressure ulcer care

▶ Collecting, delivering, and labeling specimens

▶ Assisting physicians with physical exams, foot care

▶ Postmortem procedure

▶ Policies for sterile technique procedures

▶ Blood glucose monitoring

▶ Colostomy care

▶ Nasogastric and gastrostomy tubes: flushing, feeding, administration of medications

▶ Universal precautions

▽▽▽
Medications

▶ Medication system

▶ Policy for reordering

▶ Unit stock

▶ Ordering from pharmacy

▶ Review of metric system, proportions, abbreviations

▶ Drug errors: reporting, incident reports

▶ Narcotic count

▶ References for drug administration

▽▽▽
Charting

▶ Method of charting

▶ Forms used

▶ Flowsheets used

▶ Policy for phone orders

▶ Incident reports

▶ Lists for wanderers, etc.

▽▽▽
Special Areas

▶ Emergency supplies

▶ Central supply area

▶ Physical therapy, occupational therapy

▶ Laundry

▶ Maintenance

▶ Break room
▶ Dining room
▶ Kitchen
▶ Business offices
▶ Social services
▶ Director of Nurses, staff educator
▶ Administrator of facility
▶ Conference rooms
▶ Activity department

▽▽▽
Miscellaneous

▶ Paging system
▶ Call-light system
▶ Disaster plan
▶ Routine for residents who desire CPR
▶ Chaplain service
▶ Volunteer services
▶ On-call schedule

▼▼▼
Reporting

Reports in extended care units and nursing homes, as in other health care agencies, are a way of passing pertinent information to the oncoming shift. In this way, the residents are guaranteed continuity of care.

▽▽▽
Reporting When Coming on Your Shift

The report you receive when you are coming on your shift will be the basis on which you assess resident needs. This is legally necessary so that you can adequately assign unlicensed personnel to provide care for specific residents. Reports can be taped or oral depending on agency policy.

When the report is taped, off-going personnel usually are still on duty, answering call lights and attending to residents' needs, while the oncoming shift listens to report. This will enable you to question unclear information after report is over. Nurses develop personal ways of gathering data when they are taking report, including the use of symbols and abbreviations.

▽▽▽
Reporting at the End of Your Shift

Giving report at the end of your shift requires planning. Unlicensed personnel must report to you as charge nurse before you can tape or give report. This is where the concise, clear directions that you gave to these personnel during assignment of tasks will pay off. Be sure to assess personally residents in whom changes in condition, current ongoing problems, new orders (and resident response to those new orders), and suspected side effects to medications have been noted. You will need to set priorities in deciding what information is pertinent to give the next shift. Use the same sequence of data for each resident. This will make it easier for the oncoming charge nurse to take notes from your report. An example of a suggested sequence of data for residents in an extended care unit follows:

1. Resident name, room number, and physician
2. New problems or concerns
3. Contact with physician and new orders
4. Progress of current, established problems
5. Prn medication—name of drug, time given, and reason for prn medication, need for follow-up
6. **Brief** description of resident's shift
7. Voiding, bowel movement of resident (continent vs. incontinent)

Things to avoid during report include:

1. Meaningless chatter that has nothing to do with residents' nursing care and goals
2. Routine nursing care, unless it has a bearing on current nursing problems
3. Personal opinions about residents' conditions
4. Value judgments about residents' life styles, behavior, or families

▼▼▼
Assigning Tasks vs. Delegating Duties

▽▽▽
Assigning Tasks in the Extended Care Unit

Assigning unlicensed personnel to care for specific residents follows the change-of-shift report. When practical nurses make assignments to unlicensed personnel, they are allotting tasks that are in the job description of unlicensed personnel. The assigned tasks are tasks unlicensed personnel are hired and paid to perform. The tasks are in **their** job description. These unlicensed personnel have a responsibility to complete their assignments in a safe and timely manner. The practical nurse as charge nurse shares responsibility with unlicensed personnel for the quality of the care delivered. In this situation, the charge nurse needs to evaluate the quality and effectiveness of the care that was assigned.

Assigning the Right Task

A crucial legal consideration in assigning tasks to unlicensed personnel is nursing judgment. The charge nurse must avoid real or potential harm to residents when assigning tasks to unlicensed personnel. You are *legally liable* for improper assigning of tasks. Change-of-shift report gives you an opportunity, as charge nurse, to assess the specific nursing needs of the residents during your shift and the complexity of those needs. Specific suggestions of tasks that can be assigned to unlicensed personnel include routine tasks such as bathing, feeding, ambulating, vital signs, weight, assistance with elimination, and maintaining safety factors. The actual tasks assigned depend on the needs of the residents on your unit, the training of unlicensed personnel, and the policies of the extended care unit. Assignment of more complex skills depends on what is allowed by law in your state, the needs of the unit, and advanced training of unlicensed personnel.

> *Obtain job descriptions of unlicensed personnel at the health care agencies with which you affiliated. Make a list of the tasks unlicensed personnel can perform at these sites.*

Assigning Tasks to the Right Person

Legally, you need to know the job descriptions of the unlicensed personnel to whom you assign tasks. Know their level of clinical competence. What are their strengths? What are their weaknesses? How much training have they had? What skills have they learned in their training program? Have they had orientation to your unit? Once you have worked consistently with unlicensed personnel, you will know if they are dependable and able to pursue assigned tasks. If the unlicensed staff person has had the proper training but is new to your extended care unit, make sure this person has completed orientation. Assign another unlicensed staff person who has proved to be dependable to work with this person until he or she is comfortable with the routine.

Assignment of Residents to Unlicensed Personnel In Nursing Home

Tasks to be Completed on Day Shift of One Wing of Nursing Home

Tasks

Four showers _____

_____

_____

_____

Each of the residents transfers with help of two people. Each of these residents needs to be weighed and have BP checks and complete linen change on shower day. One resident scheduled for a shower states she feels dizzy today and has a congested-sounding cough.

Nine partial baths _____

_____

_____

_____

_____

_____

_____

_____

Five residents are able to wash their own face and hands when set up. Of the remaining four, one has developed a rash over his entire body, one needs glucose monitoring two times on day shift, and two are confused and incontinent of urine and feces. Each of these residents needs the assistance of one person to transfer and ambulate.

One wet-to-dry dressing change _____ for resident on Clinitron bed (this resident is transferred by Hoyer lift and requires total care).

One PEG tube continuous feeding _____ with Jevity and drug administration two times on day shift (this resident is confused and requires two persons to ambulate).

Staff Available

Two student practical nurses, SPN1 and SPN2, who have completed half of their nursing program. Instructor makes assignments.

One nursing assistant, A, who has worked at the facility for 10 years (on state registry).

One nursing assistant, B, who has seven years' experience and has worked at your facility for 6 months (on state registry).

One nursing assistant, C, who was sent from a temporary agency to fill the position of a nursing assistant who has the flu. She completed a nursing assistant advanced course two months ago.

1. As Charge Nurse, how would you make assignments for the day shift for Wing 1? Include the reason (rationale) for your assignment decisions._____

   _____

   _____

   _____

   _____

2. Discuss your assignment plan in small groups.

Using the Right Communication to Assign a Task

Remember, the objective in assigning a task is to get the task completed safely. Give clear, concise directions to unlicensed personnel to whom you are assigning a task. Be specific about the results you expect. Make sure your directions are complete. Clarify the message by asking unlicensed staff to repeat what it is you expect them to do. Consider writing assignments in a concise, objective manner on a master assignment sheet. Explain what is expected at the unlicensed person's level of understanding. "Please" and "thank you" are in order as part of common courtesy. Use of the right communicating and motivating techniques is an excellent example of the type of leadership skills that are needed by the practical nurse first-line manager. The charge nurse's ability to motivate unlicensed personnel to carry out tasks to meet goals depends on these skills. Such skills must be learned by studying and using the techniques. Refer to Chapter 18 for hints on how to motivate personnel.

After Assigned Tasks Are Completed

When unlicensed personnel accept an assignment, they accept the primary responsibility for safely and efficiently completing that assignment. Charge nurses have the responsibility of verifying the unlicensed person's ability and success in performing the assigned task. Check the completed task. Legally, the charge nurse may not assign a task without checking the outcome of that assignment. Was the task completed? Was the task done safely? Have client goals been met?

Sometimes unlicensed personnel to whom you have assigned a task are not functioning at their highest level of competence. Document any incompetence you observe. Describe the incident objectively. Include date, time, place, and patient involved. Inform your supervisor in writing about the incident and provide this information. Request in your documentation that the staff person involved receive additional training in the specific area of observed incompetence.

> *You assigned the task of showering a resident to an unlicensed staff person. You observed that this health care worker showered the resident "unsafely." Using the above suggestions, compose a mock letter to your supervisor about the incident.*

▽▽▽
Delegating Duties

> *At this time, most states in the United States do not allow practical nurses to participate in delegating in their charge nurse positions. It is crucial that you check your state's nurse practice act to determine whether you may delegate as a charge nurse in your state. If you cannot find a clear answer, contact your state's board of nursing.*

When allowed by your state's nurse practice act, delegating duties in the extended care unit involves entrusting duties to unlicensed personnel that are in the job description of the practical nurse charge nurse. The duties being delegated are in *your* job description. The primary responsibility for the outcome of delegated acts rests with the registered nurse under whom the practical nurse charge nurse functions under general supervision. Duties can be delegated, but the responsibility that goes with that duty can never be delegated to another. See Table 19–1 for a comparison of assigning tasks and delegating duties.

If your state's nurse practice act allows practical nurse charge nurses to delegate tasks, you will have an opportunity to delegate tasks to unlicensed personnel. In addition to your state's nurse practice act, be sure to review:

1. The rules and regulations of your state's board of nursing.
2. Interpretations developed by your state's board of nursing regarding delegation.
3. Standards of your nursing organizations that apply to delegation of tasks.

Remember that most states in the United States do not allow practical nurses to delegate duties at this time.

Learning to delegate duties from your job description to unlicensed personnel, when allowed by your state's nurse practice act, can increase your effectiveness and efficiency as a charge nurse. Delegating duties to unlicensed personnel also helps these health care workers to increase and improve their job skills. Many of the suggestions in this chapter that were given for assigning tasks apply to delegating duties as well. But delegating is a complex skill. There are some important differences between assigning tasks and delegating duties.

Table 19–1
Comparison of Assigning vs. Delegating by the Practical Nurse Charge Nurse

	Assigning Tasks	*Delegating Duties*
To whom may tasks or duties be assigned or delegated?	Nursing assistants and other unlicensed personnel	Nursing assistants and other unlicensed personnel
Are tasks or duties in nursing assistant's job description?	Yes	No
May nursing assistant refuse?	No, unless staff person thinks they are unqualified for assignment	Yes. In addition, staff person must voluntarily accept delegation
Who has primary responsibility for the completion of care?	Nursing assistant	Practical nurse charge nurse

Differences Between Assigning and Delegating

Assigning tasks is done before and during your shift as a regular part of *your* job. Assigning tasks is in *your* job description. Because assigning tasks involves allocating the nursing care that is to be done by unlicensed personnel within *their* job description, these personnel cannot refuse the assignment (Wywialowski, 1993, p. 181). An exception might occur if the unlicensed personnel receiving the assignment decide they are unqualified to carry out the assigned task. These personnel would then be reassigned. Arrangements would be made for them to receive the training necessary to do the task they felt unqualified to do. Unlicensed personnel assume primary responsibility for completing tasks safely when they are assigned to them.

Delegating duties is not written in the job description for charge nurse (for example, see the job description for charge nurse at Quality Care Nursing Home, earlier in this chapter). When delegating is allowed by your state's nurse practice act, it is a voluntary function. When you delegate duties, you are asking unlicensed personnel to do part of *your* job. You are not asking them to do duties that you dislike doing. You are asking them to help you do some of your duties so that you can fulfill other responsibilities, the ultimate goal being to improve client care. Because you are delegating part of your job, the unlicensed person receiving the delegation must approve the assignment. He or she must voluntarily accept the delegation. These health care workers cannot be forced to accept the delegated duty. Delegation involves the ability to share power with another staff person. When delegating duties, the charge nurse needs to provide the unlicensed person with the authority to carry out the duty.

Legal Aspects of Delegating

In 1994 the president of the National Council of State Boards of Nursing stated that "boards of nursing must clearly define delegation in regulations, promulgate clear rules for its use, and follow through with disciplinary action when there is evidence that the rules are violated" (Rachel, 1994). *Check with the board of nursing in your state for its interpretation of delegation.*

The 1994 revised *Entry-Level Competencies of Graduates of Educational Programs in Practical Nursing* includes the following item:

> The graduate practical nurse is accountable for nursing care delegated to unlicensed health care providers.

To be legally safe when delegating duties, keep the following criteria in mind:

1. Delegate functions only if allowed to by your state's nurse practice act.
2. *Never delegate what is in your legal scope of practice.*
3. Delegate duties for which unlicensed personnel have had the educational preparation and for which they show demonstrated ability.
4. Provide clear directions to unlicensed personnel for delegated duties.
5. Provide assistance to unlicensed personnel when you delegate a duty.
6. Monitor the activities of unlicensed personnel when they carry out delegated duties.
7. Evaluate the safety and effectiveness of the duties delegated to unlicensed personnel.

When the registered nurse delegates a duty to an LPN or LVN or to an unlicensed person, the legal principle of *respondeat superior* comes into play. According to that principle, the nursing act delegated is the act of the supervising nurse, the RN, the person who delegated the act. In the extended care unit, the LPN as charge nurse is managing and directing the activities of unlicensed personnel under the *general* supervision of an RN. The RN has *ultimate accountability* for the supervision of nursing assistants. But the LPN first-line manager assists in the supervision of these health care workers and shares accountability with the RN for their actions.

▌ ***In your state's nurse practice act, find the definition of "general supervision."*** ▕

Duties That May Be Delegated

A concise list of what to delegate and what not to delegate does not exist. Employers may suggest that certain duties may be delegated, and they may suggest to whom duties may be delegated. But the person doing the delegating is ultimately responsible for (1) deciding to delegate a duty, (2) deciding to whom to delegate the duty, and (3) deciding under what circumstances to delegate the duty. Generally, necessary, routine, or repetitive duties can be delegated. Duties that are part of your legal scope of practice may never be delegated. Do not assume that more complex duties may be delegated. **Examples** of what **not** to delegate include:

1. Complex sterile technique procedures
2. Crisis situations (you be there)
3. Initial patient education by an RN

It is your license that is at stake in the matter of delegating duties.

Refer to the job description at the beginning of this chapter. Based on this job description, examples of charge nurse duties that could be delegated, if allowed in this state, would be:

1. Administers medications (no. 2). Federal regulations allow nursing assistants to administer medications after they have successfully completed a drug administration course. The duty of giving selected medications could be delegated to nursing assistants if they have successfully completed the requirements of the state in which they are employed.

2. Takes and records vital signs when necessary (no. 3). This duty refers to situations other than taking routine vital signs. In such situations, the patient has probably had a change in condition. The charge nurse may decide to delegate the duty of taking frequent vital signs to an unlicensed person who has proved competent and reliable in taking vital signs and quickly reports the results to the charge nurse. This delegation would free the charge nurse to assess or collect data from other patients with changes in condition, perform treatments that cannot be delegated, and report to physicians via phone.

3. Adjusts hours to reflect overtime and sick days (no. 11). This clerical duty could be delegated to a trusted unlicensed person. The charge nurse would review the time cards on which the unlicensed staff person recorded overtime and absences before

forwarding them for final review to the Director of Nursing.

4. Participates in orientation of all new employees (no. 16a). An experienced unlicensed person can be delegated to conduct orientation to specific aspects of the routine of the shift to which a new employee is assigned.

Examples of charge nurse duties in this job description that could not be delegated would be:

1. Calls physician when necessary (no. 5).
2. Evaluates nursing assistants (no. 12).
3. Handles grievances at the appropriate level (no. 14).
4. Interprets state and federal guidelines (no. 15).
5. Hires and fires employees (no. 16b).

> *Review charge nurse job descriptions of nursing homes/extended care units at facilities at which you affiliate. If your state's nurse practice act allows delegation, discuss charge nurse duties that could be delegated.*

▼▼▼
Collecting Data (Assessing) as a Charge Nurse

The following is a list of signs and symptoms that may indicate illness, exacerbation of a previous disease condition, injury, or decline in prior function. Be observant with each patient interaction. When unlicensed personnel report that "something does not seem right," visit the resident to assess or collect your own data. After collecting the data, record it on the proper chart form and report all abnormal observations according to agency policy. The actual parameters given are guidelines. Follow specific paramaters given for each assigned resident.

▽▽▽
Signs and Symptoms

1. Weight: Increase or decrease of 5 to 10 pounds in one week.

2. Temperature: Elevation over 100° F orally or 100° F rectally, or temperatures under 96.6° F orally.

3. Upper respiratory tract: Head congestion, headache, sore throat, ear pain, runny nose, postnasal drip.

4. Lower respiratory tract: Acute onset or worsening of: shortness of breath, dyspnea with exertion, orthopnea, cough (productive or nonproductive), wheezing or other abnormal sounds on inhalation or exhalation.

5. Heart: Blood pressure over 140/90 or below 80/50; irregular pulse (new symptom); chest, neck, shoulder, or arm pain; fatigue; increased frequency of angina; shortness of breath; orthopnea; peripheral edema, sacral edema, distended neck veins.

6. Breast: Lump found on palpation, discharge from nipple.

7. Abdomen: Localized or generalized pain, especially of acute onset, epigastric burning or discomfort, constipation, diarrhea, nausea, vomiting, bloody or tarry stools, loss of appetite.

8. Musculoskeletal system: Swollen and tender joints, loss of strength in limbs, pain, loss of motion, ecchymosis, edema.

9. Reproductive system: Vaginal discharge, abnormal vaginal bleeding.

10. Genitourinary system: Urgency, frequency, dysuria, nocturia, hematuria, incontinence. Male: Dribbling, inability to start or stop stream.

11. Sleep and rest patterns: Change from normal routine, requirement of medication for sleep, nightmares or dreams.

12. Skin: Changes in color, turgor, contusions, abrasions, lacerations, rashes.

13. Mobility and exercise: Need for support in ambulation, changes in posture, weakness of extremities, changes in coordination, vertigo.

14. Hygiene status: Mouth—condition of mucous membranes, gums, teeth, tongue, mouth odor. Body—cleanliness, odor. Hair—grooming, distribution, scalp scaling, presence of disease. Nails—color, texture, grooming.

15. Communication: Verbal and nonverbal expression, aphasia, level of understanding.

16. Sensory-perceptual: Ability to hear, condition of hearing aid; ability to see, condition of glasses; ability to feel in all extremities; ability to discriminate odors; ability to distinguish tastes.

17. Cultural and religious: Food preferences, wellness and illness beliefs, religious items (rosary, Bible, medals, icons), religious practices (communion, clergy visits, confession, sacrament of the sick).

18. Psychological status: Level of consciousness, disorientation, intelligence, attention span, vocabulary level, interests, memory.

▼▼▼
Dealing with Common Charge Nurse Problems

You have learned about the problem-solving method of nursing, the nursing process (see Chapter 2), and its benefits in planning care for clients. This same problem-solving process can be used by the first-line practical nurse manager to deal with problems that present in the clinical area. Common problem areas are absenteeism, tardiness, poor appearance, and failure to complete assigned work in a timely or satisfactory manner. Each problem differs. Problems need to be approached individually. Use the nursing process and elements of Appendix C (the Howlett style of nursing leadership) as guidelines for approaching these problems.

The following scenario may be used as a model. Actual times for observing behavior may differ depending on the specific employee. The following sequence of discipline was suggested in an article by Janet Wilson (1987, pp. 121–123). It represents a legally sound way of handling an employee problem. Be sure to follow the recommended procedure for discipline as found in your health care agency.

▽▽▽
Scenario 1: Late for Assigned Shift

Penny, a nursing assistant, is assigned to the day shift in an extended care unit. Her shift begins at 0645 with a verbal report from the night nurse.

Assessment

On May 8, 10, 15, 16, 23, and 24 Penny came to work either during the night report or after the report was finished. When questioned about this behavior, she stated that she has problems getting her teenagers up and started for school.

Problem

A record of Penny's tardiness indicates that this is a recurring problem and not an isolated incident. A pattern has been established.

Interventions

As the charge nurse, it is your responsibility to talk to Penny about this tardiness. This includes the times and days of her tardiness. Select a private spot for your discussion. Encourage Penny to determine why this behavior is inconvenient for the staff and residents. Review the extended care unit's policy on punctuality. Encourage Penny to come up with ideas for improving her home situation so she can be on time. Set limits with Penny. Make clear to her that she needs to be on time for her assigned shifts. Plan to meet with her in one month to discuss her performance. At that time, if she has not improved her performance, a written reprimand will be given and included in her personnel file. At the end of the meeting, compliment Penny on an area of her work that has been going well.

Evaluation

During the next month, continue to document Penny's arrival for her assigned shifts. If she complies, note and praise her change in performance. If she continues to be late for her shift, issue a written reprimand. Place a copy in her file, and give a copy to your supervisor. Keep a copy in your file. Be sure the warning contains objective information including:

1. Days and times late for shift.
2. Date of oral warning.

3. Seriousness of situation.
4. Consequences of failure to improve.

Be sure to discuss the written reprimand privately with Penny. At this time another interval might be set for further review. If performance has not improved, disciplinary action may be carried out.

Using the nursing process and principles found in Appendix C, the Howlett style of nursing leadership, develop a plan of action to handle the following employee problems. Suggested, but not definite, ways of handling these problems are found in Appendix D.

▽▽▽
Scenario 2: Repeated Absences

Wayne, a nursing assistant, is a full-time employee of the evening shift at the extended care unit in which you are charge nurse in the evenings. He has missed 5 of 20 scheduled shifts this month. When questioned about his absences, Wayne states that he has personal problems. Frequent absences have been a problem since Wayne was first employed.

▽▽▽
Scenario 3: Failure to Complete Assignment in a Timely Manner

Ceil completed her nursing assistant training four months ago. Since Ceil was placed on the registry, she has been employed at the extended care unit at which you are charge nurse. Since completing her orientation to the extended care unit, she has had continuing problems getting her assignment completed in an acceptable time frame. Ceil claims her resident load is always too heavy and is impossible to complete. The other nursing assistants have helped Ceil with her residents, but they tell you they are tired of carrying her load because frequently she can be seen sitting at the nurse's desk talking on the telephone.

▼▼▼   S U M M A R Y

▶ State nurse practice acts specify requirements needed by practical nurses to assume first-line manager positions. A common first-line manager position is charge nurse in an extended care unit or nursing home. Oncoming shift reports give the charge nurse the opportunity to assess resident needs and to assign unlicensed personnel duties for resident care from *their* job description. The charge nurse shares responsibility with unlicensed personnel for the quality of care that is given.

▶ Practical nurse charge nurses routinely assign care to unlicensed personnel. Charge nurses, as part of their jobs, evaluate the thoroughness and safety of all tasks they assign. *If allowed in your state's nurse practice act,* the practical nurse as charge nurse may elect to delegate duties from the *practical nurse's* job description to unlicensed personnel. Delegation gives the charge nurse time to focus on tasks that cannot be delegated.

▶ Duties can be delegated, but the responsibility that goes with those duties remains with the registered nurse under whom the charge nurse functions under general supervision. The practical nurse charge nurse shares accountability in these situations. The charge nurse position is a complex role for practical nurses. With additional education and experience, many practical nurses are doing an excellent job in this expanded role position.

▶ *It is your license that is at stake in the matter of assuming the charge nurse position. Know your state laws regulating nursing.*

▼▼▼   R E F E R E N C E S

Chornick N, Yocum C, Jacobson J. *Job Analysis: Newly Licensed Practical/Vocational Nurses.* 1994. Chicago: National Council of State Boards of Nursing, 1995 (Copyright 1995).

Entry Level Competencies of Graduates of Educational Programs in Practical Nursing. New York: NLN Council of Practical Nursing Programs, 1994.

Rachels M. President of the National Council of State Boards of Nursing (Letter). August 24, 1994.

Wilson J. Have a problem employee? Use this plan. Nursing 87 1987; April:121–123.

Wisconsin State Statutes. Chapter 441, N6.04, May 1990.

Wywialowski E. *Managing Client Care.* St. Louis: Mosby, 1993.

▼▼▼   B I B L I O G R A P H Y

Hansten R, Washburn M. What do you say when you delegate work to others? *AJN* 1992; 92(7):48, 50.

Hansten R, Washburn M. Tips for delegating to the right person. *AJN* 1992; 92(6):64–65.

Hequet M. Giving good feedback. *Training* 1994; 31(9):72–76.

Howlett H. *The Howlett Theory of Management for Nursing Instructors.* Unpublished paper, November, 1989.

Neumann T. Speaker. Update on legal matters in the state of Wisconsin. Fall Conference of Wisconsin Association of Licensed Practical Nurses, Chula Vista Resort, Wisconsin Dells, Wisconsin, November 3, 1995.

Spitzer-Lehmann R. *Nursing Management Desk Reference: Concepts, Skills and Strategies.* Philadelphia: W.B. Saunders, 1994.

How to Get There

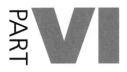

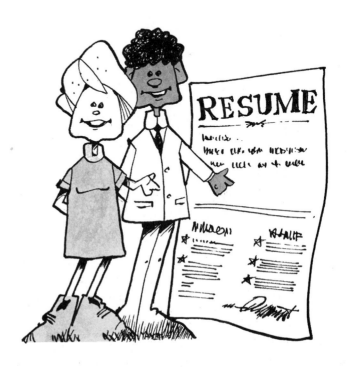

Nursing Ethics and The Law

▼▼▼ *OUTLINE*

▼▼▼ K E Y   T E R M S

autonomy

beneficence

civil action

criminal action

critical thinking

durable power of attorney

ethics

intentional torts

justice

law

liability

living will

malpractice

mandatory licensure

morals

NAPNES standards of practice

NFLPN code for practical/vocational
   nurses

NFLPN nursing standards

nonmaleficence

nurse practice act

permissive licensure

values

▼▼▼ O B J E C T I V E S

Upon completing this chapter you will be able to:

1. *Explain the relationship between nursing ethics and the law.*

2. *Discuss four principles of ethics.*

3. *Describe the difference between ethics, morals, and values.*

4. *List seven steps needed for critical thinking and ethical decision making.*

5. *Discuss legal and clinical competency.*

6. *Discuss what is meant by the client's bill of rights.*

7. *Differentiate between civil action and criminal action.*

8. *Using the correct terms, list the five steps of the legal process.*

9. *Explain the purpose of the nurse practice act, an example of statutory law.*

10. *Define terms commonly used in nurse practice acts:*
   a. basic nursing care
   b. basic nursing situation
   c. complex nursing situation
   d. delegated medical act
   e. delegated nursing act
   f. direct supervision
   g. general supervision

11. *Differentiate between mandatory and permissive licensure.*

12. *Describe how the nursing standard of care has come into being.*

13. *Review the four elements necessary to prove negligence.*

14. *Explain liability as it applies to the student nurse and instructor.*

15. *Describe three intentional torts.*

16. *List six common causes of recurring liability for nurses.*

17. *Discuss how to document client information in a legally correct way.*

18. *Differentiate between a living will and a durable power of attorney.*

Ethics in nursing deals with rules of conduct— what is right and what you ought to do in a particular situation. The *law* (legal aspects in nursing) has to do with rules and regulations that control the practice of nursing. The state nurse practice act is your legal guideline in nursing.

Sometimes ethics and the law are in conflict. For example, you may be ethically opposed to abortion; however, abortion in the United States is legally permitted under certain conditions. You may ethically refuse to assist with the abortion procedure, but you cannot refuse to give nursing care to the woman involved. "You may not abandon your patient," in the words of Sr. M. Antonette, MSC, RN, MS, Director of Nursing, School of Nursing, Sacred Heart Hospital, Allentown, PA, 1961–1964.

▼▼▼
Principles of Ethics

Four ethical principles assist in determining a right course of action: autonomy, beneficence, nonmaleficence, and justice.

1. *Autonomy* allows the competent client to maintain control over health care decisions. Clients make informed choices based on knowledge of their condition and treatment options. For example, a young woman is diagnosed with breast cancer. She has decided not to receive treatment and requests discharge as soon as possible. You will support the decision and continue to provide your finest care whether or not the client's ethics regarding treatment agree with your ethics.

Autonomy also includes client *privacy*. This is why your instructor asks the client directly for permission to allow students to observe a particular treatment or procedure. It is also the reason why the client is not exposed needlessly in the course of routine care.

Confidentiality is involved in the principle of autonomy. The client has the right to have information shared only with his or her immediate health care providers. For example, your neighbor is admitted. You are not assigned to his care. However, you want to know about his condition. Based on confidentiality, you are violating his confidentiality by reading his chart.

2. *Beneficence* involves *doing good* with your nursing actions. It may also involve preventing harm and removing harm. It does not conflict with the principle of autonomy. You provide care according to nursing care standards. For example, if you give the wrong medication, you report it as soon as you recognize your error. Your ethical concern is to prevent harm to the client. Beneficence is a greater good than concern for yourself in regard to the error. *Paternalism* is a form of beneficence that does intrude on autonomy. If you deceive, threaten, or manipulate a client into performing a therapeutic activity, the activity itself may be beneficial, but you have taken away the client's right to make the final decision (autonomy). A lactation counselor recently coached a public health nursing audience as follows: "I wish all women would breastfeed their babies. The value to the mother and the child is a scientific fact. I present the facts and respond to their questions, but the final decision belongs to the mother. I respectfully support their decision."

3. *Nonmaleficence* means *primum non nocere:* first do no harm. Nonmaleficence is the basis for many of the "rules" promoted by your instructors. Examples include the "rule of 5" in dispensing medications, checking the temperature of bathwater, checking the temperature of formula, lowering the bed to its lowest position after completing a treatment or preparing to leave the room, and not abandoning your clients when their ethical principles conflict with yours.

4. *Justice,* a fourth ethical principle, means that you must give clients their due and treat them fairly. Consider the current topic of *futility*. Health care is expensive, but medicine can often extend a life past the point of natural death. At what point is treatment considered futile and the client allowed to die?

Discuss the following statements or questions posed by a medical ethicist as part of a newspaper interview.

Health care is expensive. So is insurance. At what point do we limit what treatments insurance companies and government pay for? _____

_____

_____

Should all treatments be available to all people? Who pays? _____

_____

_____

Are we excluding from coverage worthy treatments because our ideas about medicine are too rigid?

_____

_____

_____

If the system won't provide a certain kind of treatment, should the individual look to the community for

help? _____

_____

_____

(Duluth (MN) News-Tribune 11/13/95, p. 1).

As a nurse you make daily decisions in order to give clients "their due." For example, the clients on your floor represent different levels of wealth, social status, culture, religion, and moral and value systems. All are acutely ill. The newest client has Kaposi's sarcoma, a defining component of acquired immune deficiency syndrome (AIDS). Do you classify AIDS as a life-threatening illness or as a retribution for behaviors you consider unethical? If your ethics interfere with the care you give, you may find yourself (1) giving this client more time than needed and doing less than needed for other acutely ill clients, or (2) providing minimal care for him and lavishing attention on those who "deserve the care." There are many daily care issues relating to justice. Listen to your inner talk: "He's so young—so much living left to do; she's had a full life already; she's an alcoholic—never took care of her kids"—and so on.

> At the end of your next clinical day take time to reflect on your reaction to clients and how it affected your client care. Did the word "deserve" enter in your thoughts, or did you provide justice for all?

▽▽▽
Values, Morals, and Ethics

Personal values and morals are the building blocks of ethics. *Value* means the worth you assign to an idea or an action. *Morals* refer to the customs of society or the ethical habits of a person. *Ethics* refers to our system or code of behavior. Personal values are freely chosen and are affected by age, experience, and maturity. A child usually embraces family values during childhood. The teen years are a time of trying out the family values and either incorporating them or rejecting and replacing them with new values. Values may continue to be modified throughout the one's lifetime with input from new knowledge and experience. Based on changes in values, morals can be shifted, as can one's personal code of behavior (ethics). Your personal ethics are the basis of your nursing ethics.

▼▼▼
Critical Thinking and Ethical Decisions

Critical thinking plays a major role in sorting out ethical choices and legal responsibilities in regard to the client. As a student nurse and as a LPN you rarely make a decision alone. Alfaro-LeFeure (1995) lists the following steps for moral and ethical reasoning.

1. Clearly identify the issue based on the perspective of the *players* involved.

2. Recognize your personal values and how they may influence your ability to participate in health care decision-making.

3. Identify the alternatives.

4. Determine the outcomes of the alternatives.

5. List the alternatives and rate them on the scale shown in Figure 20–1 according to which would produce the least harm or the greatest good, based on the *client's* values.

6. Develop a plan of action that will facilitate the best choices.

7. Put the plan into action and monitor the response closely.

▼▼▼
Ethical Decision Resources

Fortunately you have excellent resources to assist you in the ethical decision-making process:

► Your instructors
► Clinical nurses and physicians
► The NFLPN Code for Licensed Practical/Vocational Nurses (Table 20–1)
► The NFLPN Nursing Practice Standards (Table 20–2)
► The NFLPN Specialized Nursing Practice Standards (Table 20–3)
► The NAPNES Code of Ethics
► The NAPNES Standards of Practice for Practical/Vocational Nurses (Table 20–4)
► The philosophy, mission, and policies of your health agency
► Your job description
► The health agency staff
► The agency ethics committee

The client's knowledge of choices regarding care also affects ethical decision-making. Be sure as a student nurse and as an LPN to confirm your final ethical decisions with the RN supervisor *before* acting.

▼▼▼
General Legal Aspects

▽▽▽
Importance of Legal Aspects

As practical nursing responsibility for involvement in the nursing process and accountability for providing high-quality nursing care increase, it becomes even more important for you to understand the basic concepts of the laws that govern your nursing performance. This knowledge base will be valuable to you in making decisions. Such knowledge will also help you protect yourself against acts and decisions that could involve you in lawsuits and criminal prosecution.

▽▽▽
Client Competency

You can expect to hear increased use of the term competency in both a legal and clinical sense. The following details provide a brief framework to help you use this term correctly.

Client competency has both a *legal* meaning and a *clinical* meaning. Some client rights issues are based on proof of competency or incompetency within the court system.

Legal competency refers to a client who is:

1. Eighteen years old or older.

2. Pregnant or a married woman.

3. A self-supporting minor (referred to as a legally emancipated minor).

4. Competent in the eyes of the law (incompetency is determined by the court).

Clinical competency refers to a client who is able to:

1. Identify the problem.

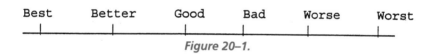

Figure 20–1.

Table 20–1 Nursing Ethics versus Personal Values		
NFLPN Code for Licensed Practical/Vocational Nurses	**A Statement of My Personal Value System**	**Adjustment Needed**
Know the scope of maximum utilization of the LP/VN as specified by the nursing practice act and function within this scope		
Safeguard the confidential information acquired from any source about the patient		
Provide health care to all patients regardless of race, creed, cultural background, disease, or lifestyle		
Refuse to give endorsement to the sale and promotion of commercial products or services		
Uphold the highest standards in personal appearance, language, dress, and demeanor		
Stay informed about issues affecting the practice of nursing and delivery of health care and, where appropriate, participate in government and policy decisions		
Accept the responsibility for safe nursing practice by keeping oneself mentally and physically fit and educationally prepared to practice		
Accept the responsibility for membership in NFLPN and participate in its efforts to maintain the established standards of nursing practice and employment policies that lead to quality patient care		

From National Federation of Licensed Practical Nurses. Nursing Practice Standards booklet. Raleigh, NC: National Federation of Licensed Practical Nurses (NFLPN), 1991.

2. Understand the options for care and the possible consequences.

3. Make a decision.

4. Provide sound reasons for the option he or she chooses.

▽▽▽
Rights of Clients

It is recognized that a personal relationship between the physician and the client is essential for the provision of

Table 20–2
NFLPN Nursing Practice Standards

Introductory Statement

Definition

Practical/Vocational nursing means the performance for compensation of authorized acts of nursing that utilize specialized knowledge and skills and that meet the health needs of people in a variety of settings under the direction of qualified health professionals.

Scope

Practical/Vocational nursing comprises the common core of nursing and, therefore, is a valid entry into the nursing profession.

Opportunities exist for practicing in a milieu where different professions unite their particular skills in a team effort for one common objective—to preserve or improve an individual patient's functioning.

Opportunities also exist for upward mobility within the profession through academic education and for lateral expansion of knowledge and expertise through both academic and continuing education.

Standards

Education

The Licensed Practical/Vocational Nurse

    1. Shall complete a formal education program in practical nursing approved by the appropriate nursing authority in a state.

    2. Shall successfully pass the National Council Licensure Examination for Practical Nurses.

    3. Shall participate in initial orientation within the employing institution.

Legal/Ethical Status

The Licensed Practical/Vocational Nurse

    1. Shall hold a current license to practice nursing as an LP/VN in accordance with the law of the state wherein employed.

    2. Shall know the scope of nursing practice authorized by the Nursing Practice Act in the state wherein employed.

    3. Shall have a personal commitment to fulfill the legal responsibilities inherent in good nursing practice.

    4. Shall take responsible actions in situations wherein there is unprofessional conduct by a peer or other health care provider.

    5. Shall recognize and have a commitment to meet the ethical and moral obligations of the practice of nursing.

    6. Shall not accept or perform professional responsibilities which the individual knows (s)he is not competent to perform.

Practice

The Licensed Practical/Vocational Nurse

    1. Shall accept assigned responsibilities as an accountable member of the health care team.

    2. Shall function within the limits of educational preparation and experience as related to the assigned duties.

    3. Shall function with other members of the health care team in promoting and maintaining health, preventing disease and disability, caring for and rehabilitating individuals who are experiencing an altered health state, and contributing to the ultimate quality of life until death.

Table continued on following page

Table 20–2
NFLPN Nursing Practice Standards (Continued)

   4. Shall know and utilize the nursing process in planning (assessing [data gathering]), implementing, and evaluating health services and nursing care for the individual patient or group.
      a. Planning (assessing [data gathering]): The planning of nursing includes:
         1) assessment of health status of the individual patient, the family, and community groups
         2) an analysis of the information gained from assessment
         3) the identification of health goals.
      b. Implementation: The plan for nursing care is put into practice to achieve the stated goals and includes:
         1) observing, recording, and reporting significant changes which require intervention or different goals
         2) applying nursing knowledge and skills to promote and maintain health, to prevent disease and disability, and to optimize functional capabilities of an individual patient
         3) assisting the patient and family with activities of daily living and encouraging self-care as appropriate
         4) carrying out therapeutic regimens and protocols prescribed by an RN, physician, or other persons authorized by state law.
      c. Evaluations: The plan for nursing care and its implementations are evaluated to measure the progress toward the stated goals and will include appropriate persons and/or groups to determine:
         1) the relevancy of current goals in relation to the progress of the individual patient
         2) the involvement of the recipients of care in the evaluation process
         3) the quality of the nursing action in the implementation of the plan
         4) a re-ordering of priorities or new goal setting in the care plan.
   5. Shall participate in peer review and other evaluation processes.
   6. Shall participate in the development of policies concerning the health and nursing needs of society and in the roles and functions of the LP/VN.

Continuing Education
The Licensed Practical/Vocational Nurse
   1. Shall be responsible for maintaining the highest possible level of professional competence at all times.
   2. Shall periodically reassess career goals and select continuing education activities which will help to achieve these goals.
   3. Shall take advantage of continuing education opportunities which will lead to personal growth and professional development.
   4. Shall seek and participate in continuing education activities which are approved for credit by appropriate organizations, such as the NFLPN.

From National Federation of Licensed Practical Nurses. Nursing Practice Standards booklet. Raleigh, NC: National Federation of Licensed Practical Nurses (NFLPN), 1991.

medical care. The traditional physician–client relationship takes on a new dimension when care is rendered within an organizational structure. Legal precedent has established that the institution itself also has a respon-

sibility to the client. It is in recognition of these factors that the rights of clients are affirmed.

   Clients have become increasingly concerned and vocal about the level of care they expect to receive.

Table 20–3
NFLPN Specialized Nursing Practice Standards

The Licensed Practical/Vocational Nurse

  1. Shall have had at least one year's experience in nursing at the staff level.

  2. Shall present personal qualifications that are indicative of potential abilities for practice in the chosen specialized nursing area.

  3. Shall present evidence of completion of a program or course that is approved by an appropriate agency to provide the knowledge and skills necessary for effective nursing services in the specialized field.

  4. Shall meet all of the standards of practice as set forth in this document.

Many agencies now issue "client's rights" statements upon admission. Some require that the client or a family member acknowledge receiving the statement by signing a form. Table 20–5 contains a summary of 24 issues addressed in the Minnesota "Patients' Bill of Rights."

▽▽▽
Legal Aspects of Nursing and the Legal System

To understand the connection between legal aspects of nursing and the legal system in the United States and Canada, a brief review of the legal system is in order. The legal system in both countries originates in the English common law system. Because it originates in the courts, common law is called judge-made law. Common law is one way of establishing standards of legal conduct. It is useful in settling disputes. Once the judge has made a decision, this decision *sets the precedent* for a ruling on a case with similar facts in the future.

  Laws developed by the legislative branch of the state and the federal government are called statutory laws. The nurse practice act, which governs the practice of nursing, is an example of a statutory law. Each state

has its own nurse practice act. States can make these laws as long as the items in their laws do not conflict with any federal statutes.

▽▽▽
Types of Legal Action

The two classifications of legal action are civil actions and criminal actions. A civil action is related to individual rights. It involves the relationship between individuals and the violation of those rights. For example, if you cause harm by administering an incorrect medication, the client can bring a civil action suit against you. Guilt on the part of the nurse can be established by a preponderance (majority) of the evidence. If the nurse is found guilty, monetary compensation is a typical punishment. A criminal action involves persons and society as a whole. It involves relationships between individuals and the government. If a nurse takes it upon herself to remove a life-sustaining device and the client dies, this is considered murder. A criminal action suit would be filed against the nurse. Guilt on the part of the nurse needs to be established by the production of proof beyond a reasonable doubt. Punishment can be death, imprisonment, fines, or restriction of personal liberties.

▽▽▽
Steps in Bringing a Legal Action

Legal actions follow an orderly process.

  1. The client believes that his or her legal rights have been violated by the nurse.

  2. The client seeks the advice of an attorney.

  3. The attorney has a *nurse expert* review the client's chart to see if the nurse has *violated the nursing standard of care*. If it is determined that a standard of care has been violated, a *lawsuit* is begun.

  4. The client (the plaintiff) files a *complaint* that documents the *grievance* (violation of rules). This is served to the defendant (the nurse).

  5. The defendant responds *in writing*.

  6. The *discovery* period (pretrial activity) begins. Statements are taken from the defendant nurse, witnesses, nurse expert, the client (plaintiff), and other care

Table 20–4
NAPNES Standards of Practice for Licensed Practical/Vocational Nurses

NAPNES has set the standards for nursing practice of LP/VNs since 1941. The following standards represent the foundation for the provision of safe and competent nursing practice. Competency implies knowledge, understanding, and skills that transcend specific tasks and is guided by a commitment to ethical/legal principles.

This statement of standards is intended for nursing educators, health-care administrators, nurses, and health-care consumers.

The LP/VN Provides Individual and Family-Centered Nursing Care by:

A. Utilizing appropriate knowledge, skills, and abilities.
B. Utilizing principles of the nursing process in meeting specific patient needs in diversified health-care settings.
C. Maintaining appropriate written documentation and utilizing effective communication skills with patients, family, significant others, and members of the health team.
D. Executing principles of crisis intervention to maintain safety.
E. Providing appropriate education to patients, family, and significant others to promote health, facilitate rehabilitation, and maintain wellness.
F. Serving as a patient advocate to protect patient rights.

The LP/VN Fulfills the Professional Responsibilities of the Practical/Vocational Nurse by:

A. Applying the ethical principles underlying the profession.
B. Following legal requirements.
C. Following the policies and procedures of the employing facility.
D. Cooperating and collaborating with all members of the health-care team to meet the needs of family-centered nursing care.
E. Assuming accountability for his/her nursing actions.
F. Seeking educational opportunities to improve knowledge and skills.

From NAPNES, 1400 Spring St, Suite 310, Silver Spring, MD 20910. Revised 1993.

givers. Policies and procedures of the health care facilities are reviewed.

7. During the *trial*, important information is presented to the judge or jury. A *verdict* (decision) is reached. The plaintiff (the client) has the burden of proof (evidence of wrongdoing) during the trial.

8. An *appeal* (request for another trial) can be made if the verdict is not considered acceptable by either the plaintiff or the defendant.

▼▼▼
Specific Legal Terms and Concepts

▽▽▽
Nurse Practice Acts

The duties and functions that nurses can perform are defined on the state level by the nurse practice act. The nurse practice act of each state defines what nursing is, what it is not, and under what circumstances it can be

Table 20–5
Patients' Bill of Rights

1. Information About Rights
2. Courteous Treatment
3. Appropriate Health Care
4. Physician's Identity
5. Relationship with Other Health Services
6. Information About Treatment
7. Participation in Planning Treatment
8. Continuity of Care
9. Right to Refuse Care
10. Experimental Research
11. Freedom From Maltreatment
12. Treatment Privacy
13. Confidentiality of Records
14. Disclosure of Services Available
15. Responsive Service
16. Personal Privacy
17. Grievances
18. Communication Privacy
19. Personal Property
20. Services for the Facility
21. Protection and Advocacy Services
22. Right to Communication Disclosure and Right to Associate
23. Isolation and Restraints
24. Treatment Plan

Summary of issues addressed in Minnesota Statute 144.651. Patients' Bill of Rights. Published by Minnesota Hospital and Healthcare Partnership. 2550 West University Ave. Suite 350 S St. Paul, MN 55114 (612-641-1121)

In 1981 a practical nursing organization, the National Association of Practical Nurse Education and Service (NAPNES), issued the following statement of responsibilities required for practice as a practical or vocational nurse:

▶ Recognizes the LPN or LVN's role in the health care delivery system and articulates that role with those of other health care team members
▶ Maintains accountability for one's own nursing practice within the ethical and legal framework
▶ Serves as a client advocate
▶ Accepts a role in maintaining developing standards of practice in providing health care
▶ Seeks further growth through educational opportunities

Statements from official nursing organizations do not carry the weight of law. They are useful as a guide for behavior and may be used in a court of law as a point of reference. *The nurse practice act of your state is your final authority.*

Terms Used in Nurse Practice Acts

Terminology remains standard in many states. As you study the standards of practice for licensed or trained practical nurses in your state, knowledge of the following terms may be helpful.

Basic Nursing Care. Nursing care that can be performed safely by the LPN or LVN, based on knowledge and skills gained during the educational program. Modifications of care are unnecessary, and client response is predictable.

Basic Client Situation. Situation as determined by the RN. Client's clinical condition is predictable. Medical and nursing orders are not changing continuously. They do not contain complex modifications. The client's clinical condition requires only basic nursing care.

Complex Nursing Situation. Situation as assessed by an RN. Client's clinical condition is not predictable. Medical or nursing orders are likely to involve continu-

practiced for compensation. The nurse practice act provides the administrative rules and regulations under which a nurse functions as an LPN or LVN.

It is necessary for practical nurses to understand that they must limit their work to the area of practical nursing defined in their state's nurse practice act. Practical nurses must realize that *no physician, registered professional nurse, or agency can give them the right to do more than what can be done legally.*

ous changes or complex modifications. Nursing care expectations are beyond that learned by the LPN or LVN during the educational program.

Delegated Medical Act.   Doctor's orders given to an RN, LPN, or LVN by a physician, dentist, or podiatrist.

Delegated Nursing Act.   Nursing orders given to an RN, LPN, or LVN by an RN.

Direct Supervision.   Supervisor is continuously present to coordinate, direct, or inspect nursing care. Supervisor is in the building.

General Supervision.   Supervisor regularly coordinates, directs, or inspects nursing care and is within reach either in the building or by telephone.

Licensure

Upon completion of a state-approved LPN or LVN nursing education program, a graduate is eligible to apply to take a national licensing examination in practical nursing (NCLEX-PN). Each state has established its own criteria for passing the examination.

States also have made arrangements for interstate *endorsements* for nurses who choose to work in other states. This means that it is possible to work in another state without repeating the NCLEX-PN if you have met that state's criteria for passing. Check Appendix A for the location of your state licensing board. All nurse practice acts address nursing licensure. Depending on the state in which you work, licensure will be mandatory or permissive.

Mandatory licensure protects, by law, the role of the nurse (that is, what nurses do). This means that anyone who practices nursing must be licensed. Permissive licensure protects the title of the nurse but not what nurses do. This means that the practical nurse may practice nursing without a license but cannot use the title LPN or LVN. Because of permissive licensure, unlicensed persons may perform nursing skills performed by the practical nurse.

> **Which kind of license is required in your state?**

Some boards of nursing are instituting on-line verification of nursing licensure. The Minnesota Board of Nursing reported in 1995 that it has contracted with the Minnesota Department of Administration to provide on-line verification of information about licensed practical nurses (Minnesota Board of Nursing, 1995, p. 4). The Board provides public information about nurses who have current registration. The verification system enables callers to obtain a nurse's license number, registration expiration date, and whether any Board action has taken place. The service is available 24 hours a day, every day. Employers will be able to use this option to comply with requirements for written verification of a nurse's registration by the Joint Commission on Accreditation of Healthcare Organizations.

The practice of licensing was instituted by nurses themselves. Nurses were concerned about the nursing care that they delivered and the safety of their clients.

All states and provinces have examining councils, which provide nursing examinations for licensure and review complaints that can lead to revocation of a license. Because of the sheer numbers of complaints received and the small number of board members, it is difficult to review all complaints. (Some states employ a compliance officer, who investigates suspected cases of drug or alcohol abuse.) Revocation (removal or elimination of) a license is a serious matter. Boards of nursing are taking a rehabilitative rather than a punitive stance to drug abuse and are limiting, suspending, or revoking licenses. Rarely are revocations due to incompetence in nursing practice or failure to update nursing skills. However, boards of nursing may limit, suspend, or deny renewal of a license because of violations of the nurse practice act.

> **What happens to the LPN whose license is revoked because of drug abuse and who remains untreated?**

▽▽▽
Standards of Care

There is a phrase used in nursing that has important legal implications: You are held to the nursing standard of care. The standard of care is based on what an ordinary, prudent nurse with similar education and experience would do or not do in similar circumstances. Resources for the nursing standard of care are

▶ Nurse practice act: Identifies the minimum level of competence necessary for you to function as a LPN or LVN in your state.

▶ Nursing licensure examination (NCLEX-PN): Tests for *minimum* competence.

▶ Practical nursing programs: Based on guidelines provided by the board of nursing, these programs guarantee a minimum knowledge base and clinical practice necessary to provide safe nursing care. Curricula, textbooks, and instructors are resources for information about the standard of care.

▶ Written policies and procedures: The agency for which you work provides a standard of nursing care for you to follow. This is the reason why it is important for you to read the policies of the agency to find out whether verbal directions are supported by written policies. If ever a question about care comes up in court, a lawyer will use the hospital policy and procedure manual as one guide to expected behavior. Remember that policies and procedures *do not* overrule your state's nurse practice act and educational preparation. However, institutional policies may be more strict than state law.

▶ Custom: An unwritten, usually acceptable way of giving nursing care. Expert witnesses would be called to testify to "the acceptable way," not your coworkers.

▶ Law: Decisions that have been arrived at in similar cases brought up before a court (judge-made law).

▶ Statements from the NFLPN and NAPNES.

▶ Nursing texts and journals.

▶ Administrative rules of your board of nursing.

▽▽▽
Tort and Tort Law

A tort is a wrong or injury done to someone that violates his or her rights. Tort law is based on the premise that in the course of relationships with each other there is a general duty to avoid injuring others. Torts are divided into unintentional and intentional torts.

Unintentional Torts

Negligence and *malpractice* are examples of unintentional torts. "Negligence is the unintentional tort of *acting* or *failing to act* as an ordinary, reasonable, prudent person with resulting harm to the person to whom the duty of care is owed" (Sorenson and Luckman, 1995, p. 52). Malpractice means negligence by a professional. In nursing, it relates to an action or lack of action, not to what you intended to do. Good intentions do not enter in. As a nurse you are held responsible for your conduct. *Student nurses are held to a level of a licensed nurse's performance.* The nurse's conduct, not his or her state of mind, is the issue.

Elements Necessary for Negligence. Duty, breach of duty, proximate cause, and damages are the four elements that must be present to cause an action for negligence against the nurse. Each of the four elements must be proved by the client to receive compensation. *Duty* refers to the nurse's responsibility to provide care in an acceptable way. The nurse has a duty based on her education as well as the expectations and standards of his or her place of employment. *Breach of duty* means that the nurse did not adhere to the nursing standard of care. What was expected of the nurse was not done (omission) or was not done correctly (commission). *Proximate cause* means that a reasonable cause-and-effect relationship can be shown between the omission or commission of the nursing act and the harm to the client. Did the nurse's negligent act cause the injury in question? *Damages* means that the client must be able to show that the nurse's negligent act injured him or her in some way. The client must prove actual damage.

Intentional Torts

Intentional torts require a specific state of mind, that is, that the nurse involved intended to do the wrongful act. Significantly, not all insurance companies cover intentional torts in their malpractice insurance policies. Check your policy. Examples of intentional torts include

▶ Assault and Battery: *Assault* is an unjustified attempt or threat to touch someone. *Battery* is actual physical harm to someone. Remember this when a client refuses a treatment or medication. The client gives implied consent (permission) for certain routine treatments by entering the institution. Clients retain the right to refuse verbally any treatment and may leave the institution when they choose unless they are there for court-ordered treatment. Nurses can protect themselves from assaultive clients but can use only as much force as is considered reasonable to protect themselves.

▶ **False imprisonment** and use of restraints: False imprisonment is keeping someone detained against his or her will. It can include use of restraints or seclusion in a room without cause and without a doctor's order. Restraint by verbal threats of physical harm is also included in this category.

How does the Patient's Bill of Rights relate to the care of an elderly confused client?

▶ **Defamation:** Defamation means damage to someone's reputation through false or unprivileged communication. **Libel** is defamation through written communication or pictures. **Slander** is defamation by verbalizing untrue or private information (gossip) to a third party. Clients have the right to expect that you will share information about them only with health care providers who are actively involved in promoting their health. This is called **confidentiality.** The client has the right to expect you to speak the truth. Additional unnecessary conversation with coworkers and those outside of the agency can result in a charge of defamation. The same is true of all documented information or of invasion of their privacy by taking unwanted photographs or showing their affliction to others, students included, without permission. The client's privacy is protected by law. Remember: Loose lips may sink your ship.

You and other health care providers have the same right to privacy. You often are privy to information about the personal lives of nurses, physicians, and other coworkers. Although the desire to repeat the information you hear may be tempting, it is best left unsaid.

▼▼▼
Common Causes of Nursing Liability

Many of the errors leading to common nursing liabilities can be avoided by following the guidelines you learned in nursing school.

In what major areas are you evaluated during each clinical rotation?

The major areas of liability can be categorized as lack of safety, knowledge, skill, observation and reporting, documentation, and acceptance of responsibility for nursing actions—all of which are part of the usual clinical evaluation. The most common errors are drug errors, most of which can be avoided if you follow the guidelines you learn in basic nursing and practice in the clinical areas. Other recurring areas of liability include falls, burns, failure to note and report changes in condition, error in client identity, infection or cross-infection resulting from lack of aseptic technique, inability to recognize and to refuse to follow improper doctor's orders, and failure to note client allergies. One of the best defenses against malpractice is development of rapport with the client. The very best defense is to not err in the first place. Always function within the standard of care.

▽▽▽
Charting

Documentation is part of your job. It is not busy work. Legal documentation is basic nursing in all institutions. The forms may be different, but the basics remain the same. The chart is a legal document and can be used in court. Be sure to review the charting procedure for your specific institution and adhere to it. Legal charting is also an opportunity for you to show that you have a legitimate knowledge base. It gives credibility to practical nursing as a vocation. Charting gives you the opportunity to show that you functioned within the standard of care.

General Guidelines for Legal Documentation

Traditional methods of charting include source-oriented (narrative charting) and problem-oriented (Subjective Objective Assessment Plan [SOAP], Subjective Objective Assessment Plan Intervention Evaluation [SOAPIE], Subjective Objective Assessment Plan Intervention Evaluation Revision [SOAPIER], and Subjective Objective Plan [SOP] charting). These traditional methods are being replaced by (1) focus charting (use of focus to label nurse's notes, categories of data, action and response, and flowsheets), and (2) charting by exception (nursing/physician order flowsheets used to document assessments and intervention). All formats are being adapted to the computer.

Regardless of which method of charting is used by an institution, the following guidelines apply:

1. Date and time should accompany each entry.

2. Each entry should be accurate, factual, specific, and objective. Nurses must consistently remind themselves to avoid subjective comments when charting. Subjective comments are judgments made by you. Avoid them. Eliminate the word "appears" except when the client is sleeping.

3. Each entry must be legible, spelled correctly, and grammatically correct. A lawyer can question your ability to give competent nursing care if you do not have command of the English language. Print, if this is an agency policy or if your handwriting is hard to read. Use correct punctuation because the meaning of a sentence can change based on punctuation. Sloppy charting may be interpreted as sloppy or unsafe nursing care. It communicates that you did not take the time to write, and a lawyer could accuse you of not taking the time to care.

4. Charting entries are always entered in chronologic order. This indicates when the event happened in the time column. If someone else charts before you are able to record an entry or if you have forgotten to record an entry, a late entry may be used. Put the actual charting time in the time column for the late entry and include the actual date and time of the events in the nurses' notes. Place entries on the chart as soon as possible after they occur. The time column indicates the time the event took place, not the time of charting.

5. For written entries, use permanent ink (no erasable pens) in the color identified in the institution's procedure manual. The trend is toward use of black ink and military time. Avoid using highlighters on any chart form. Many do not show up on Xerox or fax copies.

6. Do not leave blank lines or spaces in charting. If an item on a flowsheet does not apply, write in N/A (not applicable). If other staff persons need to make an entry, do not save lines. They can make a late entry. Write your signature immediately after the period.

7. Ditto marks are never used.

8. *Use only approved abbreviations as found in the institution's policy and procedure manual.*

9. Document medical and nursing treatments performed and the client's response to these treatments. If the client refuses these treatments, document the reason for refusal.

10. Chart physician phone orders. Document communication with supervisors by name and content of conversation.

11. As an LPN or LVN, do not co-sign for nursing students. If you must sign off a client chart that is not for one of your clients, write, "I'm signing this to complete the record; I have no knowledge of the client."

12. Do not add any notes once charting is complete unless you use a *late entry format.*

13. Do not delete notes or correct errors with "white out" on written notes. When an error is made in charting, draw a single line through the error, write in the date and time, and sign. Do not write "error" above the entry; instead, write "incorrect entry."

14. Record all abnormal observations, including changes in the client's condition and to whom these observations were reported.

15. Record care actually given, not care that will be given in the future.

16. Each dated and timed entry must be signed using your full, legal title as determined by your state.

17. If you did not chart it, you did not do it, and a lawyer will surmise that you did not care!

18. Avoid treating flowsheets casually. If you place a symbol indicating normal findings, be sure you have

reviewed the institution's parameters for normal findings. These can usually be found on the flowsheet.

▼▼▼
Additional Legal Concerns

▽▽▽
Employer Liability

The employer may be held responsible for acts performed by the nurse within the scope of employment. However, the employer may sue the nurse to recover fees and other monies involved while defending him or her.

▽▽▽
Verbal Orders

Verbal orders should not be accepted except in emergency situations. Written orders by the physician protect the doctor, the client, and the nurse. It is difficult to explain to a court why the physician, who has access to the chart, did not write the order. *Verbal orders should be repeated for accuracy.*

▽▽▽
Telephone Orders

When used, physician orders conveyed by telephone should be given directly to the nurse, who repeats the order back to the doctor. Spelling of medications or treatments is checked if necessary. So many medications sound alike, and doses can be confusing. If it is a sensitive order, meaning one that carries special risk, two people should listen to the order. (This is suggested for all telephone orders.)

Be sure to check the policy of your employer about the legality of an LPN accepting phone orders.

▽▽▽
Telephone Advice

Providing telephone advice is not part of the LPN practice of nursing in many states. Similarly, avoid calling in a reorder for medication without the explicit direction of the physician. This is considered practicing medicine and is a shortcut to a lawsuit for you.

▽▽▽
Telephone Logs

Telephone logs can be used routinely to document the time, problem, and advice received or given. Also, attempted calls to physicians or supervisors should be logged in.

▽▽▽
Discharge Instructions and Client Education

The professional nurse, physician, podiatrist, or dentist initiates health teaching for clients. The practical nurse reinforces this teaching. Teaching is the domain of the professional nurse, and LPNs play a supportive role in it, once the instruction or education has been started by the RN. Discharge instructions are given verbally and in writing, with the client signing a form indicating that he or she understands the information. Preprinted information forms are valuable and are available in many agencies. The practical nurse initiates client teaching in the area of basic health care. Examples include:

- ▶ How to avoid constipation
- ▶ Pyramid diet
- ▶ Cleanliness
- ▶ How to avoid colds
- ▶ Babysitting hints
- ▶ Parenting techniques

▽▽▽
Incident Reports

Incident reports are intended to provide in-house improvements in care. They are administration records required by federal law so that agencies can see patterns and correct them. Incident reports are written as soon as possible after the occurrences by the health providers who witnessed the incident. They are objective. Let others draw conclusions. They should be written with the thought that they may be viewed by attorneys on the "other side." The client's description of what happened should be included. The report should be legible, factual, and objective; it should be in permanent ink, and it should not be worded to accept or place blame. (If something is found on the floor, the report should state "found on floor," not "fell.") Although the incident itself is also recorded on the client's chart, avoid writing "incident report filed" on the chart.

General Consent

General consent is obtained for treating a client upon admission. It may be obtained by the LPN. The fact that a person has voluntarily sought admission to a health care agency and willingly signs a general admission form is an example of general consent. A client may revoke this permission verbally.

Informed Consent

Informed consent must be obtained for invasive procedures ordered for therapeutic or diagnostic purposes (for example, surgery). Informed consent means that the client is told in nontechnical language

- ▶ What the treatment is
- ▶ What the risks are
- ▶ What the alternative treatments are
- ▶ Who will perform the treatment
- ▶ Whether the treatment is really necessary

The client must indicate that he *understands* this information.

Parents cannot give informed consent for the treatment of their children, but they can authorize treatment for their children up to a certain age. Courts of law recognize that parents generally authorize what is appropriate for their children.

In most states informed consent is the responsibility of the doctor because he or she must explain the implications and complications of the procedure to the client before written permission is obtained. The client may revoke this permission verbally.

Access to Medical Records

The medical record belongs to the hospital. The client has the right to see the record. The practical nurse, however, does not have the authority to give the record to the client. Refer client requests to view the medical record to your supervisor and the physician.

Abandonment

You may not leave your place of employment until you can transfer the care of clients to your replacement. Notify your supervisor if you are short-staffed. Follow this with a memo because a memo is more effective than verbal notification alone. Keep a copy for yourself.

Duty to Refuse to Carry Out Improper Orders

A doctor's written or verbal order is a legal order that the nurse must carry out. However, the nurse has the responsibility to recognize whether an order may harm the client and refuse to carry it out. Deal directly with the physician first. If this is unsuccessful, use the nursing chain of command, beginning with your immediate supervisor. To avoid harm to the client, if the problem is not resolved through the nursing channels, it must reach the physician chain of command quickly. Document the order in the nursing notes and prepare an incident report identifying "inappropriate MD behavior." *Remember:* Always check out any order a client questions before carrying it out.

Standing Orders

Some states do not allow standing orders except in intensive and coronary care units. Because standing orders call for making judgments, the practical nurse must always check first with the RN before carrying them out.

No-Code Orders

No-code orders are legal orders written by the physician and do not have to be updated unless the client changes his mind. If a written no-code order does not exist and the nurse does not code the client, the nurse is in effect making a medical decision. The nurse is practicing medicine without a license and may be subject to a lawsuit. There is no such thing as a partial or slow code. All care givers must know when a written no-code order exists. Check your state and agency policy regarding no-code orders.

▽▽▽
Written Client Directives

There are two types of written directives available to clients as a way of stating their personal wishes regarding future health care. These directives are the *living will* and the *durable power of attorney*. Both are written by the client while he or she is mentally competent.

Living Will. This document is filled out by the individual and witnessed by a person who will not benefit by the death of that individual. Living wills are recognized as legal documents in 38 states in the United States and the District of Columbia. They are not recognized as legal documents in Canada. The individual generally is advised to give a witnessed copy to the health care provider and a trusted friend or relation and to keep one copy for himself in a location that is easily accessible. If a person is moving to or spending time in another state, he or she is advised to determine whether the living will is considered legal in that state. Otherwise, he may discover too late that the written directives will not be honored.

Durable Power of Attorney (DPOA). This document, sometimes known as the durable medical power of attorney, is a legal document throughout the United States. As an LPN, it is necessary for you to understand the scope and execution of the DPOA in your state or province. Choice in Dying (CID) is a national nonprofit organization dedicated to serving the needs of dying clients and their families. This organization has pio-

neered in making advanced directives for 25 years. CID advocates the right of clients to participate fully in making decisions about their medical treatment at the end of life. CID will provide one free copy of an approved directive for your state. If additional copies are desired or if a directive is desired for a different state in addition to your state, a $4.00 fee per request is suggested. Contact Choice in Dying, 200 Varick Street, New York, NY 10014 (212-366-5540, Fax 212-366-5337).

The DPOA has three major provisions:

1. It identifies who will make decisions for the person in a medical situation if he or she is unable to speak for himself or herself.

2. It identifies the extent of treatment desired by the person if the person is in a coma or a persistent vegetative state.

3. It lists the medical treatments that the person would never want performed.

The role of the next of kin in making decisions about care for the client differs from state to state.

▽▽▽
Signing a Will

Nurses may witness the signing of a will if they do not stand to gain personally from the will. Check your agency policy before doing so.

As a student, check with your instructor before you agree to witness the signing of a will. If the instructor gives approval, you must document in the client's record that you witnessed the signing of a will. Be sure you do not gain personally from the will.

▽▽▽
Removal of Life Support Systems

The doctor must pronounce the client dead and document this status *before* the nurse turns off the ventilator.

▽▽▽
Malpractice Insurance for Nurses

More nurses are being sued. Nurses are responsible for their own acts. Although the employing agency may assume responsibility for the nurse during a lawsuit, it can then turn around and sue the nurse itself. Did you know that you can also be held responsible for the "neighborhood advice" you give—for example, telling a neighbor how to care for her sick child?

Each nurse must carefully consider whether it is necessary to purchase a malpractice insurance policy. Although incidents of suing for malpractice continue, your chances of being sued as an LPN are statistically small. Look carefully at the circumstances that are a part of the agency of which you are an employee. See Table 20–6.

Table 20–6
Malpractice

Reasons for your own malpractice insurance coverage.

1. The jury's award could exceed the limits of your agency's coverage.

2. Your employing agency could pay out an award to a plaintiff and then countersue you.

3. You acted outside the scope of employment and the agency argues it is not liable.

4. Your employer's policy covers you only on the job.

5. An agency might carry a policy that covers you only while you are employed by that institution and a suit may come up years after you have stopped working for an employer. It is suggested that nurses purchase *occurrence* coverage and not *claims coverage*. For this reason, occurrence coverage protects the nurse for each incident regardless of present employer.

6. Agency may decide to settle out of court. Plaintiff could pursue a case against the nurse.

7. Has your employer paid the insurance premium?

8. After a settlement, insurers could turn around and sue the nurse.

9. With your own coverage, you will have your own lawyers, not the lawyers also defending the agency.

▽▽▽
Liability of Student Nurses and Instructors

Student nurses are held accountable for the nursing care they give. They are held to the standards of a licensed practical nurse. This emphasizes the necessity of:

1. Preparation for working in the clinical area. The instructor is held responsible for making sure that the student assigned to a client has the necessary knowledge base and skill to give safe nursing care. The instructor is also expected to provide reasonable supervision for the care given by a student.

2. Requesting additional help or supervision if needed.

3. Complying with agency and school of nursing policies.

▽▽▽
Floating

"Floating" is working in an area that is not your usual work area. In 1991, the Joint Commission on Accreditation of Healthcare Organizations (JCAHO) revised its nursing care standards that are used as a basis for making accreditation decisions. One of the standards states that nursing staff should be competent to fulfill their assigned responsibilities. Directives from the Joint Commission include the need for timely and adequate orientation and cross-training. Practical nurses need to receive adequate orientation, cross-training, and education for float duty. You are responsible for informing supervisors if you do not feel competent to work in any assigned area.

▽▽▽
Unlicensed Assistive Personnel

The use of unlicensed assistive personnel (UAP) to provide client care has grown dramatically in recent years. It is expected that the trend will continue. These unlicensed persons are trained to perform a variety of nursing tasks. Supervision of UAPs by the RN to ensure safety of client care is a major concern. The responsibility for the act delegated can never be given away. There is concern that because of the lack of licensed nurses in an agency, duties will be delegated inappropriately to UAPs. It is the RNs and LPNs who stand to lose their jobs and licenses if the care provided by UAPs does not meet the standards of safety and effectiveness. The training program for UAPs does not provide the same depth in education and experience that programs for licensed nurses provide. Licensed nurses are also accountable to both their employers and their state nursing boards.

▽▽▽
Reporting Incompetence of Other Health Providers

A drug- or alcohol-abusing nurse should be reported. Incidents supporting this report should be documented. This is a moral, ethical, and legal responsibility. A nurse must determine at the beginning of a nursing career who is the top priority, and the answer must be the client.

▽▽▽
Money and Gifts

Nurses should not accept money or gifts from clients. People in some cultures may feel that it is an insult to turn down their offer of a gift. The nurse might tactfully suggest that a gift be given to the facility instead.

▽▽▽
Good Samaritan Acts

Good Samaritan acts stipulate that a person who renders emergency care in good faith at the scene of an accident is immune from civil liability for his or her action while providing the care. The state statutes are of special concern to nurses and physicians who provide emergency care outside of the agency that employs them.

> *What does your state's Good Samaritan Act say?*

▽▽▽
Physical and Emotional Abuse

In the course of your career in practical nursing you will probably suspect or actually see the results of some type of abuse. As a practical nurse, you have a legal responsibility to report your suspicions or observations of abuse by following your facility's abuse policy. Note that a "suspicion" is a nagging doubt. Refer to your state's abuse laws for specific rules that govern your responsibility for reporting abuse. It is important to be empathetic (as opposed to sympathetic) so that your observations or reporting will be as objective as possible. Becoming a part of the client's emotions may lead you to jump to conclusions or accept a particularly convincing but untrue explanation. Whether the client is a child, woman, man, or elder, reputations are at stake. Once an accusation has been made, it is difficult to be truly free from it, even when it has been proved groundless.

Follow your facility's policy for reporting abuse. The social services department can be helpful in helping you report abuse. Offer concrete, specific observations. Quote statements made and avoid offering a personal interpretation. Let the facts speak for themselves.

▽▽▽
Euthanasia

Euthanasia is referred to as mercy killing. It is *actively* assisting with a killing or permitting the death of a person who is terminally ill. Euthanasia is not the same as a no-code order written by a physician based on a decision made by the physician and the client or the family. A no-code order is a *passive* action with the goal of avoiding prolonging life unnecessarily, not actively ending it.

The National League for Nursing news release (September 1995) stated

> President of Oregon League of Nursing to head task force. Committee will produce guidelines for nurses making decisions about assisted suicide for terminally ill clients.

This action was taken in response to legislation passed in Oregon during 1994 that permits physicians to provide "aid in dying to qualified citizens requesting such assistance." The guidelines that emerge from this task force are important to nurses because (1) the legislation is a *legal* act that can potentially affect all health care workers including LPNs and LVNs, and (2) although nurses are responsible for their own ethical choices and actions, guidelines are needed to assist nurses in making decisions in this area without recrimination.

With the permission of the instructor, divide into groups. Choose a viewpoint you do not usually hold. Be prepared to present reasons for the viewpoint. Choose a spokesperson to summarize the group views.

1. Group 1: Terminally ill clients have the right to choose death by physician-assisted suicide.
2. Group 2: Terminally ill clients must wait to die of natural causes.
3. Group 3: The nurse's personal ethic conflicts with decision (Group 1 and 2 decision). Discuss the nurse's rights, roles, and responsibilities to the client.

Refer again to the critical thinking steps on page 296, to assist you in making your decision.

▽▽▽
Organ Donation

Organ donations are voluntary. At this time they cannot be bought or sold. Although many clients and families give permission for organ donation after death, the demand for organs far exceeds supply. You may have been asked to agree to personal organ donation at the time you got your driver's license. Many states participate in this effort. It has been suggested that money be given for organs to cover funeral expenses and so on to increase the number of donors.

Body tissues that can be donated include skin, cornea, bone, heart valves, and blood. Donated body organs include the heart, liver, kidneys, lungs, and pancreas. One example of a successful body tissue transplant was the transplantation of umbilical cord blood for a rare genetic bone disease at the University of Minnesota (Duluth News-Tribune, 11/11/95). Approximately one cup of blood taken from a newborn's discarded umbilical cord and placenta was donated.

Organ donation has raised both ethical and legal questions in some instances. For example, having a baby so select organs or body tissues can be used to save a sibling.

> *What ethical and legal issues do you see in the issue of organ donation?*

▽▽▽
Accountability in Nursing

You have learned that nursing demands that you be responsible. This means being reliable and trustworthy. At no time can you expect a peer, supervisor, or client to say to you, "It's OK that you didn't come to work today because your car isn't functioning properly," or "It's OK if we talk about your interests and problems today" (rather than those of the clients), or "It's OK that you didn't do the work you were assigned because you're having a bad day." Nursing says, "I'm sorry that you have problems to cope with that are heavy, but it's up to you to deal with them because your priority, in this vocation, is the client."

The word accountability means that you are answerable. As a nursing student you are answerable to yourself, to your assigned client, to the team leader, to the physician, and to your instructor, who constantly evaluates your work. As an LPN, accountability to the instructor is replaced by accountability to the employing agency. You are held accountable for all of the nursing actions that you perform or are assigned to perform. The measures of accountability are the nursing standards of practice (see Tables 20–2, 20–3, and 20–4). Using this knowledge through theory classes to provide nursing care to clients also helps. Many of the issues of both responsibility and accountability become an integral part of you.

▼▼▼
Putting It Together: Values, Ethics, and Legal Issues

As you read the following two situations, see yourself as the LPN who has to answer the following questions:

What will you do based on your values, nursing ethics, and the legal issues involved?

How will your decision help you to maintain responsibility and accountability in nursing?

▽▽▽
Situation 1

Amanda K. Havana, age 68, has experienced a hemorrhage, resulting in a significant loss of blood. She has been rushed from the nursing home to the hospital emergency room. The physician determines that a blood transfusion is needed immediately to save her life. You have accompanied Mrs. Havana to the emergency room. You inform the physician that Mrs. Havana adheres to the beliefs of the Jehovah's Witnesses (Watchtower Bible and Tract Society). Mrs. Havana confirms this and further states that she does not want blood, and if she dies for lack of it, "so be it." Although the practical nurse does not usually administer blood, you need to be alert to the ethical and legal issues evoked by the client's refusal to have a transfusion.

What belief holds Mrs. Havana firm in her refusal of a blood transfusion? She believes that the Bible is God's word and the truth, and that all of God's laws presented in the Bible must be obeyed. Based on

Genesis 9:3-4, Leviticus 17:10, and Acts 15:28-29, Jehovah's Witnesses equate blood with life and believe that taking blood into one's body through the mouth or veins is a violation of God's law (Anderson, 1983, p. 32). Mrs. Havana accepts her possible death because of refusal to accept a transfusion as dying in accordance with her beliefs, not as suicide. She is receptive to other options that do not violate her beliefs.

According to the *Emergency Nurse Legal Bulletin* (1982, p. 2), "treating a client without consent is a battery whether or not the treatment is medically beneficial." The physician may attempt to get a court order to allow the transfusion. However, "when the client is fully competent, is not pregnant and has no children, a court is unlikely to compel a life-saving blood transfusion over the client's refusal." When faced with a similar situation, the practical nurse respects the client's belief system and notifies the supervisor for further advice or interpretation.

▽▽▽
Situation 2

You are employed in a pediatric unit. An infant admitted immediately after birth for emergency surgery is facing death. According to the parent's faith, the infant must be baptized. Because you are Baptist, you do not believe in infant baptism.

Look again at the questions presented to you at the beginning of this section. Discuss with your classmates the alternatives available to you that will fulfill the client's and parent's needs without compromising your values, nursing ethics, and nursing standards of care.

▼▼▼ S U M M A R Y

▶ Personal ethics are the building blocks of your nursing ethics. They are made up of what you believe in, value, and practice in your personal life. Your personal and professional ethics modify as you continue your personal and professional growth. Critical thinking provides the steps that allow sound ethical decisions to be made.

▶ Sometimes your ethical views differ from legal realities. In nursing, your state's nurse practice act provides the basis for the legal parameters governing your nursing practice. *Know it well.* When ethical questions arise, the legal system becomes involved in determining what can and cannot be done.

▶ Nursing ethics are based on the principles of autonomy, beneficence, nonmaleficence, and justice. Autonomy says, "the client has the right to decide." Beneficence says, "do good." Nonmaleficence says, "do no harm." Justice says, "give all clients their due." These are basic principles to keep in mind as new ethical questions arise.

▶ Tort law is based on doing no harm in relationships. In nursing it refers to the professional relationship between the client and the nurse. Torts are either unintentional or intentional. Negligence and malpractice are examples of unintentional torts—"performance less than the standard of practice." Assault and battery, false imprisonment (including use of restraints without orders), and defamation of character are all examples of intentional torts.

▶ Check out the philosophy, mission statement, and policies of your potential place of employment *before* you accept the job. You cannot abandon your client in the middle of a legal procedure because your ethics differ from those of the client.

▶ The living will and the durable power of attorney are two ways in which an individual can express his or her wishes in regard to medical interventions in a major medical event. The living will is legal in most but not all states in the United States. It is not legal in Canada. The durable power of attorney provides for a legal decision maker if the client is unable to make decisions. It is legal in all states, but each state form may differ.

▶ You have the responsibility of knowing the law—the nurse practice act of your state. It is a major resource for the nursing standards of care. Nurses are held accountable for their nursing actions, and ignorance of the law is not accepted as an excuse for illegal or unethical practices.

▶ Common areas of nursing liability most often can be avoided by following the guidelines learned in basic nursing. Medication errors are number one on the list of recurring liabilities. To avoid liability, function within the standard of care. Keep current. Take classes. Read journals. The worst questions an LPN can hear from a lawyer are, "You haven't taken *any* classes since you graduated?", "You do not subscribe to a nursing journal?", and "You do not belong to your professional organization?"

▶ Pay attention to the ethical guidelines put forth by your professional organization. Join your professional organization and take advantage of current updates. Have a voice in what becomes the law.

▶ Guidelines for nursing ethics have been developed by the International Council of Nurses (ICN), the National Federation of Licensed Practical Nurses (NFLPN), and the National Association of Practical Nurse Education and Service (NAPNES) for practical and vocational nurses.

▶ Evaluate your personal values and compare them with the accepted codes of nursing ethics. Difficult decisions about topics such as AIDS, abortion, organ transplantation, confidentiality, maintenance of life through life-support systems, and refusal of treatment due to religious convictions are some of the many ethical and legal issues facing nurses today.

▼▼▼ REFERENCES

Alfaro-LeFevre R. *Critical Thinking in Nursing: A Practical Approach.* Philadelphia: W.B. Saunders, 1995, Chapter 4.

Anderson G. Medicine vs. religion: The case of Jehovah's Witnesses. Health Soc Work 1983.

Bolander VB. *Sorensen and Luckmann's Basic Nursing: A Psychophysiologic Approach,* 3rd ed. Philadelphia: W.B. Saunders, 1994.

deWit S. *Rambo's Nursing Skills for Clinical Practice,* 4th ed. Philadelphia: W.B. Saunders, 1994.

Emergency Nurse Legal Bulletin, Westville, NJ: Med/Law Publishers, 1982, p. 2.

Hurley ML. What Do the New JCAHO Standards Mean for You? RN 1991; 54 (6):42–46.

Ignatavicius D, Workman ML, Mishler M. *Medical Surgical Nursing: A Nursing Process Approach,* 2nd ed. Philadelphia: W.B. Saunders, 1995, Chapter 6.

Iyer P, Taptich B, Bernocchi-Losey D. *Nursing Process and Nursing Diagnosis,* 2nd ed. Philadelphia: W.B. Saunders, 1991, pp. 192–208.

Majeski T. Without cord blood we wouldn't be here. Duluth News-Tribune, November 11, 1995, p. 3B.

Minnesota Board of Nursing. Board implements on-line verification. For Your Information 1995; 2 (3):4.

National Association of Practical Nurse Education and Service. NAPNES Standards of Practice for Licensed Practical/Vocational Nurses. 1976, 1981, 1993.

National League for Nursing. President of Oregon League for Nursing to head task force. News from the National League for Nursing, September, 1995.

Rachel M. President of the National Council of State Boards of Nursing. Nursing Letter. August 24, 1994.

Rosencrans K. A community cancer. Duluth News-Tribune, November 13, 1995, p. 1.

Varcarolis E. *Foundations of Psychiatric Mental Health Nursing,* 2nd ed. Philadelphia: W.B. Saunders, 1994, Chapter 3.

▼▼▼ *BIBLIOGRAPHY*

Drill J. Legal issues for licensed practical nurses. Wisconsin Association of Licensed Practical Nurses Fall Seminar, Wisconsin Dells, WI, November 3, 1995.

Kozier B, Erb G, Oliveri R. *Fundamentals of Nursing.* Menlo Park, CA: Addison-Wesley, 1991.

Moss J. Membership Services, NFLPN; Raleigh, NC, 1992.

Newmann T. State board update. Wisconsin Association of Licensed Practical Nurses Fall Seminar. Wisconsin Dells, WI, November 3, 1995.

Test Taking: The FINAL Is NCLEX-PN

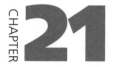

CHAPTER **21**

▼▼▼ *O U T L I N E*

▼▼▼ *K E Y   T E R M S*

▼▼▼ *O B J E C T I V E S*

Upon completing this chapter you will be able to:

1. Discuss hints for taking multiple-choice and short-answer tests.

2. Explain what is meant by NCLEX-PN.

3. Explain what is meant by computerized adaptive testing (CAT).

4. Discuss the requirements of your state board of nursing for eligibility to take the licensing examination.

5. Differentiate between a temporary work permit and licensure.

6. Discuss minimum competency.

7. Practice exercises to reduce test-taking anxiety.

8. Discuss review books and mock examinations.

Almost without exception, when student nurses are asked about their goal for the year, they respond by saying, "I want to pass the boards," meaning, pass the licensure examination.

Does the thought of having to take a test leave you feeling numb? Welcome to the club. Some anxiety about test taking is normal. It can work to your benefit. Without it you would probably watch television instead of studying. Once again the research results are on your side. Some learners blame fear and anxiety in test-taking situations for their poor test performance. Research has indicated that if you do not do well on tests, odds are that one or more of the following reasons apply to you: (1) you are less intelligent than the average student, (2) you have poor study habits, or (3) you have weak test-taking skills. The first reason does not apply in your situation because you would not have been admitted to the practical nursing program if it were true. Chapter 7 dealt with overcoming poor study habits, and this chapter will deal with test-taking skills.

In our experience, lack of preparation of the subject matter and poor test-taking skills are the most common reasons for low test scores. Occasionally a learner has such great fear and anxiety about test taking that it interferes with what was studied. This situation requires a knowledge of relaxation techniques, or even drugs, but this is the exception, not the rule.

▼▼▼
Hints for Successful Test Taking

Focus on remaining an active learner. Clarify with the instructor the types of items that will be asked. Set a goal to *understand* the information you are learning with an eye to *applying* that learning. NCLEX-PN will be testing you at the level of understanding and application. There are very few straight knowledge items. You can anticipate application type items in the practical nursing program.

Test-taking skills are divided into two general areas: preparing for the test and actually taking the test.

▽▽▽
Preparation for the Test

1. *Preparation for Test Taking Begins on the First Day of Class.* This includes (1) your system of note-making for class and assignments and (2) your goal of understanding information as a preparation for tests and for clinical performance and their focus on application.

2. *Clarify Content to Be Covered on the Test and the Form of the Test.* Specific hints for taking multiple-choice and short-answer tests are included in this chapter.

3. *Periodically Review the Material You Have Already Studied.* This is necessary to get the information into your long-term memory. Use the test step of the PQRST method frequently. Audible recitation is suggested. Make index cards of the material you are having difficulty with. Cramming—last-minute studying of new material for a test—sometimes results in short-term memory of material that might help you pass a test, but because you did not engage in repetitions spaced over days, storage in long-term memory will not occur. Application of the material to the clinical area will be difficult. Cramming for an exam is like packing your suitcase at the last minute for a vacation. You will wind up with a suitcase filled with things you do not need, and there may be a whole list of things you forgot to bring.

4. Use Time-Management Techniques to Help You Organize Your Time Before the Test. Make a schedule to help you identify study times in which you can do a grand review for each test. Do not reread the textbook. You have studied the material periodically since the last test and have used study-skill techniques. At this point, focus on your summaries, margin writings, underlinings, and index cards to check your understanding and retention of the information. The night before the test do not be tempted to watch television or go to a movie. These activities will interfere with remembering. Instead, do your grand review as described here and get a good night's sleep.

▽▽▽

Taking the Test

Arrive at the classroom in plenty of time to get your favorite seat and arrange your pencils and other materials. Beware of peers who may try to make you nervous by saying, "You didn't study that, did you?" or "You mean you didn't study that?" Keep a positive mental attitude. You organized your time and systematically reviewed for this test after clarifying the content of the exam. Silently rehearse your facts to keep out distractions. Take slow deep breaths to reduce tension. It is almost test time and you are ready!

Would you believe that some people who have organized their notes and their time, reviewed systematically, and understood the material still do poorly on tests? *They probably did not follow the directions on the test.* How well do you follow directions? Take out a blank sheet of paper and test yourself on the following directions.

How Well Do You Follow Directions?

Directions: Read the following directions carefully. You will have one minute to do the exercise after reading the directions. Be sure to write legibly. When you have finished, check your answers against the directions before handing in the paper. *Be sure to read the entire exercise before you begin.*

1. On a sheet of paper, print your name in the upper left-hand corner, last name first.
2. Under your name, write your Social Security number.
3. In the upper right-hand corner, write the name and number of the course for which you are taking this exercise.
4. In the lower left-hand corner of the paper, write today's date.
5. In the lower right-hand corner, write your instructor's name, last name first.
6. Fold your paper in half lengthwise.
7. Number the left half of your paper 1 to 6, skipping three lines between each number.
8. Number the right half of your paper 7 to 12, skipping three lines between each number.
9. Now that you have read all of the exercise, do only number one of the exercise and hand your paper to the instructor.

How did you do? If you did not follow the directions, do you feel tricked? You were not. The directions were clear, and you simply did not follow them. Listen meticulously to oral directions. Read the written directions completely before each test. To those of you who did follow the directions for this exercise: Keep up the good work! If directions are ever unclear, ask the instructor before proceeding. Clarify the time limit of the exam. Now you are ready to begin.

Quickly skim the entire exam to get an overall picture of the types of items on the test. This will help you figure out how much time you can devote to each section. Then answer the items you know well. Watch for absolutes such as always, never, all, and only. Spend a limited amount of time on difficult questions. Avoid getting upset about them. Both of these activities waste time. They do not earn points for you. Go on to the next question and return to the skipped item later.

*Keep in mind that on the NCLEX-PN you will **not** be able to skip items and then go back to them. For the NCLEX-PN you will need to answer each item as it comes up on the test.*

Take the full time allowed for the test. If you finish early, try to answer the items you skipped. This brings up the point of guessing at answers. If you are not penalized for guessing, answer all the items. But if the test is graded by subtracting the number of wrong answers from the number of right answers, generally speaking, do not guess. Make sure you have not missed an item or a group of items. Make sure your answers match up to the proper answer slot. The instructor cannot possibly know that you put the answer to number 37 in the slot for number 36. Should you change an answer? Although research has shown that test scores are generally improved by changing answers, some learners decrease their test scores by the same action. If you have given the item further thought and still believe that it should be changed, change it. Test by test, keep tabs on your test grades to see whether changing answers is helping your final score. Modify your behavior accordingly. If you are using a separate answer sheet that will be machine corrected, be sure you erase your first answer completely.

Chapter 4 discussed tests as a learning tool. When the exam is corrected and returned to you, do the following:

1. Read the items you missed. Why are they wrong? Did you make a careless mistake? Did you know the material? Can you correct the item without looking in your textbook or notes? If not, look up the answer.

2. Read the items you answered correctly. What did you do right to get credit for these items?

3. Decide which of your study skills and test-taking techniques are and are not working to your benefit. Modify your test-taking strategies accordingly.

▽▽▽
Hints for Specific Tests

The types of tests you will be taking in the practical-nursing program, including the NCLEX-PN, are achievement tests. They measure how much you have learned. Achievement tests are of two types—objective and subjective. Objective achievement tests include multiple-choice items. In objective achievement tests the answer is generally included in the test item. You must pick it out. The format of the NCLEX-PN is multiple-choice items that measure your understanding and application of nursing knowledge. Subjective achievement tests include short-answer items. In subjective tests you must answer the item by formulating the answer. We will use samples of these two test forms to help you understand them. Hints are provided for taking each of them.

Multiple-Choice Items

Here are some hints for taking the short multiple-choice test that follows. Read over all the options given before making any decision. Eliminate the options you know are definitely wrong. When a number answer is involved, choose the number in the midrange. Remember the course subject matter for which you are being tested. Eliminate options that are not related to the subject matter.

▼▼▼
Learning Exercise

Multiple-Choice Items

Choose the appropriate option for the following multiple-choice items. There is only one answer to each multiple-choice item.

1. Multiple-choice items are examples of
   a. Items for which one-word answers are required.
   b. Incomplete statements with four options for answers.
   c. Two vertical columns that must be matched item by item.
   d. Items that require a sentence to be written on the answer sheet.

2. When answering multiple-choice items, it is not necessary to
   a. Read the directions.
   b. Match lists of items.
   c. Read each of the options.
   d. Watch out for negative words.

Answers to Multiple-Choice Items

1b. A sentence or beginning of a sentence is given with four options. Usually only one option is correct. The rest of the options are distractors, that is, options that are there to test whether you really have learned the material. Option a describes fill-in-the-blank items, option *c* describes matching tests, and option *d* describes short-answer items.

2b. This multiple-choice item contains a negative word in the stem that can complicate things. Read the stem without the negative word to get some meaning out of it and read the options. One option should not fit in with the others. Now reread the original stem with the negative word and see whether the option you have already isolated fits in. Even though the test begins with directions, there may be additional directions before individual multiple-choice items. These directions may ask you to select one best answer or select all of the correct answers. **Remember, do not stop reading when you think you have the correct answer.** There may be a better option yet to come. Incidentally, options *a*, *c*, and *d* are true.

Multiple-choice items are not multiple guess questions. Think through each response thoroughly before choosing your answer. Should you ever guess? To be able to make a decision about guessing, you must know whether you will be penalized for wrong answers. Even if you are, figure out the odds. If you can eliminate one distractor for certain, you have a better chance of answering correctly. Can you eliminate two out of four distractors? Your chances are now even better. You make the decision. Remember, on the NCLEX-PN, you will have to answer every item as they come.

Short-Answer Items

1. Describe a short-answer item.

2. List five hints that the test taker should use in answering short-answer items to receive full credit for those items.

Answers to Short-Answer Items

1. A short-answer item is one in which you are given a simple command to carry out.
2. Five hints for answering short-answer items:
   a. Be sure to give the information that the item asks for. Watch the verbs in these items, and do what they ask you to do.
   b. Give objective answers.
   c. Write in complete sentences.
   d. Concentrate on packing information into your answer.
   e. Think before you write.

▼▼▼
What Is the NCLEX-PN?

The NCLEX-PN is the National Council Licensing Examination for Practical Nurses. "The NCLEX is designed to test knowledge, skills and abilities essential to the safe and effective practice of nursing at the entry level" (NCLEX-PN Candidate Bulletin, 1994). The NCLEX results provide the basis for licenses granted to practical nurses by boards of nursing. The boards of nursing are the only agencies that can release the test results to candidates.

The same examination—the NCLEX-PN—is given in the United States, American Samoa, the District of Columbia, Guam, the northern Mariana Islands, Puerto Rico, and the Virgin Islands. This makes it possible to provide licensure by endorsement from one board of nursing to another. Endorsement means that an LPN or LVN may apply for licensure without retesting when moving within this jurisdiction.

▼▼▼
Content of the NCLEX-PN

The National Council of State Boards of Nursing developed the NCLEX-PN. A document entitled Test Plan for the National Council Licensure Examination for Practical Nurses is available from the National Council of State Boards of Nursing, 676 St. Clair Street, Suite 550, Chicago, IL 60611-2921. The NCLEX-PN is a secure examination, so no actual test questions are included in this document. However, the document is helpful in explaining the general content areas of the test. It is worthwhile to send for and read the entire document.

What follows are excerpts from the document. The test plan addresses two components: (1) phases of the nursing process, (2) client needs and percentage of items on test for each component. The phases of the *nursing process* include:

> Data collection (27%–33%)
> Planning (17%–23%)
> Implementation (27%–33%)
> Evaluation (17%–23%)

The LPN acts in a more dependent role in the planning and evaluation phases of the nursing process. The data collection and implementation phases provide a more independent role for the LPN. Refer to Chapter 2 for a more detailed account of the nursing process.

The four categories of *client needs* include:

> Safe and effective care environment (16%–22%)
> Physiologic integrity (49%–55%)
> Psychosocial integrity (8%–14%)
> Health promotion and maintenance (15%–21%)

A brief review of the LPN role as it applies to each category follows.

▽▽▽
Safe and Effective Care Environment

1. *Coordinated care:* includes activities related to ethical and legal issues.
2. *Environmental safety:* includes protection of both the client and the health care worker.
3. *Safe and effective treatments and procedures:* includes preparing or caring for clients undergoing diagnostic procedures and various therapies.

The knowledge, skills, and abilities considered essential (meaning basic, initial, or necessary) that relate to a safe and effective care environment include those relating to:

▶ Advance directives
▶ Client rights
▶ Communication skills
▶ Confidentiality
▶ Environmental and personal safety
▶ Expected outcomes of various treatments
▶ General and specific protective interventions
▶ Informed consent
▶ Knowledge and use of equipment used to provide nursing care
▶ Legal accountability
▶ Quality assurance
▶ Spread and control of infectious agents
▶ Team participation

▽▽▽
Physiologic Integrity

The focus in this category is on both acute and chronic problems experienced by clients throughout the life span that have predictable outcomes. The LPN and LVN assist the authorized health care provider in caring for clients with more complex problems.

1. *Physiologic adaptation:* includes care given during acute and chronic phases of illness, including emergency situations.
2. *Reduction of risk potential:* includes reduction of the client's potential for developing complications or health problems. Examples are monitoring changes in status and administering medications.
3. *Provision of basic care:* includes assisting clients in performing activities of daily living including activities modified because of illness.

Essential knowledge, skills, and abilities needed to meet physiologic integrity needs include those related to:

▶ Activities of daily living

- Basic pathophysiology
- Body mechanics
- Comfort interventions
- Effects of immobility
- Emergency interventions
- Expected response to therapies
- Fluid balance
- Invasive procedures
- Medication administration
- Normal body structure and function
- Nutritional therapies
- Pharmacologic actions
- Skin and wound care
- Use of special equipment

Psychosocial Integrity

The focus in this category is on changes occurring throughout the life span.

1. *Psychosocial adaptation:* includes providing for needs of clients with emotional and mental health problems.

2. *Coping and/or adaptation:* includes promoting the client's ability to cope, adapt, or solve problem situations related to illness, injury, or stressful events.

Essential knowledge, skills, and abilities needed to meet psychosocial integrity needs include those related to:

- Behavioral norms
- Chemical dependency
- Common treatment modalities
- Cultural, religious, and spiritual influences on health
- Mental health concepts
- Therapeutic communication

Health Promotion and Maintenance

1. *Growth and development through the life span:* includes assisting the client through the stages of normal growth and development.

2. *Self-care and support systems:* includes (1) pro-

moting client self-care, (2) providing support to families to enhance client care, and (3) reinforcing teaching related to self-care.

3. *Prevention and early treatment of disease:* includes providing for the needs of the client in the prevention and early detection of health problems and disease.

Essential knowledge, skills, and abilities needed by the LPN or LVN to meet the health promotion and maintenance needs of the client include those related to:

- Community resources
- Concepts of wellness
- Death and dying
- Growth and development through the life span
- Human sexuality
- Parenting
- Principles of immunity
- Reproductive cycle
- Teaching appropriate to the scope of practice

Computerized Adaptive Testing

Since April 1994 practical nursing graduates (candidates) have taken the NCLEX-PN on a computer. Testing centers are located across the United States and its territories. This method is called computerized adaptive testing (CAT).

Major Benefits of CAT

The computer selects the items you will answer while you are taking the examination. This gives you the best chance to demonstrate your competence.

As you answer an item on the examination, the computer adapts the examination to your answer. This is possible because the computer has a large number of test items stored in its memory. These items are stored according to the four phases of the nursing process and the four categories of client needs. As you answer the standardized multiple-choice items, the computer chooses the next best item to measure your competence. The computer goes down a "pathway" or "branch." The item selected is neither too easy nor too difficult. The process continues until all test plan requirements have been met and a decision has been made about minimal competence.

The computer indicates that you have completed the test. Your state board of nursing is informed of the results and notifies you in approximately two to three weeks. Test results are not available over the phone. Candidates who do not pass receive a NCLEX-PN Diagnostic Profile. It identifies areas for improvement as well as areas of strength.

▽▽▽
Additional Benefits of Computer Testing

The number of items candidates answer on the NCLEX-PN varies from candidate to candidate. A five-hour time slot is scheduled. The entire time slot might not be used. Remember that success cannot be determined by the length of time one candidate spends "on the computer" compared to the next candidate. One successful candidate indicated that she answered 85 items. A friend of hers answered over 260. Both passed.

Because of the computer method, **year-round testing** is available in centers scattered throughout the United States. Your nursing instructor can identify the specific areas available in your state. Your state board of nursing gives you permission to take the licensure examination after you graduate and apply for licensure. They authorize you to make an appointment at a testing center. The testing center will schedule you within 30 days after you call to make your appointment unless you specify a later date.

Practical nursing candidates will find the computer method **less stressful**, even if they lack previous computer experience. Each testing room is limited to no more than 15 candidates. The test-taking area is quiet and relaxed. There is enough time to answer each question. Just pace yourself. There are two breaks; one is mandatory. The computer lets you know how much time you have spent on the test. The

testing time is shorter with the computer, and notification is quick.

> *A newly licensed practical nurse called her former instructor to say she passed the NCLEX-PN. "All I needed was one finger to operate the computer. The directions were easy and the sample items before the exam eased my mind."*

▼▼▼
NCLEX-PN Test-Taking Tips

▽▽▽
Types of Items

Items in the NCLEX-PN are all multiple choice. There are two types of items: (1) case scenario, and (2) stand-alone items (i.e., miscellaneous items that do not pertain to an on-going scenario). Read the scenario or stand-alone item carefully. Remember that some of the items presented may be for validation for future tests. Validation items are being tried out for use in future NCLEX-PN tests. You will not be penalized for answering them incorrectly. The only problem is, NCLEX-PN will not identify these items as validation items.

> *(Hint: Stay calm when you read a situation or item that you think you have never heard of. It could be a validation item. Or it could be a situation in which you could apply information from another area you know well.)*

▽▽▽
Answering the Items

Items appear one at a time on the computer screen. You can review the item as long as you like. However, once you have recorded your answer you cannot go back and change the answer. You may not leave an item without answering it. Answer each item even if you must guess at the answer. This permits the computer to continue and to choose the next item for you.

Recording Answers

No prior computer experience is necessary or beneficial for taking the NCLEX-PN computer test. Prior to taking the NCLEX-PN, all candidates receive instructions about how to record their answers and a practice session. The information you need to know about the computer to take your licensing examination is limited to two computer keys and an item called a cursor. A description of these three items follows. All other computer keys are locked off so that nothing will happen if you accidentally push them.

> The cursor: a blinking light that the candidate moves to each of the four choices that are provided for each item.
>
> The space bar: a long bar located at the bottom of the keyboard. The space bar moves the cursor among the answer choices when pushed.
>
> The enter key: a key on the computer marked *enter*. After the cursor is moved to the choice the candidate thinks is the right answer, the answer is recorded when this key is struck TWICE. You will not be able to go on to the next item until the answer is entered. The computer needs the entered answer to select the next item.

▽▽▽
Keeping Track of Time

Bring a watch. There are no clocks in the room. Avoid spending long periods of time on any one item. This will allow you to pace yourself.

▽▽▽
Test-Taking Etiquette

The Educational Testing Service (ETS) along with the Sylvan Learning Centers provides the test development and administration services. The testing takes place at Sylvan Learning Centers to ensure test security.

1. Call to arrange for an appointment.

2. Arrive one-half hour early. If you arrive late you may be seated if there is space. Otherwise you will have to reschedule the test and pay a new fee.

3. Present your Authorization to Test letter, which is mailed to you by ETS after your application has been processed by the board of nursing.

4. Sign in on a log, entering the time you check in and the type of test you are taking. (Sylvan Centers do all kinds of testing. The person in the carrel next to you may be someone other than a nurse candidate.)

5. Along with your Authorization to Test letter, present a picture ID and another form of identification.

6. Look to one monitor and view your demographic data (from your application) to verify data.

7. You are fingerprinted (right thumb).

8. Belongings, including the contents of your pockets, are placed in a locker; you keep the key. You may bring a snack to keep in your locker to eat at break.

9. Sit on a chair.

10. A small camera will record your facial image. You can see this on the monitor. The image is frozen and accompanies your test results and thumb prints to ETS for scoring (security purposes). If the monitor does not work, three Polaroid snaps will be taken.

11. Enter the testing room.

12. Take your seat, and adjust the height.

13. Adjust the monitor (lighter or darker).

14. Bright pink scrap paper (six sheets counted) are given to each candidate. Raise your hand if you need more. They are counted and returned at the end of the test.

15. Pencils are provided.

16. Do the practice exercise and begin the test.

17. A video and audio recording is made of the examination period. An attempt to cheat will result in expulsion from the testing area. You lose.

▽▽▽
Test-Taking Skills

All of the test taking skills discussed in this chapter are of value to you. It cannot be overemphasized that the NCLEX-PN tests the essential knowledge, skills, and abilities you have gained in your practical nursing program.

▼▼▼
Preparing for the NCLEX-PN

▽▽▽
Requirements

To help erase some of the mystique that often surrounds the licensure examination, it is worth remembering that the examination tests *minimum competence*. This means that if you have met the requirements for attending a state-board-approved school of practical nursing and have successfully completed all theory and clinical requirements, chances are excellent that you will pass the NCLEX-PN.

A detailed NCLEX-PN instruction booklet will be provided, in addition to licensing information from your board of nursing. Your instructor will assist you in applying for the licensure examination. The general rules are:

1. Submit proof of graduation.
2. Apply for licensure from the state board of nursing and submit the required fee. Some jurisdictions have additional fees.
3. Complete application for NCLEX-PN and submit fee to Educational Testing Services (ETS).
4. When you receive your Authorization to Test letter in the mail from ETS after your board of nursing has made you eligible, register with the Sylvan Center. You cannot make an appointment to take the examination until your board of nursing declares you eligible and you receive the Authorization to Test in the mail. Information regarding scheduling will be included with your Authorization to Test (NCLEX-PN Candidate Bulletin, 1994, p. 4).
5. Schedule a date and time to take the examination (within 30 days of your phone call unless you request a later date).
6. Take the NCLEX-PN.

Your instructor will also assist you with an application for a temporary permit so you will be able to work as a graduate practical or vocational nurse (GPN or GVN). Once the result of the NCLEX-PN examination is in, this permit is automatically revoked. Passing the NCLEX-PN means that you will work as a fully licensed practical or vocational nurse (LPN or LVN). If you fail the NCLEX-PN, you will have to surrender your temporary permit and will work as a nursing assistant.

▽▽▽
Reducing Anxiety Prior to Testing

Normal anxiety is your friend. It is this "cause-and-effect" type of anxiety that actually makes you sharper and more alert during a test. It is only when anxiety overwhelms you that it becomes your enemy. Accept the energy resulting from normal anxiety as your partner. Total personal comfort is not the key. Normal anxiety leaves you somewhere between too much relaxation and too much tension: perfect for testing.

Make your daydreams and positive thinking work for you. Think about what you think about. Are you in the habit of seeing yourself failing or just squeaking by? Because everyone daydreams and sets the stage for their reality, daydreaming is a natural way to practice being confident and successful. Practice the following exercise on successive days. Find a time when you can visualize without interruption.

▼▼▼
Learning Exercise

Part 1

Close your eyes. See yourself arriving at the Sylvan Learning Center one-half hour before testing begins. See yourself entering a waiting room in an officelike environment, welcoming and pleasant. Registration and sign-in go as planned. Everything including the picture-taking and fingerprinting goes smoothly. Candidates are coming in and going out continuously. You are asked to enter the testing area. As you enter you note that the room has beautiful soft-color carpeting. The carrel you are seated in reminds you of a large library carrel. Your instructor has already told you that there are 15 carrels in a room. The test room is glassed-in on two sides. Each carrel has an IBM computer with a mouse (which you do not use), a banker's lamp, and a chair with arm rests. You see yourself sitting down, adjusting the height of the chair and the monitor. You are confident and ready to begin.

Part 2

Close your eyes and imagine yourself in the same setting. Remember to include the detail. This time, the examination seems really hard for you. Rather than giving up, you do your best on every item, focusing on the item rather than on the outcome of the test. Take all the time permitted. When you get up to leave, remind yourself that you have done your best.

Remember: Your whole life does not depend on one test.

Continue to repeat the parts of the exercise in sequence until you find yourself less threatened by the idea of testing—any testing.

Spend the evening before the licensing examination relaxing. Little will be accomplished by worrying or by last-minute cramming. Read something light and entertaining, watch television, or do what you already know will relax you.

Get a good night's sleep by going to bed at your usual time (whatever meets your sleep requirements). Going to bed extra early and not falling asleep may result in a new worry for you to contend with.

Follow through with your usual morning habits. Do not force your system to adjust to a new demand.

Casual attire is appropriate. Think of comfort for sitting and writing. Wear layers of clothing that can be adjusted to your needs.

▼▼▼
A Word About Review Books and Mock Examinations

New review books based on the NCLEX-PN format have been developed by the major nursing publishing companies. Each review book basically includes an outline of practical nursing content, items with explanations, and references for the answers. Items are intended to simulate the NCLEX-PN format. Please realize that the test items of the NCLEX-PN itself are highly guarded and confidential. Actual NCLEX-PN test items are not included in any review book. Some review books contain computer discs with test items. These discs do not simulate CAT testing, but they do provide computer experience.

Review of content and test items are developed by instructors who teach specific areas of practical nursing programs. The best preparation is to study faithfully from the beginning of the program to its conclusion and also on a regular basis until you take the examination. Do not put all your eggs in one basket. Merely reading a review book without studying the content will rarely help you pass boards.

Mock examinations are available for a fee. They offer practical nursing students an opportunity to assess their level of readiness for NCLEX-PN. After taking mock examinations, a student receives a readout of his or her test performance.
This includes:

1. A percentile score for each phase of the nursing process and category of client health needs.

2. The items the student got wrong.

3. A book listing the correct answers, rationale, and explanations for correct answers and distractors for each item.

If students have an idea of their strong and weak areas, they can better focus their study efforts. Be sure to check publishers' offerings of mock examinations. Choose the one that most closely resembles the actual format of the NCLEX-PN. As a practical nursing student you can benefit from tests during the year that encourage problem solving and the application of knowledge. Some of these systems provide adaptive testing as used by NCLEX-PN. Use these experiences as additional means of preparing for your nursing licensure exam.

Good luck! Keep a positive mental attitude.

▼▼▼ S U M M A R Y

▶ Lack of preparation of subject matter and poor test-taking skills are the most common reasons for low test scores. Occasionally fear and high anxiety are involved, but these are exceptional cases.

▶ Successful test-taking involves storing information in your long-term memory. Overstudying has proved to be a successful method. Cramming may work for short-term memory in a test but is of limited value when it comes time to pass the NCLEX-PN.

▶ The NCLEX-PN is the National Council Licensing Examination taken by graduate practical nurses to become licensed. This examination is administered by computer using computerized adaptive testing (CAT).

▶ Prior to scheduling the NCLEX-PN all practical or vocational nursing course work must be completed. Proof of graduation is required. Application for licensure, accompanied by a fee, is made to your state board of nursing. Application for the examination and fee is submitted to Educational Testing Services (ETS). If the application is approved, you will receive an Authorization for Testing form from the ETS. You may register for testing at Sylvan Testing Centers throughout the United States. The NCLEX-PN test is scheduled within 30 days of your request.

▶ Each candidate takes a different track during the CAT method of testing. The track is based on your answers to previous items and provides a way for you to demonstrate your competency in practical nursing. Results are available in about two to three weeks.

▶ Remember to continue your positive mental attitude. If it needs polishing, stop and do it now!

▼▼▼ R E F E R E N C E S

Minnesota Board of Nursing. For Your Information 1994; 10(2):Winter.

Minnesota Board of Nursing. For Your Information 1994; 10(2):Spring.

National Council adopts CAT for NCLEX administration. Nurs Health Care 1991; 12(8):440–441.

Nursing Data Source 1994. Volume 3. Focus on Practical/Vocational Nursing. NLN Division of Research, New York, 1994.

NCLEX and computerized adaptive testing: New format, new challenges. Educational Assessment Q. 1992; 1(3):1, 4.

NCLEX-PN Candidate Bulletin, National Council of State Boards of Nursing, Jan. 15, 1994.

NCLEX-Using CAT material distributed by National Council during 1993-1994 school year.

NCLEX-PN Test Plan for the National Council Licensure Examination. Chicago: National Council of State Boards of Nursing, 1995.

Rafferty C. Notes on the Sylvan Center testing site visit. Wauwautosa WI, April 15, 1994.

Rayfield S. Workshop: Teaching Strategies/Test Development/NCLEX. Green Bay, WI, October 25 and 26, 1990.

▼▼▼ *BIBLIOGRAPHY*

Berkman R. *Find it Fast: How to Uncover Expert Information on Any Subject.* New York: Harper Collins, 1994.

Chenevert M. *Mosby's Tour Guide to Nursing School.* St. Louis: Mosby–Year Book, 1991.

Chornick N, Yocom C, Jacobson J. 1994 *Job Analysis Study for Licensed Practical/Vocational Nurses.* Chicago: National Council of State Boards of Nursing, 1994.

DeYoung S, Adams E. Study groups among nursing students. J Nurs Educ 1995; 34(4):190–191.

Ellis D. *Test Taking Strategies (videotape).* Rapid City, SD: College Survival, 1990.

Heaman D. The quieting response (QR): A modality for reduction of psychophysiologic stress in nursing students. J Nurs Educ 1995; 34(1):5–10.

Kent P. *The Complete Idiot's Guide to the Internet.* Indianapolis: QUE, 1994.

Meltzer M, Palau S. *Reading and Study Strategies for Nursing Students.* Philadelphia: W.B. Saunders, 1993.

Pauk W. *How to Study in College,* 4th ed. Boston: Houghton-Mifflin, 1989.

Staton T. *How to Study,* 5th ed. Circle Pines, MN: American Guidance Service Inc., 1959.

Success Through Notetaking. Del Mar, CA: Supercomp, 1987.

Finding a Job Through the Year 2005

Michael S. Hill, MS, CRC, CCM, QRC

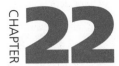

CHAPTER **22**

▼▼▼ K E Y   T E R M S

artful vagueness
conditional job offer
follow-up illusion
General Education Diploma

hidden job market
illegal questions
informational interviews
interpersonal styles

networking everyone
reference hierarchy
resignation courtesy
working a room

▼▼▼ O B J E C T I V E S

Upon completing this chapter you will be able to:

1. *List employment opportunities available to LPNs.*
2. *Determine interpersonal styles and how to use them to achieve interpersonal rapport.*
3. *Describe and use individuals within your job search network.*
4. *Effectively participate in an informational interview.*
5. *Discuss how and where to best target job leads.*
6. *Role-play employer telephone contacts and respond positively to hard interview questions.*
7. *Develop a résumé that will get an employer's attention.*
8. *Convey positive nonverbal messages at the interview.*
9. *Have an insight into the cultural and age differences of the interviewer.*
10. *Discuss the importance of employer follow-up both at the time of application and after the interview.*
11. *Anticipate and facilitate a successful prephysical examination and drug screening.*
12. *Write an effective job summary resignation letter.*

If you are reading this chapter you have probably graduated or are about to graduate with the expectation that employers will be beating down your door. You may also be concerned about your career opportunities after investing so much money in your education.

You are to be congratulated for having become a member of one of the fastest growing employment areas: health services. In *America's Top Medical and Human Services Jobs* (Farr, 1994) the author states that the job outlook for nursing has a growth rate that is faster than average through the year 2005. This is a response to the long-term care needs of a rapidly growing elderly population and the need for general health care.

Job growth and opportunities vary from region to region at different times. Employment opportunities vary according to each individual's tenacity, geographic location, and sometimes just luck. Your job search will be more successful if you consider looking into the areas of:

- ▶ Nursing homes and extended care facilities
- ▶ Home health agencies
- ▶ Physicians' offices and clinics
- ▶ Pharmaceutical suppliers
- ▶ Chiropractic offices
- ▶ Residential treatment centers
- ▶ Medical management companies
- ▶ State or federal or private prison systems
- ▶ Veterinary clinics and hospitals
- ▶ Halfway houses for the mentally ill

- ▶ Day care centers for adults and children
- ▶ Private duty homes
- ▶ Hospitals
- ▶ Insurance companies
- ▶ State jobs
- ▶ Military services
- ▶ Weight loss clinics
- ▶ Manufacturing and industry
- ▶ Social service agencies
- ▶ Ambulance and emergency medicine
- ▶ Temporary employment companies

▼▼▼
Beginning the Job Search

▽▽▽
Practical Experience

1. What type of environment do I want to work in? Business, state or federal government, private duty. . . or other?

_____

_____

2. What population, that is, type of client, do I find most rewarding to work with?

_____

_____

3. What kinds of nursing skills do I find most challenging and rewarding? Additionally, what new areas would I like to be involved in?

_____

_____

Many job ads in newspapers and professional publications require the candidate to have had prior experience. By completing your program you have gained practical experience. Now it is a matter of convincing the employer that it is to his or her benefit to hire you. Think about what your education has provided you.

It is a distinct advantage if your educational program has included clinical (hands-on) nursing experience in the areas you are most interested in. These nursing experiences include clinical rotations, special projects, internships, and/or work prior to taking the NCLEX-PN. Students involved in educational programs that do not offer such experience are encouraged to seek volunteer experiences or part-time related care jobs right away when entering school.

Your practical work experiences will lead to clarification of your school lessons, help you hone your skills, and provide valuable work references. Recruiters report that they make the best job offers to students with internships or work experiences in their field. Such students also moved up the salary ladder faster than other employees (Moreau, 1995).

Think about it: By taking advantage of the clinical rotations and work experiences available to you, a significant step in the job search has already been taken while you were finishing your education. You have had an opportunity to learn about and develop skills that are valued in the major areas of nursing employment.

▼▼▼
Using Interpersonal Styles to Your Benefit

What are interpersonal styles, and which style fits you? Think for a moment about the contacts you have made in the classroom, in the clinical areas, and among your school friends. You have the unique opportunity of making contacts with nurses at all levels who can be instrumental in helping you to obtain a job.

First, however, you must ask yourself: (1) Who am I? (2) How am I seen? The first question enables you to look at yourself in relation to your values and interests, and determine what motivates you. The answer to this question will provide you with information about which work environments to consider for employment.

Through the second question, you can learn how others see you and if what they see is congruent with the messages you think you are sending (Kuntz, 1995, p.2). A positive impression will go a long way to develop networks and work references.

Mercer (1994) suggests that to master interpersonal styles, it is necessary to foster a spirit of cooperation and to meet others on their own terms. To achieve rapport, he indicates that there were four major interpersonal styles: results-focused, detail-focused, friendly-focused, and party-focused.

▽▽▽
Results-Focused

These individuals prefer to get information quickly and act upon it immediately. Signs of this style include: "a tendency to talk fast, finish other's sentences and act irritated when others don't get right to the point."

You may want to respond to these individuals by: "making your points brief, describing what you have done and plan to do next. Speak rapidly and avoid getting sidetracked."

▽▽▽
Detail-Focused

These individuals are interested in every detail about a subject, no matter how large or how small. They are perfectionists who would rather have a task performed correctly than quickly. Signs of this type include: "speaking slowly and deliberately to absorb all information, often asking for additional details."

When responding to these individuals you will

want to bring a folder or chart full of information. "Carefully explain each element of what you have done to date and plan to do. Make sure that the individual is comfortable with every aspect of your work."

▽▽▽
Friendly-Focused

These individuals expect to have an easy-going conversation initially. Signs of this style include: "talking about themselves or conversations about your personal life along with discussing weekend plans, hobbies and nonwork activities." When the small talk is completed, they tend to shift to either a results-focused or detail-focused person.

To respond to these individuals you may want to "chat with them for two to five minutes about nonwork activities." Following this you will want to "state that you will need to return to your work and then discuss the business at hand." Then watch for clues to whether the person switches to the results- or detail-focused style.

▽▽▽
Party-Focused

"These people love to laugh, tell jokes and have a good time before getting down to business." Once this is done they, like the friendly-focused person, will shift to the results- or detail-focused style.

The best way to respond is to laugh along with them or, if you are good at it, tell a few jokes of your own. "If you are not a good joke teller, then clip cartoons from a newspaper which you can share and laugh with them about."

Mercer suggests that to make a good impression on people it is important to: (1) listen to what they have to say; (2) if you disagree with someone with whom you want to maintain rapport, use "artful vagueness." Artful vagueness is responding to another's comments without implying that either of you are wrong. An example would be to finish a statement with "You've got a point there" or "You may be right." Mercer's last recommendation is to "give out three compliments a day." He notes that the people receiving the compliments will be more likely to help you network in the future.

▼▼▼
Networking Your Way to Success

> 1. With only a year in school, who will you want to network with?
> 2. What are the best methods of networking?
> 3. What is the worst networking mistake?
> 4. What is the best way to "work a room"?

Smart networking in your school through internships or work experiences can lead to finding new jobs, better pay, faster promotions, and greater job satisfaction. Consider, for example:

► Instructors who are willing to write a positive recommendation if your work warrants it. Be sure to ask for permission prior to bringing in a form or giving out his or her name. Do not assume that an instructor will give you a positive reference. Specifically ask, "May I list your name for a positive reference?"

► Unit managers, supervisors, team leaders, staff RNs, and LPNs are sources of information about job openings in their areas and can be approached for recommendations. Some students think that they are "invisible" in the eyes of regular facility staff. Not so. Frequently staff offer feedback to instructors and nurse managers about future employees.

► School placement people are sources of information when you register with the school's career service center.

Listen carefully when feedback is passed on to you. You often have to work directly with the primary nurses or team leaders. Identify the nurses whose work you admire and ask for their evaluation and suggestions about your work.

Before completing the clinical rotation, ask select nurses if they would be willing to write a positive reference letter for you. If the answer is "yes," write down the nurse's name (spelled correctly), title, work address, and work phone number. The author strongly encourages you to ask the reference what they will say about you. When discussing your references during an interview it is to your advantage to allude to what they will say about you. If you don't ask what the person will say about you, you are risking the possibility that he or she will also discuss all of your flaws.

Send a brief courtesy letter at the time you begin your job search; follow-up telephone contact to your reference person four to five days after sending the letter will remind her of you and of her promise. Your telephone contact might sound something like this:

"Hello Ms. Anderson, this is Katelyn Bieser. I was calling to follow up on the letter I sent last week to see if you have had an opportunity to write the letter of recommendation we discussed at the end of the last rotation."

If the answer is no: "I know that you've been pretty busy lately. Would it be possible to follow up with you next week when you have had more time? Great, I will call back then. Have a good day!"

Because of their often busy schedules, offer to write a letter yourself for their review and signature. A letter to the reference person and a letter of recommendation might appear as follows:

```
May 8, 1997


Ms. Jennifer Abbinante,
Nursing Administrator
Veterans Hospital
1000 Veterans Lane
Minneapolis, MN 55402

Dear Ms. Abbinante:

Thank you again for agreeing to be a work reference for me. My experiences
on the medical-surgical unit were both challenging and rewarding. I am
pleased that I now have the opportunity to use the skills you taught me.

I am actively seeking employment in medical-surgical units at hospitals
within the metro area. A letter of reference from you is definitely an asset
to my job search.

Knowing your busy schedule, I have enclosed a possible letter of reference
for your review and signature. However, if you prefer to write your own
letter you may wish to mention my ability to work under pressure, ability
to administer medication on time, communication skills with staff and
patients, and my willingness to take on new assignments.

Your assistance in helping me to secure employment is greatly appreciated.
I will plan to give you a call next week to let you know how my job search
is going and answer any questions you may have regarding the reference
letter. I look forward to talking with you soon.

Sincerely,

Katelyn Bieser
2001 Putt Drive
Cottage Grove, MN 55016
(612) 555-2728
```

Example Letter To Be Placed On Facility Letter Head

May 15, 1997

Dear Employer:

Please accept this as a letter of recommendation for Ms. Katelyn Bieser, whom I supervised during her medical-surgical rotation. Katelyn was both enjoyable to work with and displayed a high degree of skill as a student nurse.

Specifically, she learned new tasks quickly, attended to client vital signs, diet programs and medication administration promptly. Katelyn was able to follow both physician and RN orders and had the keen sense to know when to ask for help.

I believe that Katelyn will make a positive contribution to any hospital/ company she chooses to work for. Should you have further questions about Katelyn's skills and abilities as a nursing professional please feel free to contact me.

Cordially,

Jennifer Abbinante, RN
Surgical Care Charge Nurse

Additionally, when networking, use other contacts that you have made or be willing to meet new people who can help you, such as:

▶ Family and friends with nursing contacts. Let them know that you are looking for work. Ask for job leads and names of contacts. Follow up with these people every two weeks until you get the job you want. Remember to thank these people for all of their help once you get the job. You never know, you may need their help again in the future. Job opportunities are often located not by what you know as much as by whom you know.
▶ Former health care employers. If interested in a nursing position, contact the employer.
▶ Newspapers, nursing journals, the school alumni office, telephone yellow pages, the school's career placement office, state Job Service and local county agencies. If browsing the internet, some job lines to check are:

http://www.directory.occ.com; http://www.yahoo.com; and/or http://www.career mosaic.com.

▶ Attend professional conferences or training sessions and then begin "working the room." Meissner (1995) has recommended the following steps: (1) arriving early to obtain your name badge and to see who else is attending; (2) not bringing your spouse with you; (3) avoiding sitting at tables with other students; sit instead with people already working in the field; (4) identifying the people who hire by their more professional appearance and avoidance of eye contact with others; (5) sitting down at the table and introducing yourself to the people next to you. Most people who attend conferences sit with a person they know, which may gain you an additional introduction; (6) requesting business cards; and (7) not leaving these events early or right away when the event ends. Contacts can often

Question: Who can you think of that is a part of your job network? List the individuals in the spaces below.

Name

_____

_____

_____

Phone

_____

_____

_____

be made by stating "I found Ms. _____'s comment about the _____ interesting. Have you heard about that before?"

Call a prospective employer and ask, "Are you hiring?" If the answer is no, ask "Do you know of anyone else who is hiring?" If yes, ask for the contact person's name, if known.

Networking should be a never-ending process even after you have found your dream job. You never know when that dream job might come to an abrupt end owing to reorganization and downsizing. Additionally, remember that networking is a means to job satisfaction and advancement.

Buckley (1994) stated that "the worst networking mistake [is] forgetting to network at all because you think you are immune and don't have to do it." He recommends: (1) building a good relationship with the boss, (2) building relationships with key people in different departments, (3) maintaining positive peer relationships because peers can be either strong allies or powerful enemies, (4) building long-term relationships by being ethical and focusing on others' needs, and (5) building critical relationships by being a contributor. This will lead to access to other networks.

▼▼▼
Informational Interviews

1. How might informational interviews help your career?
2. Whom do you trust to tell you how your voice sounds? Who will help you to understand how it needs to sound?

3. With whom can you practice the informational interview telephone request? List three names: _____

_____

_____

Chances are that at some time during your educational program you will be asked to visit community health facilities. Your instructor will provide objectives and questions to help make the experience worthwhile. Objectives or questions may focus on the following areas:

▶ Purpose
▶ Staffing patterns
▶ Hours or shifts
▶ Facility specialty

Viewing this assignment as an informational interview will create an additional personal focus for you. The informational interview will allow you to find out how the facility works first-hand, assist you in determining if you would want to work there, and allow you to meet the employer before you actually seek a job.

To obtain an informational interview with an employer it is important to practice with another individual prior to making the telephone contact. It may be tempting to make the phone call and read the example without practicing in advance. But if you do this, remember that is exactly how it will sound—as if you are reading!

This is the time to concentrate on how your voice sounds to the employer with respect to pitch and intonation. Franklin (1995) reported that several studies of spoken English have shown that "low-pitched, clear voices were judged to be more mature, truthful and competent than high-pitched ones." Also, "nasal voices signaled low status, were uninviting, and grated on the listener." Monotones, such as occur when reading aloud, were boring to the listener. Loud, fast talkers were viewed as dynamic but shifty. Finally, individuals with whiney voices were a definite turn-off.

The key is to find someone who will give you an honest opinion about how you sound. When you approach that person explain the reason you are asking for his or her opinion. Explain that you view it as another learning experience toward achieving your goals.

The following is an example of a telephone informational interview request:

1. Hello, my name is _____.

2. Can you give me the name of the person in charge of hiring? (Emphasis is on first learning the name of the right person. Don't begin by asking, "May I speak to the person in charge of hiring?")

3. May I speak with Mr./Ms. _____?

4. Hello, Mr./Ms. _____. My name is _____.

5. I am a student nurse at _____ (school's name).

6. As a part of my learning experience, I would like to visit your facility for an informational interview.

7. Would it be possible to set up an informational interview on _____ (day) at 9:00 A.M. or 2:00 P.M., or another time?

    7A. If yes: Great! I'll see you at _____. Thank you.

    7B. If no: Is there someone else that you recommend that I contact?

There is usually no problem with speaking directly to top nursing management during an informational interview. Management likes to "get the word out" about what their facility really is like. *However,* do not make the mistake of turning this into a job interview. No one likes to be tricked, and management tends to have a long memory.

Look sharp during the informational interview. These are not "T-shirt, shorts, sandals or jeans" side trips. Consider them as future career opportunities. Keep a copy of the information you complete with name, address, and phone number, in a safe place, for the time your job search begins. Follow up the informational interview with a thank you letter. An example follows:

January 17, 1997

Ms. LeAnn Lemberger,
Director of Nursing
St. Joseph Hospital
1000 Writers Lane
Minneapolis, MN 55402

RE: Informational Interview

Dear Ms. Lemberger:

I want to take this time to thank you for meeting with me on Wednesday, January 15, 1997. The information that you provided was both valuable and interesting. Your suggestions about areas of my schooling on which to focus were very much appreciated.

I found that the variety of programs offered was progressive and individualized to meet the needs of the client. The tour that followed supported your comments about the positive interactions between staff and clients.

I can only hope to be fortunate enough to work at such a Center following my graduation this June. Thank you again.

Cordially,

Katelyn Bieser
2001 Putt Drive
Cottage Grove, MN 55016
(612) 555-2728

▼▼▼
How to Look for a Job

1. *Is it true that it is pointless to look for work during the holidays?*
2. *Where is the most effective job search performed?*
3. *What are the advantages of working at a temporary agency?*
4. *Why is waiting for the employer to contact you a lost cause?*

It is important to begin to apply for employment approximately two months prior to graduation if you expect to work shortly after graduation. The author recommends that you obtain a telephone answering machine or use a telephone "voice mailbox" service so that you do not miss any employers' calls. If your graduation is in December, do not fret. It is a myth that the November-December holiday season is the worst time to hunt for a job. The holiday season is among the best times to look for a job.

You need to do some homework in preparation for seeking employment. Find out all you can about the facility at which you wish to work. Facilities often provide free pamphlets as part of their advertising. Obtain the "mission statement" of the facility if it is not in a pamphlet. Also remember the information you have acquired and stashed away during your education.

Your nursing program director will also have policy manuals for affiliated facilities. Ask to see those manuals. It is very important to try to find out the name of the person who does the hiring or influences hiring. This is the person whom you will want to contact. You may be referred to another department, but there is a good chance that your name will be remembered later.

According to *The Job Hunting Handbook: Job Outlook to 2005* (1995) 75% of jobs available are not advertised. Do not wait for an ad to appear to apply with an employer. Through their research, Dahlstrom & Company discovered that people use the following methods to get jobs:

Assistance from family and/or friends
Direct application to employer
Response to newspaper advertisement
State job service
Private employment agencies
Taking civil service examinations
School placement offices
Union hall hiring

Assistance from family and/or friends has the highest rate of success in getting a job. One area that was often overlooked in the past was work gained through temporary employment agencies. According to Feder (1995), "temps supplied by agencies to U.S. companies soared from 500,000 in 1983 to nearly 2 million, or 1.5 percent of the work force in 1994. This incredible growth is projected to go well into the year 2000."

Temporary employment companies may serve a useful function for graduating students and/or nurses wishing to re-enter the work force. These companies are able to enter you into the work force to gain the "work experience" desired by employers. It also allows individuals to work in a number of different clinical settings and shift situations.

"Temp" companies provide a means for individuals to determine which companies they would like to work for. The networking connections you make while working can become very valuable when a full-time position becomes available. Drawbacks do exist. Full-time hours are not always available for temporary workers. Some companies may require a minimum of 6 months of work experience. Benefits may be marginal. Individuals using the "get by" concept may obtain a temporary job to get them by until the right job comes along.

Another means of applying directly with employ-ers is sending a letter to a prospective employer. Make a follow-up telephone contact to arrange an interview or at least to use as a networking opportunity for additional job leads.

Often a brief, to-the-point letter accompanied by a résumé addressed to the director of nursing at the facility to which you are applying is helpful. Your cover letter might appear as in the following example:

<u>**COVER LETTER**</u>

April 7, 1997

Ms. Liz Murphy,
Director of Nursing
Chisago Lakes Hospital
2031 Lakeside Drive
Chisago, MN 55890

RE: LPN Staff Nurse Position

Dear Ms. Murphy:

I will graduate from the Fairview Hospital practical nursing program this June. While doing a medical nursing rotation at your hospital I was impressed by the quality of client care, staff professionalism, and learning opportunities.

In addition to this rotation, my work experiences have included: client care planning, plan review, direct client care, passing medications, and team participation.

I am interested in obtaining employment at your hospital and being able to work with your staff again. I will be contacting you on Tuesday, April 15, 1997, to see if you have received my résumé and to determine when we might arrange an interview. Should you wish to contact me prior to this time I can be reached after 3:30 P.M. I look forward to speaking with you.

Cordially,

Katelyn Bieser
2001 Putt Drive
Cottage Grove, MN 55301
(612) 843-2728

ENC: Résumé

Avoid including a personal reference list or a photograph of yourself with the cover letter. Retain the reference list for your interview and provide it only on request. *Do* follow through by calling for an interview on the day stated in your letter.

Jeffery Allen (1992) strongly recommended avoiding follow-up calls or scheduling interviews on Mondays. Traditionally, these days are filled with staff meetings and unexpected demands for the employer. He reports that "statistically, the best time to call is Tuesday through Friday, from 9:00 AM to 11:00 AM." Mark the day cited in your letter on your calendar.

As a rule, conditions in the 1990s have changed the way employers approach hiring. With hundreds of applicants and more job duties added to their personal job descriptions, employers no longer have the luxury of contacting prospective employees applying for jobs. Those candidates who wait to be contacted should prepare to be disappointed when contacts do not occur.

If your resource for a job opening is the newspaper, call for an interview (unless the ad specifically says to write). The reason for this is that others are looking at the same ad, and in such cases, "she who hesitates is lost." Ask to speak to the person in charge of hiring. Your conversation will tend to reflect the following example:

1. Hello, my name is _____.
2. "Who" is in charge of hiring?
3. May I speak with Ms. _____?
4. Hello Ms. _____. My name is _____.
5. I will be graduating from the _____ (school name) practical nursing program in _____ (city name) on _____ (date).
6. Do you have any practical nursing staff positions open?
   - 6A. If yes: Would it be possible to set up an interview on _____ (date) at 9:00 AM or perhaps 2:00 PM? If no: What would be a better time and date? . . . Great! I will see you then.
   - 6B. If the answer is no, we are under a hiring freeze, catch your breath and don't be put off. The *Job Hunting Handbook* (1995) recommends the following response:
     - 6B (1) Oh, I do understand. A lot of institutions have hiring freezes at this time of year. But those hiring freezes can't last forever. I'd like to be the first on your list when you lift your hiring freeze. Would you take a few minutes to meet with me and see where I might fit in once your hiring freeze is lifted? If yes, see 6A. If no, continue on. . .'
   - 6C. If no: Do you know of anyone who might be hiring?
     - 6C (1) If yes: Would you also know the contact person and/or have the telephone number?

       _____   _____   _____
       (facility) (contact) (telephone)
     - 6C (2) If no: I appreciate your time. Thank you.
       or
     - 6C (3) If no: Thank you for trying. Would it be possible for me to come in for an informational interview?

       If yes: See 6A.

       If no: Well, thank you again. Goodbye.

Defer the employer's questions until the interview because you do not want to be "washed out" by a phone conversation. If the employer begins to ask you questions about your background, education, or work experience, you might respond, "I have the necessary educational background and work experience required. I would like the opportunity to discuss my qualifications during our interview."

See point 6A, earlier. Say, "Would it be possible to set up an interview with you on Wednesday? . . . etc."

The tone of your voice makes a significant difference on the telephone. If you smile while talking you will project a positive tone. Practice the above suggested format in advance with a friend. Write notes for yourself if necessary.

Even if you are not ideally qualified for a job opening, apply if the job appeals to you. Advertisements often describe the ideal candidate for the job, and the ideal is usually not available. If you do lack some skills that are required and are able to obtain an interview, an employer will be impressed if you ask whether facility in-services, orientation, and continuing education courses are offered by the employer to enhance your job skills.

▼▼▼
Answers to Application Questions

> 1. What are reasonable responses to employment gaps?
> 2. What are employers doing to check on application falsification?
> 3. What are illegal questons?

You will be asked to fill out an application either before or after the interview. It is important that you answer the questions truthfully. If you have had three or more jobs in the past three years, an employer will be concerned about this and will expect you to supply good reasons for leaving. Reasons for leaving might include: work interfered with schooling, lay-off, relocation, career exploration, and job stagnation. Gaps in employment between jobs might be explained by responses such as: laid-off, job hunting, returned to school, travel, and family responsibilities (*Job Hunting Handbook,* 1995, p. 35).

If there are questions you wish to defer until the face-to-face interview, write in N/A (for not applicable) or Will explain, or leave the space blank. One such area might include expected wage and wages with former employers. For the current wage expected, write Open; don't specify a dollar amount. With wages in former employment, leave the spaces blank if you know that you were underpaid or tell the truth if the wage was fair.

Be aware that you do not have to answer questions about age, religion, marital status, children, physical data (unless these are a specific requirement for the job), and criminal record (unless it relates to security clearance, housing, or perhaps employment in schools, child facilities, and nursing homes).

An employer's eyes will naturally gravitate toward any blank spaces. Therefore, answer every question you can even if it does not apply to you (e.g., for military service, write N/A in the space).

> **If the questions asked are illegal, you need to decide whether to answer the questions or leave the space blank.**

Some employers view blanks or "Will explain" as an automatic screen for someone they do not want to employ. Should you choose to answer illegal questions, the examples below might be helpful.

Have you been hospitalized within the past five years?
Answer: I do not have any health problems that would interfere with the advertised position.

Have you ever been on workers' compensation?
Answer: N/A (not applicable)
or
I had a _____ injury in _____ (year) which I have recovered from. If I have any concerns about job assignments I am not afraid to ask for help.

Do you have a criminal record?
Answer: I made a mistake which resulted in a _____. I have paid for that mistake and am now wise enough not to get into trouble again.

Do not attempt to falsify information because this will provide grounds for dismissal after hiring. Personnel departments will contact your references, schools, former employers, and others to verify the information on your job application and résumé. The *Job Hunting Handbook* (1995) further emphasized this point when it noted that personnel departments often check your credit records to see if you are a responsible consumer. This is especially true if the job pays more than $20,000 per year.

▼▼▼
Preparing for the interview

> 1. What will the employer try to determine during the interview?
> 2. What is the best way to work with an employer when the person is different from yourself?

During an interview you are also interviewing the potential employer. If you have prepared adequately, you will be able to evaluate whether your job skills or physical abilities match the objectives of the facility. Additionally, you can evaluate whether your values about patient care and treatment of staff are close enough to establish a positive working relationship.

You should consider that interviews are often stressful for the employer. Interviewers have to fit interviews into their regular work duties, justify why one candidate should be hired rather than another, and be on constant guard not to discriminate due to age, sex, race, and so on. Knowing that there are concerns on both sides—yours and the interviewer's—will help you to be less defensive. It will also help you understand the meaning of the questions asked and help you answer them in an honest and reassuring way.

Part of your responsibility is to help the interviewer become comfortable with who you are and why you should be selected for the job. Yeager and Hough (1990) have suggested some ways to deal with the differences encountered in an interview.

If the interviewer is younger than you, statements such as "I bring a lot of experience to this position" will have a more positive effect than "I know I am older than the typical candidate, but. . . " If the interviewer is older than you, statements such as "I have always worked very hard and feel that learning is a life-long process" will help to establish your maturity.

With respect to cultural background, when there are differences between you and the interviewer, you need to remember that different groups have different norms concerning eye contact, personal distance, body language, and other subtle aspects of communication. To work through the differences, it is recommended that you follow the interviewer's lead in the course of communication. Don't mimic the interviewer's specific style, but allow her or him to establish some norms concerning how to communicate.

▼▼▼
Interview Questions and Answers: A Challenging Opportunity

> 1. **What is the best way to prepare for an interview?**
> 2. **Why is silence from an interviewer something to watch out for?**

Often the first interview question, "Tell me a little bit about yourself," is an "ice breaker" designed to make you comfortable and to determine what is important to you. Take advantage of the question to put both you and the interviewer on even ground. Practice the sample responses to typical interview questions given below as part of your preparation for the interview.

Do this as role-playing with another person in the role of the interviewer. Ask the person to mix up the order of the questions to prepare you better. You may also want the mock interview to include so-called illegal questions. This will prepare you to handle these questions effectively if they are asked. Successive practice sessions will make you appear to be confident when the time comes for the actual interview.

Also, by being prepared you will not fall victim to the interviewer's most powerful interview tool: silence. As noted by Adler (1993), "Silence makes people uncomfortable. Candidates will usually try to fill the void by providing more information—often revealing details beyond their prepared answers to standard interview questions."

▽▽▽
Sample Answers to Typical Interview Questions

Tell Me About Yourself.

Answer: Would you like to know about my work history or my personal life?

If work, provide a brief description of your recent schooling and past jobs.

If personal life: I recently graduated from school after living in this area for the past several months. I have a family, consider this my home, and plan to be here for some time. (This demonstrates stability and responsibility.)

Have You Ever Done This Type of Work Before?

Answer: Yes, in fact some of my experiences include direct care of clients during clinical rotations, volunteer work as a candy striper and. . .

Why Do You Want To Work Here?

Answer: The _____ (facility's name) has an excellent reputation in the community and job opportunities for which I am trained. Additionally, your mission statement of _____ reflects my views on _____.

Why Did You Leave Your Last Job?

Answer: As you know, I am a recent graduate and am looking for employment in my field of study.

Note: If you have worked as an LPN.

Answer: I am looking for a new position to expand my work skills, keep the job interesting, and provide better advancement opportunities.

Tell Me About Your Last Employer.

Answer: I really enjoyed my work at _____, which has an excellent reputation for _____. But it is now time to move on to new opportunities.

What Have You Done to Keep Your Clinical Skills Current?

Answer: Well, in addition to participating in several clinical rotations during school, I recently joined _____ (name of professional organization) to keep abreast of new developments in nursing.

What Kind of Salary or Wage Do You Expect?

Answer: I know that you will pay me what you feel I am worth and I can't ask for more than that.

Note: If an employer insists that you give a wage quote, give a wage range using your bottom dollar and a realistic top salary.

Answer: I would think that we could agree on a salary between $00,000 and $00,000 (Seitzer, 1995).

How Do You Compare Your Verbal Skills with Your Writing Skills?

Answer: Organizations are more dependent than ever on their employees communicating well both verbally and in writing. I am constantly taking advantage of opportunities to develop both areas by asking for and utilizing the feedback I receive.

Note: According to Yeager and Hough, (1990), this answer will avoid the booby-trap of being seen as weak in either area and acknowledge your awareness of the importance of communication.

Why Should We Hire You Instead of Someone Else?

Answer: I think that my references can best answer that question. I am sure that when you contact them they will agree that I am hard working, dependable, and get the job done right.

When Are You Available for Work?

Answer: Right away, or, I would need two weeks to resign from my current job because I owe this to my employer. This will provide time for me to tie up any loose ends and allow my employer to find a replacement.

Note: If the prospective employer insists that you terminate your position immediately, you are witnessing a power play. You need to ask yourself whether you really want to work for this individual. This could be the tip of the iceberg for future power plays.

How Is Your Health? Are There Any Parts of the Job That You Won't Be Able to Perform?

Answer: I have always been very healthy. I see myself as being able to perform all parts of the job. I think that the best approach to any job is using common sense. If I need help, I am not afraid to ask for it.

What Are Your Greatest Strengths?

Answer: I would have to say that my strengths include:
1) _____, 2)_____, 3)_____, 4)_____, and 5)_____.
Note: Your responses should be consistent with what your references say about you.

What Are Your Weaknesses?

Answer: If I make a mistake I find that no one can be harder on me than me. I want the job done right.

What Was Your Last Employer's Opinion of You?

Answer: Great! My employer always appreciated the fact that I was willing to take on new responsibilities and got the work done correctly.

Note: If you were "fired" by your last employer or if you left on bad terms:

Answer: My last employer will tell you that my work was excellent. We did not work well together. Rather than have the situation continue, the decision was made to leave. It has worked out for the best.

What Are Your Long-Term Goals?

Answer: Eventually, I would like to work as a charge nurse here at this facility. While my aim is not to replace the current charge nurse, it is my goal to learn all I can. Then I will be a contributing mem-

ber of the team, and you will feel confident that the work is being taken care of.

Can You Work Under Pressure?

Answer: Yes, I have experienced working under pressure for many years. This has meant meeting deadlines, dealing with difficult people, and having my employers know that their jobs would be done right.

Note: Be prepared to give an example because many employers will ask for one.

Will Child Care Be an Issue?

Answer: No. We have found a good day care setting for our children. If they can't go to day care my husband and I have worked out a system of alternating days on which to take care of them so that our work is minimally affected.

Note: Although some individuals believe that this is an illegal question, the author believes that the employer has a right to know. A stable staffing pattern is needed to maintain quality client care.

Do You Have Any Questions?

Answer: Yes, I would like to know if it would be possible to take a tour and to find out when I can start.

Note: Unless offered the job now, this is not the time to ask about wages. Wait until the job is offered to you, which will allow you some negotiating room. If offered the job at the time of the interview (or afterward), ask about (1) pay rate, (2) benefits, (3) vacation, and (4) starting date.

If you need a higher wage, now is the time to negotiate it because the employer has expressed a desire to hire you. One strategy to use if the starting wage is lower than you desire is to review your new job duties with the employer.

Ask the employer to agree to meet two or three times during the year to review your work performance and wage. Should you choose this strategy, ask the employer to put it into writing. Your work performance and increased wages are a goal you are both working toward.

Additional interview questions and answers that may be encountered are discussed by Allen (1990). These include:

Would You Be Willing to Work Overtime?

Answer: Yes, I believe that a job is a responsibility and not just a pay check.

May We Contact Your Current Employer?

Answer: No. I haven't informed my employer yet. Once a firm job offer has been made I would have no problem with you contacting her. However, because of our relationship, I would like the opportunity of talking with my employer first because she deserves this courtesy.

Is Your Spouse Employed? Will There Be a Conflict?

Answer: Yes, my _____ is a _____ (job) for _____ (company). Conflict? No, we've always been a two-career family and made adjustments equally to make things work.

Note: Although some individuals may believe that this is an illegal question, the author believes that the employer has a right to know the answer. A stable staffing pattern is needed to maintain high-quality client care.

Aren't You Overqualified for This Job?

Answer: I may be more qualified than other individuals you are considering, but this simply means that I will be able to hit the ground running, and make an immediate contribution. After learning your system, I hope to be eligible for advancement opportunities within the organization.

▼▼▼
Lasting Impressions

> 1. **What are the best clothes and make-up to wear for an interview?**
> 2. **What is the value of a good handshake?**

The kind of person you are is an additional concern to the interviewer. The impression you make includes everything that has been discussed previously plus your appearance and habits during the interview. Suggestions for all nurses include the following.

▽▽▽
Personal Hygiene

Bathe. Hair should be clean and arranged in a moderate style. Men's hair and beard should be neatly trimmed. Nails should be clean and nicely manicured (avoid bright polish). If you are a smoker, yellow finger stains may be removed with bleach and water. A nonperfumed deodorant should be used.

Recent mouth care may be needed to remove bad breath (remember not to indulge in food or drink with a heavy unpleasant odor near the time of the interview). Floss and brush your teeth, tongue, palate, and inner cheeks with a soft toothbrush. Use a breath freshener. Go easy on the aftershave or perfume, and don't sprinkle any on your clothing. Limit yourself to light perfume (a "clean" look goes a long way).

▽▽▽
Clothing

Dress conservatively. When choosing clothing, both men and women should try on many different suits or blazers to determine which fits best and hangs right. A poorly fitting suit looks bad and wears out faster. When buying clothing, the reality is that students may not always be able to afford the ideal. You can always look your best in clothes that are clean and ironed and shoes that are polished. Check out thrift stores and consignment shops, because they are resources waiting to be discovered. Additionally, you might check out community organizations such as Clothes Closets, which will loan clothing (i.e, the YWCA). When looking for clothing, consider the following points:

Men. Wear a long-sleeved white shirt, a solid or pin-stripe navy blue or gray suit, and a medallion pattern red or navy tie that is 3½ inches wide. Dark shoes, long dark socks, and a belt that matches the shoes are also a must.

Women. Choose solid or pin-stripe navy or blue dresses, jacket dresses, or suits. Look for simple straight or pleated skirts that reach at least knee level and are comfortable to sit in. Remember that a skirt that is too short may be viewed as being "too sexy." Wear dark low-heeled shoes with closed toes.

Women with larger hips may want to avoid wearing short jackets. Short jackets flatter women who are petite. Additionally, women who wear gray jackets will want to keep the gray away from their faces by wearing a crisp white blouse or a soft beige sweater. Gray clothes near your face may "drain your complexion."

▽▽▽
Make-up

Conservative make-up is always appropriate. Make-up should be kept to a minimum; wearing too much is the most common mistake. Remember that it is the confidence you display in the interview that makes you attractive to the employer.

▽▽▽
Accessories

Wear simple jewelry or none at all. Simple necklaces such as pearls and colored beads work well. Avoid hanging earrings and bracelets that clank or rhinestones and fake rubies. Plan ahead what purse or briefcase you will carry. You will want to limit yourself to one or the other and have it small enough to avoid getting in your way, yet big enough to hold any papers. If you have a coat or umbrella, ask politely where you can hang or lay them. The main point is to avoid holding items or balancing them on your lap. The fewest distractions will help keep you calm and focused on the interview.

▽▽▽
Posture

Walk tall and sit erect but not entirely at the back of your chair. Both feet should rest on the floor, and your head should be upright. Arms and hands should be in an open position and not crossed (remember, you have nothing to hide). Keep your hands inactive. If you must fidget consider bringing a paper clip to the interview to hold in your hands.

▽▽▽
Manner

Your manner should be assured. Do not interrupt the interviewer. Pause to think as needed, then answer without hesitating. Ask for an explanation or repetition of any questions you do not understand. Eye contact is essential, especially when answering questions. If you are uncomfortable with making eye contact, two techniques can be used to correct this—looking at the employer's nose or looking at the space between the eyebrows. Both give the illusion of eye contact. Remember to look away periodically. Avoid making negative statements or comments about school, former jobs, or personal problems.

▽▽▽
Courtesy

When meeting the employer, smile and extend your hand for a firm handshake. Do not use a "bone crusher" grip or a limp "dead fish" handshake. Find someone to practice with prior to the interview to get your handshake right. Additionally, if your palms tend to sweat, rub your hand along the top of your thigh when standing up. It will remove the moisture while appearing very natural.

After the handshake, say, "Mr. (Ms.) Smith, my name is _____." Similarly, when the interview is over, stand up, look the person in the eyes, and offer your hand for a firm handshake. Address the employer by his surname: "Mr. (Ms.) Smith, thank you for the opportunity to interview with you. Based on what I have learned here today, I know that I can do the job. I would like to call you in four days to see if you have made a decision. Would that be all right?" If you want the job, give the employer a list of your work references or letters of recommendation.

▽▽▽
Habits

Do not chew gum or smoke while in the waiting room or during the interview. Also, don't smoke outside the building and then come in for the interview. Although the nicotine may make you feel calm, you will be bringing in the fresh smell of smoke, which is often offensive to nonsmokers. Politely refuse an offer for coffee or tea or cigarettes. In addition, do not read any materials on the employer's desk.

▼▼▼
References: A Treasure

■ *What is a reference hierarchy?*

Prospective employers will be more interested in some work references than in others. There is a *hierarchy* of individuals who act as references. Ranging from most to least important are:

1. Current or former supervisors from work and volunteer experiences, unit managers, and teachers.
2. Coworkers who have seen your work.
3. Personal references or friends.

(Note: Employers generally don't bother to contact personal references and put little value in their opinions.)

On reference sheets include the person's name, job title, address, and work phone number. Three is the usual number of references requested. Pick and choose from your list of resources for maximum impression.

The statement "References on Request" can be placed at the end of your résumé. It is a matter of personal choice. References should be listed on the reference list and given to the interviewer if he or she requests them. References, however, are "treasures." Avoid giving them out if you are not interested in the position.

▼▼▼
Résumés: The Contributions You Will Make

> 1. *What items should not be included in a résumé?*
> 2. *Why are job duties written in sentence form not used?*
> 3. *Why is a GED more valuable than was first thought?*

Development of a résumé is a must! It focuses on your work skills, experiences, and qualifications. Résumés are not used as a confession or "tell-all" script. They should not include such items as reasons for leaving past jobs, salary requirements, personal photographs, and personal data including marital status, race, religion, height, weight, or number or age of children.

Ethridge (1995) also recommends cutting out a statement of your "Objective," often located at the top of the résumé. Additionally, it has been noted that employers don't care about your "personal goals" and that statements like "excellent health" are a waste—who would report that their health was bad?

Unfortunately, many résumés are never read because they are too cluttered or wordy or contain the areas noted earlier that have turned the interviewer off. The initial impression made by the résumé is significant. Basic factors to consider include:

▶ Length: Two pages is maximum. One page is preferred.

▶ Paper: Quality bond. Stay with colors such as white, cream, beige, or gray. Use matching paper for the cover letter and envelope.

▶ Typing: Absolutely no spelling or grammatical errors or extra marks. Type your résumé on a computer and use a laser printer. The computer allows for painless corrections. Updating is performed quickly. It is worth going to a quick print shop to make résumé copies. Standard copy machines provide poorer-quality copies.

▶ Faxing: Copy your résumé onto white paper. By sending the fax on white paper the transmission will be faster and the faxed copy will be clearer and easier to read.

▶ Balance and space: An uncluttered, balanced design is desirable so that the résumé is easy to read. Because most managers don't have time to read, a "bulleted" style is recommended when listing job skills and past duties.

▶ Emphasis: Depends on whether you have a strong or a limited work history.

A suggested format follows. It may be varied according to the job you are seeking. Remember, you want to let the employer know that you can fill the job before he has met you.

1. Personal data. Include your legal name, address, phone number, or message phone number.

2. Education. If you are a recent graduate, list this area before your work experience. If you are already working in the field, it is recommended that education be listed *after* work experience to emphasize your experience. Education should include: diplomas, certificates, honors, scholarships, continuing education classes, and the institutions granting these degrees.

   Hint: For individuals who did not finish high school but went on to obtain their General Education Diploma (GED), spread the GED name out on the résumé so that employers will focus on the fact that you have a diploma (see example résumé).

   This author's experiences with people who have earned a GED is that they often feel apologetic because they did not finish traditional high school. As a result, they think that their degree "does not count for anything." Individuals who obtain a GED should be proud of having the courage to go back to school and proud of passing tests that are significantly harder than those given in any high school.

3. Licenses and professional memberships. List these after the Work Experience section if you are a recent graduate or after the Education section if you have worked for a period of time.

4. Work experience. This section is organized by listing your most recent job or duties first. List the job title, employer's name, city and state, and the duration of the job or years you were employed. Review what tasks you actually performed including operation of any computer or medical device or management responsibilities, no matter how minor. Management responsibilities might include participation on work committees like "quality assurance" or "assisted with experimental Alzheimer's medication studies."

   4a. *Homemakers are domestic managers.* Remember that you have several valuable skills that deserve comment. Skills include: bookkeeping, scheduling, transportation, home management, inventory control, purchasing, quality control, supervision, and training.

   4b. *Older workers.* Substitute years of experience for dates. Don't dredge up your entire work history; stop at ten years. Avoid listing skills in outdated technology, and take some classes to update your skills (Shrieves, 1995).

   4c. *Uncovering résumé lies.* According to Half (1992), employers may read your résumé from the bottom up because "most applicants put unflattering material at the end." Keep your résumé consistent and well-balanced.

5. Military service. List your last station of active duty and its location by state. Indicate your area of specialization (e.g., infantry) and rank (e.g., E-4). It is recommended that you do not list dates or wars fought in.

Two sample résumés and a work reference sheet are provided to give you an idea of how to make these suggestions work for you.

KATELYN BIESER

2001 Putt Drive, Cottage Grove, MN 55301   (612) 555-2728

EDUCATION

Fairview School of Nursing   <u>Practical Nursing</u>   **Diploma**
Minneapolis, Minnesota   1997

* Nursing Care Principles   * Medication Administration   * Med-Surgical Principles
* Clinical Nursing   * Professional Communications   * Health Care Delivery
* Maternal/Child Nursing   * Psychosocial Development   * Nutritional Care

Cottage Grove High School   **Diploma**
Cottage Grove, Minnesota   1992

WORK EXPERIENCE

Forest View Nursing Home   <u>Certified</u>   **Nursing Assistant**
Hastings, Minnesota   Two Years

* Assisted Physicians/Staff   * Direct Patient Care   * Obtain/Chart Vital Signs
* Personal Health Intervention   * Injury Prevention   * Promote Daily Living Skills

Bieser & Associates   **Domestic Manager**
Cottage Grove, Minnesota   1993 to present

* Budgeting/Inventory Control   * Health Care Management   * Quality Control
* Coord. Daily Living Activities   * Mediation/Planning   * Crisis Intervention

LICENSES/MEMBERSHIPS

State of Minnesota Board of Practical Nursing   **License**
St. Paul, Minnesota   (In Progress)

National Practical Nursing Association   **Membership**
Silver Springs, Maryland   1997 to Present

REFERENCES

Available Upon Request

KATELYN BIESER

2001 Putt Drive, Cottage Grove, MN 55301   (612) 555-2728

WORK EXPERIENCE

KESA Temporary Health Care Agency Plymouth, Minnesota	Contracted Services	**Licensed Practical Nurse** 1998 to Present

* Personal Care Services   * Administered Medications   * Responded to Patient Calls
* Assisted Medical Staff   * Flexible Shift Scheduling   * Quality Assurance
* Medical Equipment Operation   * Charted Observations   * Computer/Dictaphone Use

Forest View Nursing Home Hastings, Minnesota	Part Time To Attend School	**Certified Nursing Assistant** Two Years

* Assisted Physicians/Staff   * Direct Patient Care   * Obtain/Chart Vital Signs
* Personal Health Intervention   * Injury Prevention   * Promote Daily Living Skills

The Small Town Cafe Bloomington, Minnesota	**Waitress** 2 ½ Years

* Direct Customer Service   * Time Management   * Cashiering
* Assisted w/Food Preparation   * Cleaned Tables/Dishes   * Maintained Work Area

EDUCATION

Fairview School of Nursing Minneapolis, Minnesota	Practical Nursing	**Diploma** 1997
Cottage Grove High School Cottage Grove, Minnesota	General Education	**Diploma** 1992

LICENSES/MEMBERSHIPS

State of Minnesota Board of Practical Nursing St. Paul, Minnesota	**License** 1997 to Present
National Practical Nursing Association Silver Springs, Maryland	**Membership** 1997 to Present

WORK REFERENCES

Ms. Shirley Zaic Nursing Supervisor Forest View Nursing Home 1995 Seattle Avenue Hastings, MN 55751 (612) 555-1234	Mr. Peter Hinkkanen, Owner The Small Town Cafe 3006 Deer Blvd. Bloomington, MN 55179 (612) 555-2104	Ms. Terry Illmari Nursing Instructor Fairview School of Nursing 2401 Riverside Drive Minneapolis, MN 55401 (612) 555-2222

▼▼▼
Cover Letters: Tailor-Made to Fit the Job You Want

▌ *Why do cover letters need to be sent in with résumés?*

It is essential to include a cover letter with each résumé. The cover letter may be submitted by mail or dropped off with an application for the employer. Cover letters respond directly to newspaper ad quali-fications or the unsolicited phone calls you made inquiring about job openings. Neatness, correct spelling, and proper grammar are mandatory. Each letter should be one page long, an original (never photocopied) with no "whiteout applied," and in a block letter format.

If an employer asks for supervisory experience or other specific experience, be sure to list these in your cover letter even if your experiences are not listed on the résumé. Sample cover letters to an employer contacted through an unsolicited telephone call and through a newspaper ad appear as examples.

August 11, 1997

Ms. Valerie George, RN
Director of Nursing
St. Helen General Hospital
8354 177th Lane
St. Paul, Minnesota 55000

RE: LPN Staff Nurse Position

Dear Ms. George:

Thank you for taking the time to speak with me about the Practical Nurse staff position. As we discussed, I have enclosed my résumé for your review.

I am a recent graduate of the Fairview Nursing Program and will be taking my State Board examination on September 20, 1997. My clinical work experience includes: client care planning, plan review, direct client care, administering medications, and team participation. Additionally, I have worked as a Nursing Assistant for two years at the Forest View Nursing Home in Hastings, MN and I am listed with the state nursing assistant registry.

I will be contacting you on Tuesday, August 19, 1997, to see if you have had an opportunity to review my résumé and determine when an interview may be arranged. I look forward to speaking with you soon.

Cordially,

Katelyn Bieser
2001 Putt Drive
Cottage Grove, Minnesota 55301
(612) 555-2728

ENC: Résumé

August 11, 1997

Ms. Valerie George, RN
Director of Nursing
St. Helen General Hospital
8354 177th Lane
St. Paul, Minnesota 55000

RE: LPN Staff Nurse Position

Dear Ms. George:

Please accept my résumé as application for the Licensed Practical Nurse
position advertised in the Minneapolis Star & Tribune newspaper. I believe
that my work experiences through the Fairview Nursing Program and my
nursing home are a good match for the position.

As a recent graduate of the Fairview Nursing Program, I will be taking my
NCLEX-PN on September 20, 1997. My clinical work experience includes: client
care planning, plan review, direct client care, administering medications,
and team participation. Additionally, I have worked as a Certified Nursing Assistant for two years at the Forest View Nursing Home in Hastings, Minnesota
performing the above duties, plus more.

I will be contacting you on Tuesday, August 19, 1997, to see if you have
had an opportunity to review my résumé and determine when an interview may
be arranged. I look forward to speaking with you soon.

Cordially,

Katelyn Bieser
2001 Putt Drive
Cottage Grove, Minnesota 55301
(612) 555-2728

ENC: Résumé

▼▼▼
Proactive Follow-up Today

> 1. What is the percentage of people who
>   do not follow up with employers after
>   submitting résumés or participating in
>   interviews?
> 2. When is the best time to make a
>   follow-up call?
> 3. How might you get past the secretary
>   to find out if you have been hired?

Follow-up after a job interview is essential. It is a
constant source of amazement to employers that 90%
of the people who interview never follow up to see if
they will get the job. Recent graduates and even nurses
who have been working in the field for some time are
under the illusion that it is the employer's responsibility to contact them. She who hesitates will be disappointed!

While the information is fresh in your mind, write
a thank you letter to the interviewer the same day you
interviewed. Write before you become distracted by
other projects. Remember, the more often the employer
sees or hears your name, the better your chances of
being hired rather than the person waiting for the
phone call. A thank you letter may be as simple as the
following example:

August 26, 1997

Ms. Valerie George,
Director of Nursing
St. Helen General Hospital
8354 177th Lane
St. Paul, Minnesota 55000

RE: LPN Staff Nurse Position

Dear Ms. George:

I want to thank you for meeting with me today to discuss the LPN staff
position. Following our conversation about the job duties and the tour of
the hospital floor, I feel that my work experiences and education are a good
match.

Specifically, I look forward to the opportunity to work on the pediatric
floor as this is a special interest area of mine. Through our work together
the clients will receive timely, quality care.

I remain very interested in the position. I will contact you on Wednesday,
September 3, 1997, to see if you have made a decision and/or if a second
interview should be arranged. I look forward to speaking with you soon.

Cordially,

Katelyn Bieser
2001 Putt Drive
Cottage Grove, Minnesota 55301
(612) 555-2728

Remember to follow up with the employer! Call the employer on the date stated in your letter. Make it a practice not to make follow-up contacts on Mondays. These days are traditionally reserved for staff meetings and other duties and are just plain full. The best times to make your follow up calls are 9:00 AM and 2:00 PM. Allen (1992) recommends that you be courteous but firm with the secretary. Ask to speak with the person in charge of hiring. The following is a sample conversation:

Secretary: Good morning. Ms. George's office.
You: This is Katelyn Bieser calling. May I speak with Ms. George, please?
Secretary: I'm sorry, she's away from her desk/on another line/in a meeting. May I take a message?

You: Ms. George and I met last week for the LPN staff position and said that I should follow up.
Secretary: One minute, please.

Allen notes that although the boss might be away from her desk, or on another line, the secretary was probably checking to see whether your call should be taken. If the employer is not available, ask the secretary to tell you the best time to reach the employer.

▼▼▼
Prephysical Examinations and Drug Screening

1. Does a conditional job offer mean that you got the job?

| **2. If you fail a drug test, does it mean that you have a chemical abuse problem?**

More and more employers are requiring prephysical examinations as a part of conditional job offers. A conditional job offer states that you have been offered the job contingent upon your passing a physical examination or drug screening. If you fail, the job offer is withdrawn.

You will be required to meet with a physician specified by the employer, who will perform a physical examination and ask you about your past medical history. Think about any past surgeries, work injuries, allergies, and family history including cancer and heart trouble. Be prepared to provide the dates of these occurrences and the names of the physicians who provided treatment. If you have any personal concerns about the answers your physician might provide, call your own doctor prior to the exam. Discuss the job and obtain the doctor's opinion.

If you are required to participate in a drug screening examination, and are taking medications, be sure to notify your employer prior to the screening. You will want to reaffirm in the employer's mind that you are taking a medical prescription that will not interfere with your work. Be aware that although drug screening accuracy is improving, it is not 100% accurate.

According to Sakson (1995), "many legal drugs will trigger a positive result including common foods such as a poppy seed bagel for breakfast." Any positive test should be followed by a second and more rigorous test. The manufacturer of the First Stage drug screening test admits a 5% error rate, but independent research companies estimate a rate closer to 25%. Typically, second tests are not performed by the employer because of the cost involved.

Therefore, it is easier for the employer to say that you are out. If you fail the first test, contact the employer about your concerns. In your conversation with the employer you may want to offer to take a more rigorous test with the same company doctor at your own expense. The key is sincerity; if you want the job, let the employer know that you are willing to go the extra mile.

▼▼▼
Discussing Pregnancy

| *If you are pregnant, what do you need to consider before talking with an employer about it?*

When do you tell a new employer that you are pregnant? Even if your job is protected by the Pregnancy Discrimination Act and the Family and Medical Leave Act, when do you discuss the pregnancy so that it doesn't interfere with career advancement? Kleiman (1995) reported that waiting a couple of months is okay. She indicated that the "real issues are your comfort level and professionalism."

When you are ready to talk about your pregnancy, be prepared to discuss (1) how long you plan to work, (2) how long you intend to be gone, and possibly, (3) how your work will be covered while you are away. Then talk with your coworkers about the pregnancy and enlist their moral support. Expectant mothers may have both good and bad days during the pregnancy; friends can be a great help.

▼▼▼
Resignation with Style

| *Is there a difference between "burning bridges" and "untying the connection"? What is the value of recapping your accomplishments with a resignation letter?*

If you have made the decision to leave your employer, it is important to leave the job with class. Perhaps the best expression I have heard is "Untie, don't sever, the connection." You never know who may call your former employer as a part of their follow-up. You may wish to return to their employ again in the future.

It is strongly recommended that you have a position secured prior to leaving. Some employers will let you go the day they are informed even though the policy requires a two-week notice (Sixel, 1995). Either way, it is recommended that the employer be given written notice of your intention to leave, allowing adequate time to hire a replacement. It is a courtesy to give two weeks' notice even if there is no policy in place. (It is expensive for an employer to hire and orient a new person and for the new person to become a productive team member.)

Use a business format and plain paper, and type the letter. Even if you are leaving because of unhappy circumstances on the job, do not vent these feelings in the letter. As mentioned before, you may need this employer as a work reference in the future. Additionally, your current supervisor may also leave in the future, and all that is there to remind the employer about you is your personnel file.

Because resignation is part of your permanent record, it provides you with an opportunity to recap your accomplishments or special recognition. The employer may refer to the letter when he or she is contacted by employers with whom you are seeking employment. See the following sample resignation letter.

September 13, 1999

Ms. Barbara Bauer,
Director of Nursing
Brown County Hospital
1515 Placebo Lane
Minneapolis, Minnesota 55401

Dear Ms. Bauer:

Please accept my resignation as Charge Nurse on Unit 3 to be effective on September 27, 1999. My association with the Brown County Hospital has been rewarding professionally and personally. It is satisfying to have been able to contribute to the positive reputation of client care.

I am especially pleased to have been a member of the Quality Assurance committee which furthered my professional growth. In addition, I remain appreciative of having been honored as ''Employee of the Month.'' Please accept my thanks for the support you have provided me during the past one and a half years of employment. I wish the members of this hospital the very best.

Cordially,

Katelyn Bieser, LPN
Alzheimer Unit

▼▼▼ *S U M M A R Y*

- ► To be successful in your job search, it is important to begin it with the first day of classes and not stop from that day on. Opportunities present themselves to those who are willing to put forth a little effort and realize that the world does not owe them a living.
- ► The methods presented in this chapter have proved to be successful for graduates, people wishing to make career changes, or those wanting to institute a change in their work. Remember to treat the job search like a job.

▶ Make your contacts by telephone, by forwarding résumés or cover letters, or by physically going to the employer to apply and schedule an interview. Explore the hidden job market via networking or using the telephone book and then calling employers whether an ad has been placed or not.

▶ Actively follow up on all interviews! Let the employer know that you are interested. Remember, the more often the employer hears your name, the better your chances will be. If you are hired, send thank you notes to those who helped you. You may need them again. Remember, you are responsible for making your own luck.

▼▼▼ *R E F E R E N C E S*

Adler E. Powerful interview tool: Silence. Boardroom Reports 1993; 22(8):15.
Allen J. *Jeff Allen's Best Win The Job.* New York: John Wiley & Sons, 1990.
Allen J. *The Perfect Follow-Up Method To Get The Job.* New York: John Wiley & Sons, 1992.
Baker W. How to make the right friends inside your company. Bottom Line Personal 1994; 15(17):13–14.
Dahlstrom & Company. *The Job Hunting Handbook: Job Outlook to 2005.* Holliston, MA: Dahlstrom & Company, 1995.
Ethridge M. Keep ahead of the curve when seeking jobs; rules for the hunt are evolving. St. Paul Pioneer Press 1995; May 28, 1K.
Farr J. *America's Top Medical and Human Services Jobs.* Indianapolis, IN: JIST Works, Inc., 1994.
Feder B. Corporate giants' attitude toward temps changing. Star Tribune 1995; April 9, 13J.
Franklin D. What your voice says about you. Health Magazine 1995; 19(2):38, 41.
Half R. Tells how to protect the company from résumé fraud. Boardroom Reports 1992; 21(23):11.
Kleiman C. Planning leaves for pregnancies eases interim for moms, employers. St. Paul Pioneer Press 1995; June 4, K1.
Kuntz S. Critical career questions. Twin Cities Employment Weekly 1995; 2(44): 2.
Meissner J. How to work a room. Twin Cities Employment Weekly 1995; 3(7): 2, 8.
Mercer M. How to make a great impression on anyone. Bottom Line Personal 1994; 15(21): 13–14.
Moreau D. Good jobs for fresh grads. Kiplinger's Personal Finance Magazine 1995; 49(3): 110–114.
Sakson S. Positive drug tests post decline. St. Paul Pioneer Press 1995; June 30, B3.
Seitzer D. Salary negotiations. Twin City Employment Weekly 1995; 2(43): 2–3.
Shrieves L. "Temping" can become permanent career. St. Paul Pioneer Press 1995; Aug. 20, K1.
Sixel L. When to tell boss you're planning to quit. St. Paul Pioneer Press 1995; January 22, K1.
Yeager N, Hough L. *Power Interviews: Job-Winning Tactics from Fortune 500 Recruiters.* New York: John Wiley & Sons, 1990.

▼▼▼ *B I B L I O G R A P H Y*

Feder B. More large firms viewing temps as permanent answer. St. Paul Pioneer Press 1995; April 9, K1.
Shrieves L. For older workers, the right résumé will lessen age as a factor in hiring. St. Paul Pioneer Press 1995; Aug. 27, K1.

▼▼▼
Appendix A: State Boards of Nursing

Alabama

Alabama Board of Nursing
P.O. BOX 303900
Montgomery, Alabama
 36130-3900
Phone: (334) 242-4060
Fax: (334) 242-4360

Street Address
RSA Plaza, Suite 250
770 Washington Avenue
Montgomery, Alabama
 36130-3900

Alaska

Alaska Board of Nursing
Department of Commerce and
 Economic Development
Div. of Occupational Licensing
3601 C Street, Suite 722
Anchorage, Alaska 99503
Phone: (907) 561-2878
Fax: (907) 562-5781
NCNET: NCZ026

Alaska Board of Nursing
P.O. Box 110806
Juneau, Alaska 99811-0800
Phone: (907) 465-2544
Fax: (907) 465-2974

American Samoa

American Samoa Health Service
 Regulatory Board
LBJ Tropical Medical Center
Pago Pago, American Samoa
 96799
Phone: (684) 633-1222 Ext. 206
Fax: 011-684-633-1869
Telex No.: #782-573-LBJ TMC

Arizona

Arizona State Board of Nursing
1651 E. Morten Ave., Suite 150
Phoenix, Arizona 85020
Phone: (602) 255-5092
Fax: (602) 255-5130

Arkansas

Arkansas State Board of Nursing
University Tower Building,
 Suite 800
1123 South University
Little Rock, Arkansas 72204
Phone: (501) 686-2700
Fax: (501) 686-2714

California-RN

California Board of Registered
 Nursing

P.O. Box 944210
Sacramento, California
 94244-2100
Phone: (916) 322-3350
Fax: (916) 327-4402
NCNET: C.Puri 132:NCZ030

Street Address
400 R Street, Suite 4030
Sacramento, California
 95814-6200

California-VN

California Board of Vocational
 Nurse and Psychiatric Tech-
 nician Examiners
2535 Capitol Oaks Drive,
 Suite 205
Sacramento, California 95833
Phone: (916) 263-7800
Fax: (916) 263-7859

Colorado

Colorado Board of Nursing
1560 Broadway, Suite 670
Denver, Colorado 80202
Phone: (303) 894-2430
Fax: (303) 894-2821

Connecticut

Connecticut Board of Examiners
  for Nursing
Department of Public Health
  Nurse Licensure
150 Washington Street
Hartford, Connecticut 06106
Phone: (860) 566-1041
Fax: (860) 566-1032

Delaware

Delaware Board of Nursing
Cannon Building, Suite 203
P.O. Box 1401
Dover, Delaware 19903
Phone: (302) 739-4522
Fax: (302) 739-2711

District of Columbia

District of Columbia Board
  of Nursing
614 H. Street, N.W.
Washington, District of Columbia
  20001
Phone: (202) 727-7468
Fax: (202) 727-7662

For Exam Information:
Phone: (202) 727-7454

Florida

Florida Board of Nursing
4080 Woodcock Drive, Suite 202
Jacksonville, Florida 32207
Phone: (904) 858-6940
Fax: (904) 359-6323

For Exam Information:
Same as above

Georgia-PN

Georgia State Board of Licensed
  Practical Nurses
166 Pryor Street, S.W.
Atlanta, Georgia 30303
Phone: (404) 656-3921
Fax: (404) 651-9532

For Exam Information:
Exam Development
  & Testing Unit
Phone: (404) 656-3903

Georgia-RN

Georgia Board of Nursing
166 Pryor Street, S.W.
Atlanta, Georgia 30303
Phone: (404) 656-3943
Fax: (404) 651-7489

Guam

Guam Board of Nurse Examiners
P.O. Box 2816
Agana, Guam 96910
Phone: 011-(671) 475-0251
Fax: 011-(671) 477-4733

Hawaii

Hawaii Board of Nursing
P.O. Box 3469
Honolulu, Hawaii 96801
Phone: (808) 586-2695
Fax: (808) 586-2689

Idaho

Idaho Board of Nursing
P.O. Box 83720
Boise, Idaho 83720-0061
Phone: (208) 334-3110
Fax: (208) 334-3262
NCNET: ID NC2022

Illinois

Illinois Dept. of Professional
  Regulation
320 West Washington Street
  3rd Floor
Springfield, Illinois 62786
Phone: (217) 785-9465
(217) 785-0800
Fax: (217) 782-7645

Illinois Dept. of Professional
  Regulation
100 West Randolph Suite 9-300
Chicago, Illinois 60601
Phone: (312) 814-2715
Fax: (312) 814-3154

For Exam Information:
Application Requests
Licensure Information
Asst. Nursing/Act Coordinator
Phone: (217) 782-0458
(217) 782-8556
(217) 785-9465

Indiana

Indiana State Board of Nursing
Health Professions Bureau
402 West Washington Street
Room #041
Indianapolis, Indiana 46204
Phone: (317) 232-2960
Fax: (317) 233-4236

Iowa

Iowa Board of Nursing
State Capitol Complex
1223 East Court Avenue
Des Moines, Iowa 50319
Phone: (515) 281-3255
Fax: (515) 281-4825

Kansas

Kansas State Board of Nursing
Landon State Office Building
900 S.W. Jackson, Suite 551-S
Topeka, Kansas 66612-1230
Phone: (913) 296-4929
Fax: (913) 296-3929

Departments:
General Information
Continuing Education
Practice or Disciplinary
Phones: (913) 296-4929
(913) 296-3782
(913) 296-4325

Kentucky

Kentucky Board of Nursing
312 Wittington Parkway,
  Suite 300
Louisville, Kentucky 40222-5172
Phone: (502) 329-7000
Fax: (502) 329-7011

Louisiana-RN

Louisiana State Board of Nursing
912 Pere Marquette Building
150 Baronne Street
New Orleans, Louisiana 70112
Phone: (504) 568-5464
Fax: (504) 568-5467
NCNET: NCZ018

Louisiana-PN

Louisiana State Board of Practical
  Nurse Examiners
3421 N. Causeway Boulevard
  Suite 203
Metairie, Louisiana 70002
Phone: (504) 838-5791
Fax: (504) 838-5279

Maine

Maine State Board of Nursing
State House Station #158
Augusta, Maine 04333-0158
Phone: (207) 624-5275
Fax: (207) 624-5290
NCNET: NCZ010

Maryland

Maryland Board of Nursing
4140 Patterson Avenue
Baltimore, Maryland 21215-2299
Phone: (410) 764-5124
Fax: (410) 358-3530

Massachusetts

Massachusetts Board of
  Registration in Nursing
Leverett Saltonstall Building
100 Cambridge Street, Room 1519
Boston, MA 02202
Phone: (617) 727-9961
Fax: (617) 727-2197

Michigan

Bureau of Occupational and
  Professional Regulation
Michigan Department
  of Commerce
Ottawa Towers North
611 West Ottawa
Lansing, Michigan 48933
Phone: (517) 373-1600
Fax: (517) 373-2179

For Exam Information:

Office of Testing Services
Michigan Department
  of Commerce
P.O. Box 30018
Lansing, Michigan 48909
Phone: (517) 373-3877
Fax: (517) 335-6696

Minnesota

Minnesota Board of Nursing
2829 University Avenue SE, #500
Minneapolis, MN 55414-3253
Phone: (612) 617-2270
Fax: (612) 617-2190

Mississippi

Mississippi Board of Nursing
239 N. Lamar Street, Suite 401
Jackson, Mississippi 39201
Phone: (601) 359-6170
Fax: (601) 359-6185

Missouri

Missouri State Board of Nursing
P.O. Box 656
Jefferson City, Missouri 65102
Phone: (314) 751-0681
Fax: (314) 751-0075

Street Address

3605 Missouri Blvd.
Jefferson City, Missouri 65109

Montana

Montana State Board of Nursing
111 North Jackson
P.O. Box 200513
Helena, Montana 59620-0513
Phone: (406) 444-2071
Fax: (406) 444-7759
NCNET: NCZ032

Nebraska

Bureau of Examining Boards
Nebraska Department of Health
P.O. Box 95007
Lincoln, Nebraska 68509
Phone: (402) 471-2115
Fax: (402) 471-3577

Street Address

301 Centennial Mall South
Lincoln, Nebraska 68508

Nevada

Nevada State Board of Nursing
P.O. Box 46886
Las Vegas, Nevada 89114
Phone: (702) 739-1575
Fax: (702) 739-0298

Street Address

4335 S. Industrial Road, Suite 430
Las Vegas, Nevada 89103

Nevada State Board of Nursing
  (2nd Office)
1755 East Plumb Lane, Suite 260
Reno, Nevada 89502
Phone: (702) 786-2778
Fax: (702) 322-6993

New Hampshire

New Hampshire Board of Nursing
Health & Welfare Building
6 Hazen Drive
Concord, New Hampshire
   03301-6527
Phone: (603) 271-2323
Fax: (603) 271-6605

New Jersey

New Jersey Board of Nursing
P.O. Box 45010
Newark, New Jersey 07101
Phone: (201) 504-6493
Fax: (201) 648-3481

Street Address:
124 Halsey Street, 6th Floor
Newark, New Jersey 07102

New Mexico

New Mexico Board of Nursing
4206 Louisiana Blvd., NE
   Suite A
Albuquerque, New Mexico 87109
Phone: (505) 841-8340
Fax: (505) 841-8347

New York

New York State Board of Nursing
State Education Department
Cultural Education Center,
   Room 3023
Albany, New York 12230
Phone: (518) 474-3843/3845
Fax: (518) 473-0578

For Exam Information:
Division of Professional
   Licensing Services
State Education Department
Cultural Education Center
Albany, New York 12230
Phone: (518) 474-6591

North Carolina

North Carolina Board of Nursing
P.O. Box 2129
Raleigh, North Carolina 27602
Phone: (919) 782-3211
Fax: (919) 781-9461
NCNET: NCZ014

Street Address
3724 National Drive
Raleigh, North Carolina 27612

North Dakota

North Dakota Board of Nursing
919 South 7th Street, Suite 504
Bismarck, North Dakota 58504-
   5881
Phone: (701) 328-9777
Fax: (701) 328-4614

Northern Mariana Islands

Commonwealth Board of Nurse
   Examiners
Public Health Center
P.O. Box 1458
Saipan, MP 96950
Phone: 011-670-234-8950
   thru 8954
Fax: 011-670-234-8930

Telex Number is 783-744,
Answer back code is PNESPN744.
When calling, ask for Public
   Health Center
(ext. 2018 or 2019)

Ohio

Ohio Board of Nursing
77 South High Street, 17th Floor
Columbus, Ohio 43266-0316
Phone: (614) 466-3947
Fax: (614) 466-0388

Oklahoma

Oklahoma Board of Nursing
2915 North Classen Blvd.,
   Suite 524
Oklahoma City, Oklahoma 73106
Phone: (405) 525-2076
Fax: (405) 521-6089

Oregon

Oregon State Board of Nursing
Suite 465
800 NE Oregon Street, Box 25
Portland, Oregon 97232
Phone: (503) 731-4745
Fax: (503) 731-4755

Pennsylvania

Pennsylvania State Board
   of Nursing
P.O. Box 2649
Harrisburg, Pennsylvania
   17105-2649
Phone: (717) 783-7142
Fax: (717) 787-7769

Street Address:
124 Pine Street
Harrisburg, PA 17101

*For Exam. Program/Contract
   Requirements*
Use same address as Penn. Bd.

Puerto Rico

Commonwealth of Puerto Rico
   Board of Nurse Examiners
Call Box 10200
Santurce, Puerto Rico 00908
Phone: (809) 725-8161 or
   (809) 725-7904
Fax: (809) 725-7903

Rhode Island

Rhode Island Board of Nurse Reg-
istration & Nursing Education
Cannon Health Building
Three Capitol Hill, Room 104
Providence, Rhode Island
02908-5097
Phone: (401) 277-2827
Fax: (401) 277-1272

South Carolina

South Carolina State Board
of Nursing
220 Executive Center Drive,
Suite 220
Columbia, South Carolina 29210
Phone: (803) 731-1648
Fax: (803) 731-1647
NCNET: NCZ023

Departments
Legal & Disciplinary Services
Education/Examination/
Accounting/Computer Services
Phone: (803) 731-1667
(803) 731-1648

South Dakota

South Dakota Board of Nursing
3307 South Lincoln Avenue
Sioux Falls, South Dakota
57105-5224
Phone: (605) 367-5940
Fax: (605) 367-5945

Tennessee

Tennessee State Board of Nursing
283 Plus Park Blvd.
Nashville, Tennessee 37217-1010
Phone: (615) 367-6232
Fax: (615) 367-6397

Texas-RN

Texas Board of Nurse Examiners
P.O. Box 140466
Austin, Texas 78714
Phone: (512) 305-7400
Fax: (512) 305-7401

Street Address
William P. Hobby Building,
Tower 3
333 Guadalupe, Suite 460
Austin, Texas 78701

Departments:
Practice & Compliance
Administration/Education/
Examination
Phone: (512) 835-8686
(512) 835-8650

Texas-VN

Texas Board of Vocational
Nurse Examiners
William P. Hobby Building,
Tower 3
333 Guadalupe Street, 3-400
Austin, Texas 78701
Phone: (512) 305-8100
Fax: (512) 305-8101

Utah

Utah State Board of Nursing
Division of Occupational & Prof.
Licensing
P.O. Box 45805
Salt Lake City, Utah 84145-0805
Phone: (801) 530-6628
Fax: (801) 530-6511

Street Address
Heber M. Wells Building,
4th Floor
160 East 300 South
Salt Lake City, Utah 84111

Vermont

Vermont State Board of Nursing
109 State Street
Montpelier, Vermont 05609-1106
Phone: (802) 828-2396
Fax: (802) 828-2853
81 River Street
Montpelier, Vermont 05602-1106

Virgin Islands

Virgin Islands Board of Nurse
Licensure
P.O. Box 4247, Veterans Drive
Station
St. Thomas, U.S. Virgin Islands
00803
Phone: (809) 776-7397
Fax: (809) 777-4003

Street Address
Plot #3 Kongens Gade
St. Thomas, U.S. Virgin Islands
00803

Virginia

Virginia Board of Nursing
6606 West Broad Street, 4th Floor
Richmond, Virginia 23230-1717
Phone: (804) 662-9909
Fax: (804) 662-9943

Washington

Washington State Nursing Care
Quality Assurance Com-
mission
Department of Health
P.O. Box 47864
Olympia, Washington
98504-7864
Phone: (360) 753-2686
Fax: (360) 586-5935

West Virginia-RN

West Virginia Board of Examiners
for Registered Professional
Nurses
101 Dee Drive
Charleston, West Virginia
25311-1620
Phone: (304) 558-3596
Fax: (304) 558-3666

West Virginia-PN

West Virginia State Board of Examiners for Practical Nurses
101 Dee Drive

Charleston, West Virginia
25311-1688
Phone: (304) 558-3572
Fax: (304) 558-3666
(Please indicate for PN BD.)

Wisconsin

Wisconsin Department
of Regulation & Licensing
1400 East Washington Avenue
P.O. Box 8935
Madison, Wisconsin 53708-8935
Phone: (608) 266-0257
Fax: (608) 267-0644

For Application Information:

Examinations:
Phone: (608) 266-0070

Endorsement:
Phone: (608) 266-8957

Wyoming

Wyoming State Board of Nursing
2020 Carey Avenue, Suite 110
Cheyenne, Wyoming 82002
Phone: (307) 777-7601
Fax: (307) 777-3519

▼▼▼

Appendix B: Learning Exercises for Chapter 5

Time Management: Sample Personal Roles and Activities

Below is an example of one person's listing of personal roles and activities. Using the blank page provided on the next page, list your personal roles and activities for each category. (Explanations for notations appear below.*)

School	Job	Family
A Be at school 40 hours per week.	A School is my job.	A Principal organizer for family of three.
A Be prepared to teach three courses each week (total of 25 hours in class and clinical).		(A) Spend time with son.
		(A) Prepare dinner seven evenings per week.
Community		(B) Prepare one special breakfast on weekend.
(A) Lector at church.		(A) Do one load of laundry per day.
(B) Member of library board.		(A) Do several loads of laundry on weekend.
(B) Member of homemaker's group.		(A) Food shop several times a week.
Recreation		B Major housecleaning one time per year.
A Write a book.		(A) Daily straightening up of house.
A Attend symphony five times per year.		(A) Perform errands as necessary.
A Attend Civic Music five times per year.		(B) Attend PTA.
B Periodically attend movies and watch television.		(B) Attend Boy Scout activities.
B Night out with husband.		
A "Special" activities with son.		
(B) Selected activities that come up in community during year.		

*A = priority items (These items *have* to be done.);
 B = nonpriority items (These items *do not have* to be done.);
Circled items = delegated items.

My Personal Roles and Activities

School	Job	Family	Community	Recreation

Use of Personal Time

In order to record personal time most accurately, be sure to pick a school day that includes usual activities. A blank page has been provided on p. 366 so you can record your activities in chronologic order. When you total up the minutes spent in each activity, they should total 1440, the number found in each 24-hour day. A sample day's activity log has been provided below. This example does not reflect how you actually spend your time. It merely reflects one person's use of time in a 24-hour period. You will see as many different one-day logs as there are students in your personal issues class.

Sample Personal Time and Activity Log for Monday

Time Span	Activity	Total Time
5:45– 6:00 A.M.	Shampoo and blow-dry hair	15 minutes
6:00– 6:30 A.M.	Breakfast and make "to do" list	30 minutes
6:30– 6:45 A.M.	Dress	15 minutes
6:45– 7:05 A.M.	Drive to school	20 minutes
7:05–7:30 A.M.	Prepare for first class	25 minutes
7:30– 9:00 A.M.	Class	90 minutes
9:00– 9:20 A.M.	Break	20 minutes
9:20–10:20 A.M.	Class	60 minutes
10:20–10:30 A.M.	Break	10 minutes
10:30–11:20 A.M.	Class	50 minutes
11:20–12:30 P.M.	Lunch	70 minutes
12:30– 1:20 P.M.	Class	50 minutes
1:20– 1:30 P.M.	Break	10 minutes
1:30– 2:20 P.M.	Class	50 minutes
2:20– 2:30 P.M.	Break	10 minutes
2:30– 3:30 P.M.	Study	60 minutes
3:30– 3:50 P.M.	Drive home	20 minutes
3:50– 4:30 P.M.	Start laundry, dinner, "pick up" house	40 minutes
4:30– 5:45 P.M.	Talk to son, study	75 minutes
5:45– 6:15 P.M.	Dinner	30 minutes
6:15– 8:00 P.M.	Study	105 minutes
8:00– 8:30 P.M.	Bathe, set out clothes for tomorrow	30 minutes
8:30– 9:45 P.M.	Watch TV/study	75 minutes
9:45– 5:45 A.M.	Sleep	480 minutes
		1440 minutes

Personal Time and Activity Log for _____

(Day/Date)

Time Span	Activity	Total Time

Setting Personal Priorities

Review all the activities you have listed on page 364 of Appendix B under the five categories of roles you play in everyday life, and rank them according to the following directions:

1. Place an "A" beside the activities you have to do without question. Remember, "A" activities are those you HAVE to do, not necessarily WANT to do. These are your priority activities. For example, you might not want to get up on rainy mornings and go to school, but you have to if you want to graduate.
2. Place a "B" beside those activities that DO NOT have to be done. These are nonpriority items as far as your long-term goal and your well-being are concerned. You might want to do these activities, but you don't have to do them.

Many of you came to the practical nursing program while filling a variety of roles in your family and community. As much as you hate the idea, you will not be able to do everything you did before starting school. Are all the "A" activities really "A" activities? Can some of them be moved to the "B" category while you are in school? This is like moving them to the back burner for now. Take a few minutes and review the "A" and "B" status of the roles you have listed. The sample roles and activity list on page 363 has examples of setting priorities with activities.

Delegating Activities

Review your list of personal activities on page 364 of Appendix B with the goal of determining if the activity can be delegated to someone else while you are a student, and make the following notations:

1. Read over all your "A" activities (your "have-to" activities).
2. Circle the activities that can realistically be delegated while you go to school.

Are the "B" activities still on your mind? Can any of these be delegated while you go to school? If so, circle them also. The "Sample Personal Roles and Activities" on page 363 also has examples of activities that were chosen to be delegated. The only thing left to do is to contact the appropriate person to ask about delegating or assigning an activity.

Time Management: Weekly Schedule

Time	Sun	Mon	Tue	Wed	Thur	Fri	Sat
6–7:00 AM							
7–8:00 AM							
8–9:00 AM							
9–10:00 AM							
10–11:00 AM							
11–12:00 noon							
12:00 noon–1:00 PM							
1–2:00 PM							
2–3:00 PM							
3–4:00 PM							
4–5:00 PM							
5–6:00 PM							
6–7:00 PM							
7–8:00 PM							
8–9:00 PM							
9–10:00 PM							
10–11:00 PM							

Appendix C: The Howlett Style of Nursing Leadership

The idea for this management style was found in the *One Minute Manager* and *Putting the One Minute Manager to Work* and was originally written as *The Howlett Theory of Management for Nursing Instructors*.

1. Never assume employees know what is expected of them. Employees are informed of what is expected of them in their job descriptions. They are held accountable for these expectations. Expected performance needs to be stated objectively. This will make employees aware of the appropriate behavior to reach the institution's goals.

2. Reward employees for their "good" behavior (doing what is expected or going beyond the call of duty). This will encourage them to repeat good behavior. But do not ignore bad performance; to do so will have a negative effect. Most employees know what it is like to be caught doing something "bad." Surprise the heck out of them and catch them doing something good. Let them know how you feel about the "good" behavior. Praise them in some way (name on bulletin board, note indicating you caught them doing something "good," and list the behavior).

3. Employees, being human beings, will sometimes make mistakes, for example, they may not follow rules/policies, etc. When these situations arise, determine if it involves something the employee *cannot* or something he/she *will not* do. If the employee *cannot* do

something, it is a training problem. Skill development is the suggested way of handling the situation. If the employee *will not* do something, it is an attitude problem. A reprimand may be in order, according to the policies of your institution. See #6.

4. Employees who feel good about themselves produce good results. Let your employees know they are the best group in the world to work with because . . . (identify reason). Wear an apron that says you work with the best staff in the world.

5. Written and oral feedback about behavior and its consequences, whether positive or negative, needs to be objective. Unemotionally, indicate what they did. Relate feedback as closely as possible to the event. Do not save feedback until clinical performance evaluation time. Point out the consequences of positive and negative behavior. For positive behavior, give praise in measurable terms so the behavior can be repeated. Blanchard and Johnson suggest reprimanding negative behavior in such a way that the person will think about the *reprimand* after the episode and *not* the manner in which it was delivered. Offer praise at the end of a reprimand so that the reprimand is heard more clearly and does not ruin the impact of the praising. Focus reprimands on behaviors, not on the individual.

6. Sometimes employees do not respond to support or assistance and need to be disciplined or terminated. Refer to the policies of your institution.

▼▼▼

Appendix D: Problem-Solving Leadership Scenarios

Scenario 2*

Wayne, a nursing assistant, is a full-time employee on the evening shift of his local nursing home. He has missed five out of twenty scheduled shifts this month. When questioned about his absences, Wayne states he has personal problems. Frequent absences have been a problem since Wayne was first employed.

Assessment	Problem	Intervention	Evaluation
Absent on 9/12, 9/13, 9/20, 9/22, and 9/30. Scheduled to work evenings on these dates. States he has personal problems.	Five absences in one month. States he has personal problems.	1. Meet in private with Wayne for oral warning. 2. Review attendance record for month. 3. Review attendance and sick leave policy. 4. Review existence of the Employee Assistance program for help with personal problems. 5. Set limits. Wayne's attendance will be documented for one month. Absences will be recorded for inclusion in a written warning and placed in his file.	Evaluate Wayne's compliance with set limits.

*The interventions presented are an example of suggested actions in this situation. Actual handling of the situation depends on the established policies of the health care institution and experience of the first-line nursing leader. This scenario presents one legal way of handling an absentee problem.

Assessment	Problem	Intervention	Evaluation
		6. Schedule meeting for the end of October to review attendance.	
Absent on 10/14, 10/15, 10/19, 10/20, 10/25, and 10/26. States he has personal problems. Has not made arrangements to see Employee Assistance.	Continues to be absent from assigned shift (six absences since last meeting) for personal reasons.	1. Objectively document absences in writing. 2. In private, discuss written warning with Wayne. Have Wayne write his comments on warning and sign it, indicating he has read the written warning. 4. Distribute copies of written warning to supervisor and employee. Keep a copy in your file. 5. Set date, in writing, for desired change in behavior (attend when scheduled). 6. Refer situation to supervisor and discuss appropriate actions if Wayne is not present.	Evaluate Wayne's compliance with set limits.

Scenario 3*

Ceil completed her nursing assistant training four months ago and has been employed at a nursing home since she became registered. Since completing her orientation at the nursing home, she has had continuing problems getting her assignment completed in an acceptable time frame. Ceil states her patient load is too heavy and is impossible to complete. The other nursing assistants have helped Ceil with her patients, but they tell you they are tired of carrying her load because she can frequently be seen sitting at the desk making personal phone calls.

Assessment	Problem	Intervention	Evaluation
9/14—employed in May after being registered as a nursing assistant. Unable to finish patient load since orientation. States her patient load is too heavy.	Unable to finish patient assignment. Possible problem with time management.	1. Review patient load as to number of residents assigned and degree of need for assistance and compare to assignments of peers. 2. In private, discuss findings with Ceil. 3. Ask Ceil for suggestions for improving her performance. 4. Suggest that Ceil observe and assist a successful peer for one week to learn how to prioritize care and complete assignment. 5. After observing and assisting for one week, try Ceil with patient assignment.	Assignment equal to peers in number and degree of need for assistance. Is able to get assignment completed.
9/28—Resident A states he did not receive oral hygiene or his bath today. Was assigned to Ceil. 9/29 and 9/30—Resident B states her bed was not made and she was not helped to bathroom when she asked. Assigned to Ceil. From 9/28 to 9/30 Ceil was observed sitting at nurse's desk frequently.	Possible lack of skill development versus attitude problem.	1. Document dates and complaints from residents. 2. Document time sitting at desk. 3. Meet privately with Ceil, and present written documentation. 4. Through discussion, determine if problem is due to lack of skills or an attitude problem. 5. If problem is due to lack of skills, TRAIN. 6. If problem is due to attitude problem, proceed according to policies of institution.	Determine through discussion if problem is due to lack of skills or an attitude problem.

*The interventions presented are examples of suggested actions in this situation and reflect one legal way of handling a problem dealing with inability to complete assignments. Actual handling of this situation depends on the established policies of the health care institution and experience of the first-line manager.

▼▼▼ *Glossary*

▼

Accountability Obligation to answer for your actions.

Acculturate To adopt the culture of a different group.

Accumulative exercise Current recommendation for moderate exercise permits adding short periods of exercise to equal 30 minutes per day most days of the week.

Active learner Takes charge of his or her own education.

Active listener A person who hears sounds and searches for information relevant to those sounds so that the sounds may be understood.

Adult ADD Adult form of attention deficit disorder (ADD).

Advanced practice Post-registered nurse (RN) degree or special education resulting in an expanded role (e.g., clinical nurse specialist, nurse practitioner, certified nurse midwife, nurse anesthetist).

Affirmations Positive statements to oneself that set the stage for changing negative images and behaviors.

Aggressiveness An attacking type of behavior that occurs in response to frustration and hostile feelings.

Alliances New partnerships among hospitals, clinics, laboratories, health care systems, and physicians. Coordinate the delivery of care, contain costs, and attempt to provide a seamless system.

Answer Response by the defendant to the plaintiff after the formal charge has been made.

Appeal Request for another trial or hearing before a regulatory board.

Assault An unjustified attempt or threat to touch someone.

Assertiveness A way of accepting responsibility for oneself by expressing thoughts and feelings directly and honestly without blaming oneself or others.

Assessment Step 1 of the nursing process, which involves gathering as much significant information about a patient as is possible. See Data Collection.

Assigning Allotting tasks that are in a job description for workers. Assigned tasks are those that these workers are hired and paid to perform.

Assisting Maintaining a dependent role under the supervision of an RN.

Associate degree nurse An RN who has received his or her education in a two-year community college or technical school program.

Attitude How you project yourself to others; described as being either positive or negative. Expressed both verbally and nonverbally.

Auditory learner Talks to himself or herself or hears sounds when he or she thinks. Learns best by hearing.

Automatic responses Both passive and aggressive responses result from being caught by an emotional hook, and these responses are not based on choice.

Autonomy Control over personal decisions.

▼

Baccalaureate nurse An RN who has received his or her education in a four-year college or university program.

Battery Actual physical harm to someone.

Beneficence Doing good.

Bilingual Using or ability to use two languages fluently.

Biomedical (Western medicine) Belief that abnormalities in structure and function of body organs are caused by pathogens, biochemical alterations, and environmental factors.

Body language Nonverbal communication of one's thoughts and feelings.

Bucket theory Suggests that merely by lecturing, the teacher can transfer knowledge from the teacher's mind to the student's mind.

▼

CAI Computer-aided instruction.

Capitation Set fee paid annually regardless of the number of health services provided.

Career ladder Nursing program planned to avoid duplication of content. The student may progress from a position as a nursing assistant to a practical nurse to an associate degree nurse to a baccalaureate nurse in about four years.

Case nursing A method of client care in which one nurse is assigned to give total care to one patient.

Certification Certificate awarded to an RN after passing a comprehensive examination in a select area of practice.

Charting by exception (CBE) Normal events charted by placing a check mark on a flow sheet. Abnormal events or changes are charted in narrative form.

Civil action related to individual rights Involves the relationships between individuals and the violation of those rights.

Clinical area An area, such as a hospital or nursing home, where nursing students can apply classroom learning.

Clinical evaluation The task, shared by an instructor and a student, of identifying positive behaviors and behaviors that need to be modified as they relate to meeting one's goal.

Clustering An unstructured method of mapping.

Co-dependency Situation in which a person allows another person's behavior to affect him or her and is obsessed with controlling that person's behavior.

Common law Judge-made law, which has its origins in the courts.

Communication Conveying a thought or idea from a sender to a receiver or from one person to another.

Compensation A coping/mental mechanism whereby the individual covers for a real or imagined inadequacy by developing or exaggerating what some consider to be a desirable trait.

Computer simulation Learning activities on a computer that make use of an imaginary client situation. The student uses the nursing process as he or she would in an actual clinical situation.

Confidence The ability to look at oneself and respect what one sees projected in a positive manner through verbalization and body language.

Confidentiality A client's right to privacy.

Constructive evaluation Critique directed toward performance and behavior; has no bearing on one's value as a person.

Continuous quality improvement (CQI) Searches for new ways to improve client care, prevent errors, and identify and fix problems.

Cooperative learning Emphasis on individual accountability for learning a specific academic task while working in small groups.

Co-payment Percentage of the bill that is paid by a subscriber who is enrolled in a health insurance plan.

Copyright laws Permit a single copy of an article for personal use. Instructors may not make copies of articles, chapters, or books for distribution to students.

Cost containment Holding costs within fixed limits.

Cost effectiveness Getting the most for your money.

Creative communication A method of dialogue in which each segment of the conversation is checked out between the sender and the receiver. If the communication is understood, the dialogue continues; however, if the communication is not understood, the segment is re-explained until understanding takes place. The process continues to repeat.

Criminal action Involves persons and society as a whole; for example, murder.

Critical pathways Also called care maps and care guides. Show a sequence of care to be delivered within a definite time frame. Include potential problems and expected outcomes. Help the client to be discharged from the hospital in the fastest time possible.

Critical thinking Used to resolve problems and find ways to make improvements even when no problem exists.

Cross-training Health care workers trained to provide specific skills when needed by clients in an attempt to improve care.

Cultural bias Prejudice.

Cultural sensitivity Learning about other cultures and being respectful of their customs, rites, and beliefs.

Culture The total of all the ideas, beliefs, values, attitudes, and objects that a group of persons possesses. Culture includes ways of doing things.

Custom Ways of doing things that are common to a group of people of the same culture.

▼

Data collection Step 1 of the nursing process for practical nurses, which involves gathering significant information about the client to assist the RN in the assessment process.

Decentralized Locate centralized service departments such as the x-ray department and the laboratory on client units. Health care workers are cross-trained to provide a variety of services for the client. The goal is client-focused care.

Deductible Amount the subscriber must pay before health insurance begins to cover costs.

Defamation Damage to someone's reputation through false or unprivileged communication.

Defendant Individual whom the plaintiff claims is at fault.

Delegating Generally necessary routine or repetitive tasks within your job description can be delegated. Duties that are part of your *legal* scope of practice cannot be delegated. The LPN as charge nurse cannot delegate.

Diagnostic related groups (DRGs) Prospective payment system. A hospital is paid a fixed fee for Medicare services regardless of the client's length of stay.

Diploma nurse An RN who has received his or her education in a three-year hospital-based program.

Discipline Internal source of control for one's behavior.

Discovery period Pretrial period during which the defendant and the plaintiff attempt to get all the facts.

Distraction Anything that draws attention away from the task at hand.

Durable power of attorney (DPOA) In this case durable **medical** power of attorney. Written while the person is mentally competent. Identifies who will make decisions regarding future care, extent of treatment, and kinds of treatment if the person is unable to make his or her own decisions.

▼

Effectiveness Choosing the most important thing to do and doing it as soon as possible.

Efficiency Getting tasks done in the shortest time possible.

Empathy Respectful, detached concern.

Endorsement An agreement between some state boards of nursing to accept an LPN for licensure in that state, without written examination, if the LPN's score is at or above the score established by the board of nursing in the state to which application is made.

Ethics Rules or principles that govern correct conduct.

Ethnic group Special type of cultural group composed of people who are members of the same race, religion, or nation or who speak the same language.

Ethnocentrism The belief that one's own culture is best; the belief

that one's way of doing things is best.

Evaluation Step 5 of the nursing process; involves taking a critical look at the effectiveness of a nursing action.

Extended family The nuclear family plus all other relatives.

External distractions Interruptions in concentration from outside oneself, such as background sounds, lighting, peers, and so forth.

Eye contact Cultural interpretation varies. Eye contact may be a sign of respect or disrespect in some cultures or may imply sexual consent.

▼

Facilitator Teacher who creates a learning environment by arranging for a variety of activities and experiences. The student is expected to participate actively in his or her own learning.

False imprisonment Keeping someone detained against his or her will without cause.

Fat gram budget Number of fat grams recommended daily to maintain, lose, or increase body weight.

Fee-for-service Client pays a fee to the physician for each service provided.

Functional nursing A method of client care that is task-oriented and involves dividing the tasks to be done among staff members according to their abilities.

▼

GED General education diploma. A high school equivalency diploma may be earned by persons who did not complete high school by taking a special course of study.

Generalizations Broad, sweeping statements made about a group.

Genes Structures in the body cells that pass on inherited traits.

Goals Realistic, measurable, time-limited statements of resolution of a problem or need.

▼

Health care setting An agency or facility that provides health care and to which the client goes for care.

Health care team The various individuals who provide the services needed for the comprehensive care of patients.

Health maintenance organization (HMO) A managed care system developed to provide health care with cost controls. Members pay a set annual fee regardless of the number of services provided.

Hispanic Americans Residents of the United States whose country of origin is Mexico, Cuba, Puerto Rico, or Central or South America.

Holistic The adjective for holism, a philosophy that looks at a person as a complete unit.

▼

"I" messages Sender takes responsibility for his or her own thinking, feeling, and actions. This is conveyed in the sender's verbalization.

Idea sketch Representing a verbal concept with a picture.

Imagery A way deliberately to "picture" future encounters.

Impaired nurse One who is addicted to alcohol or other drugs.

Implied consent Assumed permission given by a client by entering an institution for certain routine treatments. The client retains

the right verbally to refuse any treatment and may leave the institution when he or she chooses, unless he or she is there for court-ordered treatment.

Implementation Step 4 of the nursing process, which uses the client-care plan as a guideline for daily care and carrying out planned activities.

Incongruous Inconsistent with expected behavior.

Incremental changes Occur here and there without affecting the system as a whole.

Information interview By appointment, meet with an administrator to learn about a facility. This is not a job interview, although it is treated with the same courtesy.

Intentional tort Intent to do a wrongful act.

Interaction An action between two or more persons.

Internal distractions Interruptions in concentration from inside oneself, such as daydreaming and boredom.

Internship A program of clinical experiences to complete the requirements for licensure as a practicing physician.

Interpersonal style Four major styles: (1) results focused, (2) detail focused, (3) friendly focused, and (4) party focused.

Intonation Tone of voice.

▼

Joint Commission of Accreditation of Health Care Organizations Sets the standards of care for hospitals and long-term care agencies. Agencies receive accreditation if they meet standards or are cited if standards are not met.

Justice Giving clients their due and treating them fairly.

▼

Kinesthetic (tactual) learner Experiences feelings in regard to what is being thought about.

▼

Leadership Manner in which the leader gets along with coworkers and gets the job done.

Learning The active process of acquiring new knowledge and skills.

Left brain dominant More ordered; logical; reads and writes well, and excels at analytical thinking.

Liability Legal responsibility of a person to account for wrongful acts by making financial restitution.

Liability insurance Insurance to protect the nurse from the consequences of negligent acts and from malpractice costs.

Libel Damage to someone's reputation through written communication or pictures.

Linguistic learner Learns best by reducing the number of words included in class notes.

Living will Written directive stating personal wishes regarding future health care. Not recognized as a legal document everywhere.

Logical learner Learns best by using an organized method of study.

Long-term goal A general realistic statement of what one hopes to attain ultimately.

Long-term memory A function of the brain that allows one to store information over time; for example, knowledge of what one wore on one's first date (synonym—permanent memory).

▼

Malpractice A part of negligence that relates to lack of skill or misconduct by professional persons.

Managed care See Health Maintenance Organization as an example of managed care.

Management Organization of all care required for clients in a health care setting for a specific period of time.

Mandatory licensure Licensure required to practice nursing.

Manipulation An indirect way of dealing with issues that may be positive or negative. Negative (maladaptive) manipulation occurs if the feelings of others are disregarded or other people are treated as objects.

Mapping A form of notemaking in which information and its relationships are put in a visual pattern.

Medicaid (medical assistance) Financial assistance provided by the federal government for states and counties to pay for medical services for eligible poor.

Medical asepsis Being free from germs and infection.

Medicare Federally sponsored and supervised health insurance plan for persons 65 years of age and older.

Message Idea being conveyed or the question being asked.

Mini task Simple to do and takes no more than five minutes of time. An unpleasant, difficult time-consuming task can be divided into a series of mini tasks.

Minimum competency The least amount of knowledge and skill needed to attain something.

Mnemonic device Memory aid such as rhymes or acronyms.

Morals Ethical habits of a person.

Motivation An internal or external push that makes one do what needs to be done.

Musical learner Learns best by humming, singing, or playing an instrument.

▼

NANDA North American Nursing Diagnosis Association.

NAPNES National Association for Practical Nurse Education and Service.

Naturalistic system Beliefs developed from the traditional medical practices of the ancient civilizations of China, India, and Greece. Believe illness is due to imbalance of body elements caused by excessive heat or cold.

NCLEX-PN National Council Licensing Examination—Practical Nursing.

Negligence Conduct that falls below the standard of care established by law for the protection of others and that involves an unreasonable risk of harm to the patient.

Neural trace A record of information in the brain.

NFLPN National Federation of Licensed Practical Nurses.

Nightingale, Florence Founder of modern nursing who is often known as "The Lady with the Lamp" because of her after-hours rounds with her lamp during the Crimean War.

NLN National League for Nursing.

No-code order Written order by a physician not to resuscitate a client.

Nonmaleficence First, do no harm.

Nonverbal communication Sending or receiving information by facial expressions or body language.

Norm A standard by which to measure something; the expected way to do things.

Notemaking The act of condensing the words of a speaker or narrator into the main ideas presented.

Note taking The act of trying to capture every word of a speaker or narrator.

Nuclear family Mother, father, and children.

Nurse Practice Act Governs the practice of nursing. Developed by each state and provincial board of nursing.

Nursing The diagnosis and treatment of human responses to actual or potential health problems (ANA definition). Assisting sick or well individuals in performing activities that contribute to health or its recovery (Henderson's definition).

Nursing process RN's orderly way of developing a plan of care for the individual client. Usually broken down into five steps: assessment, nursing diagnosis, planning, implementation, and evaluation. The LPN or LVN assists the RN in four steps of the nursing process: gathering data (assessment), planning, implementation, and evaluation.

Nursing team The individuals who carry out the client's plan of care 24 hours a day, seven days a week. This team includes registered and practical nurses, nursing assistants, ward clerks, unit managers, and unlicensed persons.

▼

Objective Data that can be observed and verified. Helps to support or cast doubt on subjective information.

On-line catalog Computerized card catalog in the library.

Optimism The ability to see problems as challenges with solutions that can be attained through problem solving.

Organizational chart Picture of the hierarchy of responsibility in an employment situation.

▼

Passive (nonassertive) behavior Dishonest, self-defeating behavior, that is an attempt to avoid conflict by not dealing with issues.

Passive listener A person who receives sounds with little recognition or personal involvement.

Pastoral care team Members of the health team who assist nurses in meeting the spiritual needs of the patients.

Patient-focused care Attempt to improve the quality of care by using hospital resources more efficiently to meet the client's needs (e.g., decentralizing services).

Performance evaluation Evaluation of clinical performance that involves both the teacher and the student.

Permissive licensure May practice nursing without a license but cannot use the title of LPN.

Personalistic system Belief that the sick person is being punished by a deity, ghost, god, evil spirit, witch, or angry ancestor.

Philosophy of individual worth The belief in the uniqueness and value of each individual.

Physiologic needs According to Maslow's human needs theory, the most powerful needs are those of physical survival: air, water, food, shelter, sleep, and sex.

Plaintiff An individual who claims to have had his or her legal rights violated.

Planning Step 3 of the nursing process, which involves setting priorities, establishing goals, determining approaches to achieve the goals, and documentation of a plan of care. A blueprint for action.

PQRST A method of reading to increase understanding by developing comprehension.

Practical nurse A person who performs, for compensation, any simple acts in the care of convalescent, subacutely or chronically ill, injured, or infirm persons, or any act or procedure in the care of the acutely ill, injured, or infirm under the specific direction of a registered nurse, physician, podiatrist, or dentist. An individual on the nursing team who functions dependently regarding decision-making in nursing care of the client.

Preferred provider organization (PPO) Similar to HMOs, except that physicians maintain their own practice and continue to be part of their own physician group. Part of the day is spent treating clients enrolled in a PPO.

Prejudice The opinion that a person has about something, even though facts dispute the opinion.

Presenting complaint The health care problem or symptom for which the client is seeking care.

Primary care The point at which a person enters the health care system.

Primary-care nursing A method of client care in which one nurse is responsible and accountable for care given to clients on all shifts from admission to discharge. Primary-care nursing places emphasis on meeting the total needs of clients.

Private health care agencies Agencies that are generally proprietary (for profit) and that charge a fee for service. The primary focus is curing illness. Recently a disease prevention and wellness promotion component has been added.

Private pay The client pays out of pocket for services received.

Procrastination Putting off tasks that must be done.

Projection A coping or mental mechanism whereby an individual attributes his or her own weaknesses to others.

Punishment External source of control provided by others, circumstances, or events.

▼

Rapport A harmonious relationship.

Rationalization A coping or mental mechanism in which the individual offers a logical, but untrue reason as an excuse for his or her behavior.

Reactive learner Expects to be taught.

Reading efficiency Rate of speed and degree of comprehension.

Receiver Person receiving the message, idea, or question.

Recycled adult learner Starting a new cycle in a career by enrolling in practical nursing.

Reference hierarchy Potential employers rate references: (1) current and former supervisors from work and volunteer experiences, unit managers, and teachers; (2) workers who have seen your work; and (3) personal references or friends.

Registered nurse A member of the nursing team who has gone to nursing school for two, three, or four years and has passed an examination to be registered. The person on the nursing team who functions independently in decision-making regarding the nursing care of clients.

Religious denomination An organized group of persons with a philosophy that supports their particular concept of God.

Representational   As used in this textbook, refers to a system corresponding to the three senses—vision, hearing, and feeling—in which people think.

Responsible   Reliable and trustworthy.

Resume   Summary of what you have accomplished—work, skills, education, experience, and sometimes personal achievements. Used to persuade an employer that you are the right person for the job. Limited to one or two pages.

Returning adult learner   A learner in the age bracket of the mid-20s or older who has entered an educational program and has not experienced formal education for a period of time.

Revocation of license   Nursing license taken away because of illegal or unethical nursing actions.

Right brain dominant   More creative; exhibits ability in the fine arts and fantasy.

Rite   A system of ceremonies.

▼

Script   Dialogue or self-talk.

Self-directed learner   Takes responsibility for own learning and performance.

Self-image   The way that one views one's personal strengths and weaknesses.

Self-talk   The constant talk that goes on in one's head, which is thought to be as high as 1200 words per minute.

Sender   Person conveying an idea or asking a question.

Serving size   Portion size recommended in USDA guidelines. Serving sizes in restaurants and bakeries often exceed the recommended amount.

Short-term goal   A smaller, more reasonable and manageable unit of a long-term goal; that is, the small step toward attaining a long-term goal.

Short-term memory   A function of the brain that allows one to store information for a short time; for example, a telephone number (synonym—temporary memory).

Skill mix   Cross-trained health care workers. See cross-training.

Slander   Damage to someone's reputation by verbalizing untrue or confidential information.

Social class   A person's standing in society that sociologists base on economic level and educational background. Ancestry is also sometimes used as a criterion for social class standing.

Social conversation   Between friends; focuses on personal issues.

Socialization   Learning the ways of a group.

Spacial learner   Learns best by studying diagrams, boxes, and special lists.

Spiritual   Pertaining to the soul; pertaining to the immaterial.

Spiritual needs   Requirements that arise out of the desire of human beings to find meaning in life, suffering, and death.

Standard of care   How an ordinary prudent nurse would perform in the same or a similar situation.

Standards of care   Used instead of care plans in many institutions. Standards provide minimum guidelines for a consistent approach to delivering client care.

Statutory law   Law developed by the legislative branch of state and federal governments.

Stereotyping   The fixed notion that all individuals in a cultural group are the same.

Stress management   Maintenance of stress at a moderate level. The re-action to both high and low levels of stress be overwhelming.

Subjective   Information based on a client's opinion.

Syllabus   Up-to-date course document distributed at the beginning of a course. This document usually includes a course description, course objectives, course requirements, required text, grading scale, and instructor information.

Sympathy   Identifying with the issue and experiencing the same emotion as the other person.

▼

Team nursing   A method of client care in which small teams of nursing personnel are assigned to give total care to groups of patients.

Temporary work permit   Permission to practice nursing during the interval between graduation and when results of the NCLEX-PN are received. The permit is revoked if licensure is unsuccessful.

Territoriality   The geographic area that a person assumes is his or hers.

Therapeutic   Having healing properties; results of treatment.

Therapeutic blocks   Responses that halt the flow of conversation.

Therapeutic communication   Between the client and the nurse. The focus is on the client.

Therapeutic techniques   Ways that are learned and that encourage communication.

Time management   The effective use of time to meet goals.

Tort   A wrong or injury done to someone that violates his or her rights.

Total quality management (TQM)   A method by which continuous quality improvement (CQI) is carried out.

Traditional adult learner   A learner who comes to an educational program directly from high school or from another program of study, usually in the late teens or early 20s.

▼

Universal coverage   Health insurance coverage for all persons that is usually paid through taxes.

Unlicensed assistive personnel   Trained by health care organizations to function in an assistive role to RNs and LPNs. Also known as patient care technicians, patient care associates, nurse extenders, multi-skilled workers, and so on.

▼

Values   Personal beliefs learned from one's family and significant others that influence one's perception of right and wrong.

Verbal communication   Use of words or language to convey messages that are written or spoken.

Verdict   Decision reached by a judge or jury after a trial is over.

Visual learner   Generates visual images, that is, thinks primarily in pictures. Learns best by watching a demonstration first.

Voluntary health care agencies   Not-for-profit nonofficial health care agencies that complement official health agencies and meet the needs of persons with a specific disease.

▼

Walk the walk   To be congruent in one's thinking, feeling, and doing (actions).

Wellness promotion   Use of disease prevention strategies to promote wellness. Modify life style: nutrition, exercise, weight management, smoking, drinking, and so on.

Index

Note: Page numbers in *italics* refer to figures; those followed by t refer to tables.